# Encyclopedia of Neurodegenerative Diseases: Prevention and Management

## Volume IV

# Encyclopedia of Neurodegenerative Diseases: Prevention and Management Volume IV

Edited by **Natalie Theresa**

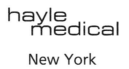

hayle
medical

New York

Published by Hayle Medical,
30 West, 37th Street, Suite 612,
New York, NY 10018, USA
www.haylemedical.com

**Encyclopedia of Neurodegenerative Diseases:**
**Prevention and Management**
**Volume IV**
Edited by Natalie Theresa

International Standard Book Number: 978-1-63241-179-2 (Hardback)

Printed in the United States of America.

# Contents

**Permissions**

**List of Contributors**

# Preface

Information regarding neurodegenerative diseases has been provided in this all-inclusive book. It concentrates on prevention as well as monitoring of the disease growth. Although the main etiology for distinct neurodegenerative diseases is not same, there is a great level of similarity in the disease processes. The book provides an assessment of how metabolic and hormonal controls modulate disease progression. Some preventive techniques using natural products and novel pharmacological targets are also given. The process of facilitation of patient monitoring with the help of medical devices is also explored. This book will serve as a good source of information for college students, researchers, health care professionals and even patients' families, relatives as well as friends.

The information shared in this book is based on empirical researches made by veterans in this field of study. The elaborative information provided in this book will help the readers further their scope of knowledge leading to advancements in this field.

Finally, I would like to thank my fellow researchers who gave constructive feedback and my family members who supported me at every step of my research.

Editor

# Part 1

# Hormonal Control and Metabolism in Neurodegeneration

# Hormonal Signaling Systems of the Brain in Diabetes Mellitus

Alexander Shpakov, Oksana Chistyakova,
Kira Derkach and Vera Bondareva
*Sechenov Institute of Evolutionary Physiology and Biochemistry*
*Russia*

## 1. Introduction

Diabetes mellitus (DM) is nowadays a major global health problem affecting more than 200 million people worldwide. It is one of the most severe metabolic disorders in humans characterized by hyperglycemia due to a relative or an absolute lack of insulin or the action of insulin on its target tissue or both. Many neurodegenerative disorders, such as diabetic encephalopathy and Alzheimer's disease (AD), are associated with the type 1, insulin-dependent, and the type 2, non-insulin-dependent, diabetes mellitus (DM1 and DM2). Manifestations of these disorders in diabetic patients include alterations in neurotransmission, electrophysiological abnormalities, structural changes and cognitive deficit (Biessels et al., 2001). In the recent time attention to the neurological consequences of DM in the CNS has increased considerably.

Many approaches and tools have been used to study etiology and pathogenesis of DM and DM-associated neurodegenerative disorders, and their diagnostics and treatment. The most perspective approaches are based on a combined use of the methods of biochemistry, molecular biology and physiology, they include clinical investigations of diabetic patients and the experimental models of DM and their complications, such as the model of DM1 induced by streptozotocin (STZ) treatment of young or adult rodents, the neonatal model of DM2 induced by the STZ treatment of newborn rats, and also the models of spontaneous DM and nutritional background causing DM2, as well as the models produced by transgenic manipulations or gene knockout techniques are all successfully used to study the molecular, cellular and morphological changes in diabetic brain (Shafrir, 2010).

A severe hyperglycemia in DM1, mild hyperglycemia typical of DM2, and recurrent hypoglycemia induced by inadequate insulin therapy are the major factors responsible for the development of CNS complications in DM. The brain is mainly a glucose-dependent organ, which can be damaged by hyper- as well as by hypoglycemia (Scheen, 2010). Being a major problem in clinical practice, hypoglycemia unawareness is associated with an increased risk of coma. Note that low blood glucose level induces negative mood states, primarily self-reported "nervousness" (Boyle & Zrebiec, 2007). Moreover, patients with a history of severe hypoglycemia show a much higher level of anxiety compared to other DM patients (Wredling, 1992). The prolonged influence of mild hypoglycemia on the brain leads to deregulation of many processes in CNS, which underlines the importance of scrupulously avoiding even mild hypoglycemic episodes in patients with DM. Hypoglycemia induces progressive reduction in cerebral glycogen and glucose, which is due to an increase in gene expression of GLUT3, the glucose transporter rather abundant in the brain (Antony et al., 2010b). Alteration of expression of GLUT3 in the cerebral cortex in hypoglycemia is the evidence for impairment of neuronal glucose transport during glucose deprivation. The impaired transport and utilization of neuronal glucose in hypoglycemia is likely to be an important factor contributing to an increase of neuronal vulnerability. The disturbances of neuronal glucose transport and metabolism in hyperglycemia are similar to those in hypoglycemia and also induce neuronal damages and CNS disorders. For example, chronic diabetic encephalopathy leading to cognitive dysfunctions and dementia may be the result of recurrent hypoglycaemia and/or chronic hyperglycaemia, both inducing cerebral vascular damages (Scheen, 2010).

A new view of the nature and pathogenesis of DM-induced cerebral complications shared by many specialists nowadays has been prompted by the results of study of functional activity of hormonal signaling systems regulated by insulin, insulin-like growth factor-1 (IGF-1), leptin, biogenic amines, purines, glutamate, and peptide hormones controlling the fundamental processes in the neuronal and glial cells. The data were obtained showing that the alterations and abnormalities of hormonal signaling systems regulated by these hormones and the changes in expression of hormones and signal proteins, the components of these systems, induce disturbances of growth, differentiation, metabolism and apoptosis in neuronal cells and contribute to triggering and development of neurodegenerative processes in the diabetic brain. The present review is devoted to the achievements in the study of the functional state of hormone-sensitive signaling systems of the brain in human and experimental DM, to the alterations and abnormalities in these systems, and to the search of new approaches in the therapy of cerebral complications of DM based on restoration of normal functioning of some signaling systems and overall integrative signaling network in the diabetic brain.

## 2. Insulin, insulin-like growth factor-1 and leptin in the diabetic brain

Polypeptide hormones insulin, IGF-1 and leptin, the principal players responsible for pathogenesis of DM and its central and peripheral complications, are to a large extent affected in the diabetic brain. The abnormalities in numerous signaling pathways regulated by insulin, IGF-1 and leptin lead to disturbances of the biochemical and physiological functions of the neuronal and glial cells. It was shown by many investigators that the level of these hormones in the brain is decreased in DM, and the signaling pathways regulated by insulin, IGF-1 and leptin and involving a large number of effector proteins, such as insulin receptor substrate (IRS) proteins, phosphatidylinositol 3-kinase (PI 3-kinase), protein phosphotyrosine phosphatases, AKT kinase, ERK1/ERK2 kinases and glycogen synthase kinase 3β (GSK3β), are impaired (Fig. 1). Therefore, the treatment of diabetic patients with insulin, IGF-1 and leptin, and the restoration of activity of the signaling pathways they regulate are a reliable approach in the therapy of central and neuroendocrine dysfunctions in DM.

### 2.1 Insulin and insulin-like growth factor-1
Insulin and IGF-1 are genetically related polypeptides with similar three-dimensional and primary structures. Insulin is synthesized predominantly in pancreatic β-cells, while IGF-1 is synthesized primarily in the liver and also in the brain. Peripheral insulin penetrates

the blood-brain barrier (BBB) and binds to brain insulin receptors (IRs), which leads to the triggering of their intrinsic tyrosine kinase activity and, as a result, to tyrosine phosphorylation and activation of IRS proteins (Boura-Halfon & Zick, 2009). Phosphorylated IRS proteins then activate p110/p85 heterodimeric PI 3-kinase, protein phosphotyrosine phosphatase and adaptor Shc/GRB2 dimer complex, which triggers the intracellular signaling cascades controlling the gene expression and, thus, regulating growth,

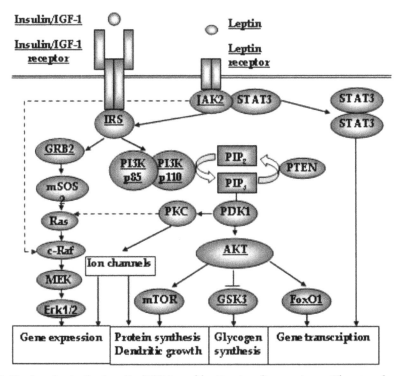

Fig. 1. Critical nodes in the insulin/IGF-1 and leptin signaling systems. The signal components of the systems whose expression and functional activity are significantly changed in DM are underlined. These changes are brain area-specific, they depend on the type of human DM, its severity and duration, DM-induced complications, and on the model of experimental DM. Abbreviations: IRS, insulin receptor substrate proteins; GRB2, growth-factor-receptor-bound protein-2; mSOS, mammalian *son of sevenless* nucleotide exchange factor; Ras, small G protein of Ras family; c-Raf, cytoplasmic serine/threonine-specific protein kinase Raf; MEK, mitogene-activated protein kinase; ERK1/2, extracellular signal-regulated kinases 1 and 2; p85/p110 PI 3K, heterodimeric p85/p110 phosphatidylinositol 3-kinase; PTEN, phosphatase and tensin homologue; PDK1, phosphoinositide-dependent kinase 1; PKC, protein kinase C; AKT, protein kinase B; mTOR, mammalian target of rapamycin; GSK3, glycogen synthase kinase 3; FoxO1, forkhead box O1 protein; JAK2, Janus kinase-2; STAT3, signal transducer and activator of transcription of the type 3; $PIP_2$ and $PIP_3$, phosphatidylinositol 3,4-diphosphate and phosphatidylinositol 3,4,5-triphosphate, respectively

differentiation and the other processes in neuronal cells. The activation of PI 3-kinase leads to phosphorylation and activation of AKT kinase that regulates the metabolism and cell survival via numerous downstream proteins in the peripheral insulin-sensitive tissues as well as in the CNS, primarily in hypothalamic neurons (Iskandar et al., 2010). AKT kinase partly facilitates signal transduction via phosphorylation and cytoplasmic sequestering of forkhead-box protein O1, a negative regulator of insulin signaling, whose nuclear translocation is associated with obesity and hyperphagia (Kitamura et al., 2006). The same signaling network is regulated by IGF-1 that specifically binds with cognate IGF-1 receptor demonstrating a close structural homology and sequence identity with IR and also possessing the tyrosine kinase activity and triggerring IRS-dependent signaling pathways.

Both IRs and IGF-1 receptors are widely expressed in the brain and are localized preferably in neuron rich structures in many brain areas, such as the granule cell layers of the olfactory bulb, hippocampal formation and cerebral cortex. The fact that these receptors are localized in the brain accounts for the role of insulin and IGF-1 in CNS functioning. Since the main function of insulin is to regulate glucose homeostasis, central insulin and brain IRs specifically recognizing the hormone modulate the energy, glucose and fat homeostasis in the brain, being involved, in addition, in the regulation of metabolism in the peripheral tissues. However, in the brain insulin performs some other functions specific of the CNS. Interacting with the other regulatory peptides and neurotransmitters, central insulin participates in controlling the feeding behavior, learning and memory, and is involved in the intercellular communication within brain structures, the hypothalamus and the limbic system in particular (Gerozissis, 2008). IGF-1 is involved in neuronal development, stimulates neurogenesis and synaptogenesis, facilitates oligodendrocyte development, promotes neuron and oligodendrocyte survival, and stimulates myelination. All this speaks about a very important role it has in preserving the integrity of neuronal cells and in protecting the brain structures from damages and injury (D'Ercole et al., 2002).

The alterations of proteins, the components of brain insulin- and IGF-1-regulated signaling cascades, typical of DM and pre-diabetic states, are the causes of the DM-associated neurodegenerative diseases. It should be emphasized that the abnormalities in brain insulin/IGF-1 signaling can be provoked by DM, being a result of the systemic changes of integral signaling network in the diabetic brain, and, on the other hand, the disturbances of the functioning of insulin/IGF-1 signaling systems of the brain induced by neurodegenerative disorders can also lead to DM. In the latter case we can talk about the central genesis of DM.

The initial component of insulin/IGF-1-regulated cascades is a hormonal molecule, insulin or IGF-1, whose brain concentrations are significantly reduced in DM (Gelling et al., 2006). A significant decrease of the IGF-1 level was found in the cerebellum of insulin-deficient rats with STZ-induced DM with poorly controlled glycemia, whereas there were no changes in cerebellar IGF-1 mRNA level, which indicates the abnormalities of hormone processing and secretion in the diabetic brain (Busiguina et al., 1996). The appropriate glycemic control with insulin completely restored IGF-1 concentration in the cerebellum (D'Ercole et al., 2002). Since IGF-1, the same as insulin, crosses the BBB, a decrease of serum IGF-1 in human DM1 and STZ-induced DM also contributes to brain IGF-1 deficit leading to attenuation of IGF-1 signaling (Busiguina et al., 2000). The children with DM1 had a 50% decrease of peripheral IGF-1 level compared with control group, and in diabetic children with poor glucose control it was decreased even more compared with moderate metabolic control. In the patients with DM2 the peripheral level of IGF-1 at the early stages of the disease did not change significantly, but began to decline markedly in prolonged DM2 and in long-term hyperglycemia (Clauson et al., 1998). It indicates the temporal dynamics of a decrease of IGF-1 and the impairments of its signaling in the diabetic brain, correlating with an increase of neurological disorders in prolonged uncontrolled DM2.

Central administration of insulin and IGF-1 restores to a great extent the function of the CNS, being in some cases the most effective co-administration of insulin and IGF-1, the latter refers mostly to the cases of much lower concentrations. It is shown that in DM1, in the case of insulin deficit, a concomitant decrease of insulin and IGF-1 levels in the brain leads to atrophy of some brain areas inducing impaired learning and memory. A combined infusion for 12 weeks of insulin and IGF-1 into the brain lateral ventricles of STZ rats prevents a decrease of the brain weight, and leads to normalization of the level of DNA and the content of proteins associated with neurons and glial cells, whose level and activity are significantly decreased in the diabetic brain. As a result, the brain DNA loss in DM1 is prevented (Serbedzija et al., 2009). The administration of IGF-1 to STZ rats prevents irrespective of the severity of hyperglycemia IGF-1 reduction in the brain and the DM-associated cognitive disturbances (Lupien et al., 2003). Anti-IGF-1 antibody infused into the lateral ventricles led, on the contrary, to deterioration of learning and memory functions of diabetic as well as non-diabetic rats. Quite often DM and its complications in human are associated with the changes in IGF-1 binding proteins, which contribute to the concentration of peripheral and central IGF-1 (Busiguina et al., 2000). The alterations of the content of these proteins are responsible for a decline in memory and for many DM-associated neurodegenerative disorders, such as AD and vascular dementia (Zhu et al., 2005).

The second component of insulin/IGF-1 signaling is IR or IGF-1 receptor. According to some reports, mice with a neuron-specific disruption of the IR gene increased food intake and diet-sensitive obesity with an increase in body fat, mild insulin resistance, elevated plasma insulin and leptin levels, and hypertriglyceridemia typical of DM2 (Bruning et al., 2000). These mutant mice also exhibited impaired spermatogenesis and ovarian follicle maturation due to deregulation of luteinizing hormone-releasing factor secretion caused by attenuation of insulin signaling in the hypothalamus. The restoration of IRs in the brain of these mice maintained energy homeostasis, improved functions of the CNS and prevented DM (Okamoto et al., 2004). The expression of IRs in the brain of mice lacking the genes encoding IR and the glucose transporter GLUT4 also improved their survival, but did not completely eliminate the symptoms of DM2 due to dysfunction of GLUT4 (H.V. Lin & Accili, 2011). The study of expression of IRs and IGF-1 receptors in the frontal cortices of 8-month-old diabetic rats with spontaneous onset of DM1 and DM2 showed that the IR expression was decreased in DM1 only, whereas IGF-1 receptor expression was decreased in both models (Z.G. Li et al., 2007). The disruption of IR expression in discrete hypothalamic nuclei led to hyperphagia and increased fat mass, which was a result of disturbances of regulation of hepatic glucose production by central insulin (Obici et al., 2002). The mice lacking the brain IR had severe hypoleptinemia as well as more severe hyperinsulinemia and hyperglycemia than the mice lacking the receptor in the peripheral tissues, which demonstrates the major role of central insulin in regulating white adipose tissue mass and glucose metabolism in the liver (Koch et al., 2008). Both neuron-specific IR knockout (NIRKO) mice and the rats with spontaneous DM exhibited a complete loss of insulin-mediated activation of PI 3-kinase and inhibition of neuronal apoptosis, and had markedly reduced phosphorylation of AKT kinase and GSK3β, leading to substantially increased phosphorylation of the microtubule-associated Tau protein at sites associated with neurodegenerative diseases (Z.G. Li et al., 2007; Koch et al., 2008). This is one of the molecular mechanisms responsible for the altered insulin signaling and insulin resistance in the brain to be predisposed for the development of neurodegeneration, creating a clinical link between DM2 and AD and other CNS dysfunctions (Schubert et al., 2004).

The third component of insulin/IGF-1 signaling is IRS proteins. They have a key role in linking IR and IGF-1 receptor to the intracellular signaling cascades and in coordinating signals from these receptors with those generated by other neurotransmitters, peptide hormones, pro-inflammatory cytokines and nutrients. The alterations of the IRS protein functions are responsible for the failure of insulin/IGF-1 signaling not only in the peripheral tissues, but also in neuronal cells, they induce insulin resistance and, finally, cause DM and neurodegenerative diseases associated with it (Lee & White, 2004). The deletion of gene encoding IRS-2 protein leads to the weakening of hypothalamic insulin signaling and increases both food intake and hepatic glucose production (X. Lin et al., 2004). Conversely, over expression of IRS-2 in the mediobasal hypothalamus was found to significantly enhance the glycemic response to systemic insulin treatment in STZ rats (Gelling et al., 2006). It was shown that in *Irs2* gene knockout mice the embryonic brain size is 55% of that in normal animals due to the reduced neuronal proliferation in the course of development, indicating IRS-2 to be involved in the brain growth. It seems likely that IRS-2 are involved in neuroprotective effects of insulin and IGF-1, because in the hippocampus of old *Irs2* knockout mice there are formed neurofibrillary tangles containing phosphorylated Tau protein, a hallmark of neurodegenerative processes (Schubert et al., 2003). No direct evidence for IRS-2 being involved in human brain growth and differentiation is available, but breaks at the distal end of human chromosome 13 (13q) near the *Irs2* gene between micro satellites D13S285 and D13S1295 are frequently associated with microcephaly, while very distal deletions between D13S274 and D13S1311 with microcephaly and neural tube defects, suggesting a possible contribution of partial *Irs2* deficiency to microcephaly (J. Luo et al., 2000). Based on these data, the conclusion was made that the regulation of activity of IRS-1 and IRS-2 controlling the growth, metabolism and survival of neuronal cells is a new strategy aimed at prevention or cure of DM and its CNS complications. However, according to the recently obtained data, the deletion of gene encoding IRS-2 improves the functioning of the brain of mutant mice, because IRS-2 act as negative regulators of memory formation by restricting dendritic spine generation (Irvine et al., 2011). The above may be due to the fact that various groups of scientists are engaged in the study of mutant lines of animals with a large number of alterations of insulin/IGF-1 signaling, and these alterations induce different changes in the brain signaling network. With this in mind, it is clear why the functions of IRS-2 can be redistributed among the other types of IRS proteins or described as depending on the activity of upstream or downstream signal proteins interacting with IRS-2. The downstream components of insulin/IGF-1 signaling, such as PI 3-kinase, AKT kinase and protein phosphotyrosine phosphatase 2A (PP2A) are also changed in DM and greatly contribute in etiology and pathogenesis of DM-induced neurodegenerative diseases. The main molecular mechanism in this case is a rapid and significant increase of phosphorylation of Tau protein (Clodfelder-Miller et al., 2006). The hyperphosphorylation of Tau was detected in the mouse cerebral cortex and hippocampus within 3 days after STZ treatment and can be rapidly reversed by peripheral insulin administration. The increase of Tau phosphorylation in the brain in DM partly depends on the fact that the activity of PP2A, the major protein phosphatase acting on Tau, was decreased by 44% in the cerebral cortex and by 55% in the hippocampus. This indicates that a significant decrease in PP2A activity is likely to account for a majority of cases of a significant increase in Tau phosphorylation caused by STZ treatment. The decreased PP2A activity and Tau hyperphosphorylation on the background of insulin deficiency may increase the susceptibility of the diabetic brain to insults associated with AD, thereby contributing to the relationship between DM and heightened susceptibility to AD (Clodfelder-Miller et al., 2006).

To study the role of PI 3-kinase in the diabetic brain, it was shown by making i.c.v. infusion of LY294002, a specific inhibitor of the enzyme, into the 3rd cerebral ventricle of STZ rats that the inhibition of PI 3-kinase activity and downstream effector AKT kinase in this case leads to attenuation of the glycemic response to systemic insulin treatment (Gelling et al., 2006). The glucose-lowering effect of insulin in STZ rats after adenovirus delivery of *Irs-2* gene into the hypothalamic arcuate nucleus was increased 2-fold compared to diabetic rats receiving a control adenovirus. The same results were obtained after injection of adenovirus encoding a constitutively active AKT kinase. These findings indicate that the response to adenovirus encoding IRS-2 involves signal transduction via PI 3-kinase and AKT kinase, and the increased hypothalamic signaling either upstream or downstream of PI 3-kinase is sufficient to enhance insulin-induced glucose lowering in diabetic rats (Gelling et al., 2006). Hence, being the most insulin-responsive brain area, the hypothalamus contributes to whole-body glucose homeostasis via IRS–PI 3-kinase signaling.

The prime function of the other mechanism of neuroprotective action of insulin and IGF-1 realized via PI 3-kinase is to control the oxidative stress and susceptibility of the brain endothelium, the important contributing factors in the development of CNS disorders in DM (Okouchi et al., 2006). It was found that chronic hyperglycemia exacerbated apoptosis of human brain endothelial cells in accordance with exaggerated cytosolic and mitochondrial glutathione and protein-thiol redox imbalance. Insulin activates the PI 3-kinase/AKT kinase/mTOR kinase cascade, increases serine phosphorylation and nuclear translocation of nuclear NF-E2-related factor 2 (Nrf2), and enhances the expression of catalytic subunit of Nrf2-dependent glutamate-L-cysteine ligase, a heterodimeric enzyme participating in glutathione metabolism, and, hence, attenuates hyperglycemia-induced apoptosis via the restored cytosolic and mitochondrial redox balance. Inhibitors of IR tyrosine kinase, PI 3-kinase, AKT kinase and mTOR kinase abrogate insulin-induced Nrf2-mediated glutamate-L-cysteine ligase expression, redox balance, and the survival of human brain endothelial cells (Okouchi et al., 2006). Insulin-regulated PI 3-kinase-dependent pathways are involved in the prevention of endoplasmic reticulum stress that contributes to DM and neurodegenerative disorders (Hosoi et al., 2007). It was found that PI 3-kinase regulates the expression of CHOP protein, an endoplasmic reticulum stress-induced transcription factor involved in control of neuronal cell survival.

The important role in regulation of insulin level in the diabetic brain belongs to the insulin-degrading enzyme (IDE). In addition to insulin, it also degrades β-amyloid peptide. Thus, in the case of hyperinsulinemia in DM2, insulin competes with β-amyloid peptide for IDE and this leads to an increase in β-amyloid peptide concentration and provokes neurodegenerative processes and the development of AD (Qiu & Folstein, 2006). The genetic studies indicate that *IDE* gene variations are associated with the clinical symptoms of AD as well as with the risk of DM2. In DM1 it was shown that the activity of IDE and the level of mRNA encoding IDE were significantly decreased in the temporal cortex of STZ rats. Since the activity of two other β-amyloid peptide-degrading enzymes, neprilysin and endothelin-converting enzyme 1, was also decreased though to a different extent in the brain of diabetic rats, the level of the β-amyloid peptide 1–40 was markedly elevated, which induced DM-associated AD and other abnormalities of CNS (Y. Liu et al., 2011). The other authors reported a significant reduction of IDE expression in the brain of STZ mice after 9 weeks of hyperglycemia (Jolivalt et al., 2008). The treatment with insulin partially restored phosphorylation of IR and downstream components of insulin signaling system and led to restoration of IDE activity. Based on these data the conclusion was made that in both types of DM the level of β-amyloid peptides was increased, although the molecular mechanisms and the role of IDE in this case may be different.

## 2.2 Leptin

Leptin, the product of the *ob* gene, is mainly secreted by peripheral adipocytes, it regulates energy metabolism and body weight. Leptin deficiency in rodents and humans leads to severe obesity. Leptin penetrates into the brain through the BBB as a result of receptor-mediated endocytosis, binds to the leptin receptors located on neurons in the hypothalamus, where the density of receptors is high, and in some extrahypothalamic regions including the cortex, thalamus, cerebellum, choroid plexus and olfactory bulb (Mutze et al., 2006, Marino et al., 2011). The leptin receptor belonging to the cytokine family receptors has several isoforms, but only the full-length isoform generates an intracellular signal. Activated leptin receptors trigger the stimulation of JAK2 tyrosine kinase that phosphorylates the intracellular domain of the receptor to create a binding site for IRS proteins activating PI 3-kinase and the MEK/ERK signaling pathway (Hegyi et al, 2004). JAK2 kinase also activates the transcription factor STAT3, and the JAK/STAT pathway plays the major role in leptin signaling via the membrane receptors (Mutze et al., 2006).

Central leptin interacts with the hypothalamic nuclei and regulates energy expenditure and food intake through production of agouti-related protein (AgRP), the antagonist of melanocotin receptors (MCRs), and neuropeptide Y (NPY), and α-melanocyte-stimulating hormone (α-MSH) (M.W. Schwartz et al. 2000; Signore et al., 2008). Leptin, like insulin, is involved in the control of the excitability of hypothalamic neurons, modulates the synaptic plasticity and promotes the learning and cognition. Leptin facilitates the presynaptic transmitter release and postsynaptic sensitivity to the transmitters in the hippocampal neurons and regulates hippocampal synaptic plasticity and neuronal development. The rodents with dysfunction of leptin signaling display impaired hippocampal synaptic plasticity, and the application of leptin restores the functions of hippocampus (X.L. Li et al, 2002). In neuronal cells leptin activates JAK/STAT, MEK/ERK and PI 3-kinase signaling pathways and functions as the antiapoptotic factor regulating cell survival. The central effects of leptin are mainly mediated via PI 3-kinase and AKT kinase (Morton et al., 2005). Leptin also serves as neurotrophic factor, because it reverses the loss of dopaminergic neurons and dopamine (DA)-mediated behavior induced by the toxin destroying these neurons (Weng et al., 2007). Therefore, leptin not only protects the rescuing dopaminergic neurons from toxicity, but also preserves the DA-regulated signaling network in neurodegenerative diseases, which might prove useful in the treatment of DM-associated neurodegenerative diseases.

Some time ago in the CA1 hippocampal region of leptin receptor-deficient rodents (Zucker *fa/fa* rats and *db/db* mice) the impairments of hippocampal long-term potentiation (LTP) and long-term depression (LTD) were detected (X.L. Li et al., 2002). The animals showed deficiencies in neuronal and behavioral plasticity and, as demonstrated by the impairment of spatial memory in the Morris water-maze test, had memory deficit due, at least in part, to a deficiency in leptin receptors. The leptin administration gave no results probably because of insensitivity of the hippocampus to the hormone. Since the deficiency in hippocampal plasticity in diabetic patients and STZ-treated animals is independent of insulin level, it can be assumed that the cause for these abnormalities is the concert functioning of leptin and insulin signaling systems and their ability to modulate other neuronal systems regulated by γ-aminobutyric acid (GABA), DA and melanocortin (Van der Heide et al., 2005). A close interrelation between the signaling pathways controlled by leptin and the dopaminergic and peptidergic signaling systems is supported by the following data obtained with experimental DM and obesity. The leptin deficiency in the obese mice lacking leptin (Lep$^{ob/ob}$ mice) led to a decrease in the content of somatodendritic vesicular DA and the amount of DA to be released (Roseberry et al., 2007). One possible cause is related to a decrease of the number of functionally active DA transporters controlling the synaptic level of DA. I.c.v. and parenchymal hypothalamic administration of leptin into MKR mice, a model of non-obese DM2, lacking IGF-1 receptor and having hyperglycemia, hyperinsulinemia, and hyperlipidemia, significantly increased the rate of disappearance of glucose. These effects were mediated by brain MCRs, as central administration of SHU9119, the antagonist of MCRs of the types 3 and 4 (MC$_3$R and MC$_4$R), blocked the ability of hypothalamic leptin to increase skeletal muscle glucose metabolism, glucose uptake and fat oxidation, while in the presence of the agonists of the receptors the anti-diabetic effects of leptin were retained and intensified even more (Toda et al., 2009). The involvement of hypothalamic signaling systems regulated by neurotransmitters in the regulatory effects of central leptin on the energy balance and peripheral glucose homeostasis is supported by the results of the study of non-obese diabetic MKR mice, where i.c.v. administration of leptin dramatically improved insulin sensitivity both via the hypothalamus and direct contact with the peripheral tissues (X. Li et al., 2011).

Studying the action of i.c.v. administered leptin on metabolic imbalance caused by experimental DM1 it was found that leptin normalizes the glucose homeostasis and ameliorates the functioning of CNS in STZ-treated rodents (Kojima et al., 2009; Wang et al., 2010). I.c.v. infusion of leptin reversed lethality and greatly improved hyperglycemia, hyperglucagonemia, hyperketonemia, and polyuria in STZ mice. The leptin therapy improved the expression of the metabolically relevant hypothalamic neuropeptides pro-opiomelanocortin (POMC) and NPY, and also the expression of AgRP in the brain of diabetic mice and restored their signaling cascades impaired in DM1. For the effects of leptin to be long-term, the technique of i.c.v. administration of recombinant adeno-associated virus vector (rAAV) encoding leptin gene (rAAV-lep) was developed and used in adult STZ-treated mice. The injection of rAAV-lep gene markedly increased the level of hypothalamic leptin, rescued the STZ mice from early mortality, gradually decreased hyperphagia to normalize food intake by the 20th week, and maintained body weight within significantly lower than the control range. The blood levels of glucose in these mice started to recede dramatically by the 2nd-3rd week to normalize by the 8th week, and euglycemia was sustained during 52 weeks of experiment. rAAV-lep gene injected mice did not exhibit any discernible untoward behavioral changes, nor diabetic complications (Kojima et al., 2009).

The addition of low-dose insulin to the leptin therapy provides physiological insulin level for the peripheral targets of STZ rats and leptin in this case suppresses the hyperglucagonemia, avoiding high doses of insulin required to decrease the elevated glucagon level (Wang et al., 2010). Thus, leptin administration has multiple short- and long-term advantages over insulin monotherapy of DM1, and the combined application of leptin and insulin can be recommended for the treatment of human DM1. A high efficiency of the combined action of insulin and leptin suggests that the brain signaling systems sensitive to these hormones have the common components enabling their interaction which takes place in the hypothalamus or the other brain areas sensitive to insulin and leptin. This view finds support in the fact that leptin directly governs glucose homeostasis via activation of leptin receptors in neurons within the hypothalamic arcuate nucleus enriched by IRs (Huo et al., 2009). Summing up, the brain is a critical site for mediating leptin metabolic-improving actions in DM and the action of central leptin is in concert with the action of insulin and, probably of IGF-1.

## 3. Neurotransmitter signaling systems in the diabetic brain

The various neurotransmitter systems, including dopaminergic, serotonergic, cholinergic, glutamatergic, and GABAergic, undergo a significant change in DM (Jackson & Paulose, 1999; Gireesh et al., 2008; Antony et al., 2010a; Anu et al., 2010; T.P. Kumar et al., 2010) (Fig. 2). The well-coordinated activation and inhibition of different neurotransmitter systems in normal brain are disrupted in DM-associated hyper- and hypoglycemia and in the case of insulin and leptin deficit. The synergistic effect of alterations of neurotransmitter receptors leads to neurodegenerative changes in different brain areas and to the development of CNS disorders and dysfunctions.

### 3.1 Dopamine signaling

DA is the predominant catecholamine neurotransmitter in the brain of mammals, where it controls a variety of functions including locomotor activity, cognition, emotion, positive reinforcement, food intake, and endocrine regulation. DA also plays multiple roles in the periphery as a modulator of cardiovascular function, catecholamine release, hormone secretion, vascular tone, and gastrointestinal motility. The results obtained with diabetic animals and the clinical study of patients with DM2 showed that reduced dopaminergic activity in the brain is involved in the pathogenesis of DM2 and metabolic syndrome and is responsible for DM-induced changes in the CNS (Pijl & Edo, 2002).

The treatment of diabetic patients with selective ligands of dopamine receptors (DARs) is a promising approach to improve the functions of CNS in DM. In the recent years a selective $D_2$-DAR agonist bromocriptine, an ergot derivative, has been widely used in the treatment of DM, especially DM2, and obesity. Bromocriptine acts on a central target in the brain, mainly in hypothalamus, and reduces ventromedial, arcuate and paraventricular hypothalamic drive for increased hepatic glucose production, lipid synthesis and mobilization, and insulin resistance, which decreases the risk of damage of neuronal cells and the cardiovascular system in patients with DM2 (Scranton et al., 2007). It is very important that bromocriptine reduces fasting and postprandial glucose without increasing insulin level and its therapeutic effects are not associated with weight gain or hypoglycemia. The main mechanism of action of bromocriptine is based on its ability to bind with $D_2$-DAR coupled with the adenylyl cyclase (AC) via $G_i$ protein, which provides the utility in resetting hypothalamic circadian organization of monoamine neuronal activities in patients with DM2. The other mechanisms include the influence of bromocriptine on signaling pathways regulated by α-adrenergic ligands and prolactin, as well as its inhibitory effect on serotonin (5-hydroxytryptamine, 5-HT) turnover in the CNS, and may also be involved in glucose-lowering effects of bromocriptine (Kerr et al., 2010).

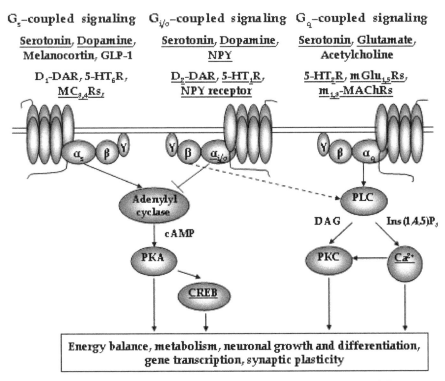

Fig. 2. $G_s$-, $G_{i/o}$- and $G_q$-coupled signaling pathways including the receptors of the serpentine type regulated by biogenic amines, glutamate, acetylcholine and peptide hormones. The signal components whose activity and expression are significantly altered in DM are underlined. Abbreviations: NPY, neuropeptide Y; GLP-1, glucagon-like peptide-1; $D_{1,2}$DARs, dopamine receptors of the types 1 and 2; 5-$HT_{1,2,6}$Rs, 5-hydroxytryptamine receptors of the types 1, 2 and 6; $MC_{3,4}$Rs, melanocortin receptors of the types 3 and 4; $mGlu_{1,5}$Rs, metabotropic glutamate receptors of the types 1 and 5; $m_{1,3}$-MAChRs, muscarinic acetylcholine receptors of the types 1 and 3; $\alpha_{s,i/o,q}\beta\gamma$, heterotrimeric $G_s$-, $G_{i/o}$- and $G_q$-proteins; PKA, protein kinase A; CREB, cAMP response element-binding; PLC, phosphoinositide-specific phospholipase C; PKC, protein kinase C; cAMP, 3′,5′-cyclic adenosine monophosphate; DAG, diacylglycerol; Ins(1,4,5)P$_3$, phosphatidylinositol 1,4,5-triphosphate

The treatment with bromocriptine can reverse the metabolic abnormalities in humans with DM2 and obesity and in obese experimental animals. Using 22 obese patients with DM2 it was found that bromocriptine significantly reduces both glycosylated hemoglobin level and fasting and postprandial plasma glucose concentrations, it decreases the mean plasma glucose concentration during oral glucose tolerance test, which indicates the improvement in glucose tolerance (Pijl et al., 2000). There are also reports that administration of Cycloset (bromocriptine mesylate) either as monotherapy or adjunctive therapy to sulfonylurea or insulin markedly reduces glycosylated hemoglobin, plasma triglycerides and free fatty acid levels (Scranton et al., 2007). The effects of once-daily morning Cycloset therapy on glycemic control and plasma lipids are demonstrable throughout the diurnal portion of the day (7 a.m. to 7 p.m.) across postprandial time points. Recently it was shown that the bromocriptine therapy of 4328 patients with DM2 during 6–24 weeks leads to a significant decrease of glycosylated hemoglobin and plasma glucose levels (Kerr et al., 2010).

Bromocriptine improved the functional state of obese glucose-intolerant Syrian hamsters, inducing a decrease in their insulin resistance and markedly lowering the plasma levels of insulin and free fatty acids (S. Luo et al., 2000). These anti-diabetic effects of bromocriptine are associated with its influence on the daily rhythms of metabolic hormones and daily monoamine profiles within the hypothalamic suprachiasmatic nuclei that modulate circadian neuroendocrine activities and, thus, regulate metabolism of seasonal animals. The bromocriptine significantly reduced DA turnover during the light period and shifted daily peaks of the content of 5-HT and 5-hydroxy-indoleacetic acid (5-HIAA), the main metabolite of 5-HT, by 12 h from the light to the dark period of the day within the hypothalamic suprachiasmatic nuclei, it also increased extracellular 5-HIAA in the brain of diabetic hamsters during the dark phase toward levels observed in normal glucose-tolerant animals.

Using animal models it was found that a combined administration of agonists of $D_1$- and $D_2$-DARs is a successful approach for decreasing appetite in both STZ rats and ob/ob mice (Bina & Cincotta, 2000; Kuo, 2006). The anorectic response induced by $D_1/D_2$ agonists is due to their antagonistic action on hypothalamic neurons containing NPY, the most potent appetite transducer in the CNS, and on NPY-dependent signaling. In DM the NPY system is up-regulated due to increased expression of both NPY and its receptor and to enhanced release of NPY. The co-administration of $D_1/D_2$ agonists normalized the elevated NPY content and hyperphagic effect observed in STZ rats and *ob/ob* mice (Bina & Cincotta, 2000; Kuo, 2006). However, the response of $D_1/D_2$ agonist-induced appetite suppression was attenuated in diabetic rats compared to normal animals, which can be ascribed both to a decreased inhibitory action of central dopaminergic system and to enhanced activity of hypothalamic NPY neurons in DM. The insulin treatment in DM normalized the response to $D_1/D_2$ agonists owing to the restoration of NPY content in the hypothalamus and DA signaling.

The reduction of activity of the brain dopaminergic system in DM is mainly due to changes of the initial stages of DA-induced signal transduction which involves DARs, $G_i$ or $G_s$ proteins and effectors, AC and phospholipase C (PLC), generating second messengers. In many brain regions the activity of DARs and signal proteins coupled to them has DAR-specific differential alterations. The studies in this area are mostly devoted to the functional state of DARs in DM. In the early 1980s it was found that the binding of [$^3$H]-spiperone, antagonist of $D_2$-DAR, to striatal membranes is significantly increased in rats with DM induced by alloxan or STZ treatment, and insulin therapy leads to normalization of functioning of central dopaminergic system (Lozovsky et al., 1981). Recently it was shown that the expression of $D_1$- and $D_2$-DARs and total DAR binding ($B_{max}$) are increased in the cerebral cortex of STZ rats (T.P. Kumar et al., 2010). In the cerebellum $D_1$-DAR was down regulated and $D_2$-DAR up regulated, a total number of DARs being however decreased. The treatment with insulin or curcumin, an active component in rhizome of *Curcuma longa*, reduced DM-induced alteration of $D_1$- and $D_2$-DARs in the cerebral cortex and increased $D_1$-DAR expression in the cerebellum to near control, thereby improving the cognitive and emotional functions associated with these regions. In the hypothalamus and brainstem of STZ rats a significant decrease in the DA content and the number of $D_2$-DARs, and an increase in affinity of the latter were found, and the insulin therapy did not completely reverse the DM-induced changes of $D_2$-DAR functions (Shankar et al., 2007). The hypothalamus and brainstem are two parts of the brain very important for monitoring the glucose status and the regulation of feeding. The hypothalamus, in addition, controls the release of pituitary hormones having a key role in regulation of the CNS and the periphery. These data indicate that the activity of the dopaminergic system in different areas of the diabetic brain either increases or decreases, which must be taken into consideration in clinic practice for successful management of DM and its cerebral complications.

The alteration of DA-regulated signaling cascades in DM is associated with their downstream components, such as the transcription factor CREB playing a pivotal role in DAR-mediated nuclear signaling and neuroplasticity (Finkbeiner, 2000) and $D_1$-DAR-coupled PLC involved in the neuromodulation of hippocampal LTD (J. Liu et al., 2009). It was found that STZ-induced DM produces a significant attenuation of functional activity of CREB and PLC in the cerebral cortex and cerebellum of diabetic rats and these alterations are largely eliminated by the treatment with insulin and curcumin (T.P. Kumar et al., 2010).

We showed that in the brain of rats with STZ-induced DM1, duration one month, as well as with neonatal model of DM2, duration 3 to 6 months, the sensitivity of AC to regulatory action of bromocriptine was decreased (Shpakov et al., 2006, 2007a). The inhibitory effect of bromocriptine on forskolin-stimulated AC activity and its stimulating effect on GppNHp binding of $G_i$ proteins in synaptosomal membranes of diabetic rats were significantly decreased, predominantly in DM1. As the binding characteristics of DARs and the catalytic activity of AC did not change essentially, a suggestion was made that the impairment of bromocriptine-induced signaling in the diabetic brain was due to the reduced function of $G_i$ proteins (Shpakov et al., 2007b). This view finds support in the fact that the regulatory effects of somatostatin and 5-$HT_1R$ agonists acting, like bromocriptine, on AC via $G_i$ protein-coupled receptors were decreased in the brain of diabetic rats (Shpakov et al., 2007a). The attenuation of $D_2$ agonist-induced suppression of appetite in STZ rats (Kuo, 2006) is also likely to be the result of reduction of $G_i$ protein activity in the diabetic brain.

Another cause why the activity of dopaminergic system in the diabetic brain is decreased is the reduction in DA uptake and the DA transporter (DAT) expression that depend on the activity of PI 3-kinase and AKT kinase (Garcia et al., 2005). The uptake by DAT is the primary pathway for the clearance of extracellular DA and hence for regulating the magnitude and duration of dopaminergic signaling. Insulin activates PI 3-kinase and AKT kinase, increases DA uptake and blocks the amphetamine-induced DAT intracellular accumulation leading to a decrease of the number of active transporters. In DM1, which is characterized by hypoinsulinemia, the available cell surface DATs are reduced, and this leads to decrease of synaptic DA level. As a result, the DM-induced alterations in DA uptake and transport induce attenuation of synaptic DA signaling. Actually, the impairment of DA uptake and transport systems in the hippocampus of both STZ and spontaneously diabetic *WBN/Kob* rats leads to a significant decrease in the basal level of DA (Yamato et al., 2004).

### 3.2 Serotonin signaling

The brain serotonergic system regulates several behaviors (e.g., feeding, locomotion, reproduction, sleep, pain, aggression and stress responses) as well as some autonomic functions (e.g., thermogenesis, cardiovascular control, circadian rhythm and pancreatic function). The changes of serotonergic transmission in the diabetic brain provoke disturbances in neuronal processing and the altered plasticity of neurotransmission, and play an important role in DM-induced behavioral abnormalities. This is due first of all to the alteration of the brain sensitivity to 5-HT, which depends on the functioning of 5-HT-regulated signaling pathways and the disturbances in the biochemical conversion, reuptake and transport of 5-HT and its metabolites. These changes cause a distorted response of neuronal cells and the CNS as a whole to 5-HT and its analogs, as well as to the drugs that increase the level of central 5-HT.

Selective 5-HT reuptake inhibitors are widely used in the pharmacological treatment of depression typical of both DM1 and DM2 and have a significant effect on the course and outcome of this medical illness (Lustman & Clouse, 2005). The 5-HT reuptake inhibitors contribute to lowering the level of hyperglycemia, decrease the rate of hemoglobin glycosylation, improve metabolic control through their positive effect on weight loss, thereby improving insulin resistance, and restore cognitive functions impaired in DM (Van Tilburg et al., 2001). It was shown that the treatment of 60 patients with depression associated with DM1 and DM2 by fluoxetine, selective 5-HT reuptake inhibitor, significantly reduces depressive symptoms and increases the sensitivity of the brain and the peripheral tissues to insulin (Lustman et al., 2000). Consequently, the approach leading to an increase of the brain 5-HT level and, thus, improving 5-HTR signaling in the CNS is a successful strategy to treat DM (Zhou et al., 2007).

In the late 1970s, it was shown that STZ-induced DM and hyperglycemia have a significant influence on the brain tryptophan (Trp) and 5-HT metabolism (MacKenzie & Trulson, 1978). The content of 5-HT and 5-hydroxyindoleacetic acid (5-HIAA), the main metabolite of 5-HT, as well as 5-HT turnover (5-HIAA/5-HT) is decreased in different brain areas of STZ rats with long-term hyperglycemia and in the hippocampus of spontaneously diabetic *WBN/Kob* rats (Sandirini et al., 1997; Jackson & Paulose, 1999; Yamato et al., 2004). A decrease in 5-HT level is due to the decreased uptake of Trp, the precursor of 5-HT, by the brain (Mackenzie & Trulson, 1978). An increase in the level of insulin can result in decreased plasma concentrations of large neutral amino acids (phenylalanine, valine, leucine, isoleucine, tyrosine) competing with Trp for uptake by the brain, which accounts for a low availability of plasma Trp. The other cause of a decrease of the biosynthesis of 5-HT is a long-lasting inhibition of the rate-limiting enzyme tryptophan-5-hydroxylase 2 (Herrera et al., 2005). It was shown that the Trp level and the free/total Trp ratio in the plasma and in the brain of children and adolescents with DM1 and in women with DM2 were also significantly decreased (Manjarrez-Gutierrez et al., 2009). Free fraction and free fraction/total Trp ratio were also decreased in adolescents with metabolic syndrome, although to a small extent (Herrera-Marquez et al., 2011). In the case of diabetic adolescents two groups of patients, with and without depression, were studied and it was shown that diabetic patients with depression had a lower level of Trp compared with diabetic adolescents without depression (Manjarrez-Gutierrez et al., 2009). Diabetic patients with depression had the most expressed hypoinsulinemia and more extended episodes of hyperglycemia than patients without depression. These results indicate that the degree of disturbances of brain serotonergic activity is likely to correlate with the degree of metabolic disturbances induced by DM1.

Hypoglycemia caused by fasting or by treatment of diabetic patients with peripheral insulin, like hyperglycemia associated with STZ DM, leads to disturbances in serotoninergic system of the brain (Das, 2010). Hypoglycemia increases turnover of 5-HT and decreases the level of 5-HT precursor 5-HIAA in both ventromedial and lateral hypothalamic areas, which induces a decrease of central 5-HT concentration (Shimizu & Bray, 1990). At the same time, i.c.v. administered insulin at doses 50 and 100 μUnits, which induced minimal hypoglycemia, increased 5-HT concentration in the midbrain and ponsmedulla oblongata of hyperglycemic rats with alloxan DM and partially restored 5-HT-regulated functions of the CNS (Bhattacharya & Saraswati, 1991). It indicates the importance of the appropriate glycemic control for restoration of 5-HT metabolism in the diabetic brain.

With a decrease of concentration of 5-HT and 5-HIAA in the diabetic brain the number of different types of 5-HTRs and their affinity to available 5-HT increases inducing alteration of 5-HT neurotransmission. Thus, in the frontal cortex of STZ rats the density of 5-HT$_{2A}$R, coupled to PLC via G$_q$ proteins, was significantly higher than in control group of animals (Sandrini et al., 1997). An increase in affinity of 5-HT$_{2A}$Rs in the cerebral cortex without any change in the number of receptors, and a significant increase in B$_{max}$ for these receptors in the brainstem with a decrease in affinity during STZ-induced DM were also shown (Jackson & Paulose, 1999). The alterations of 5-HT$_{2A}$R in the cerebral cortex and brainstem are a compensatory mechanism responsible for a decrease of 5-HT level in these brain areas in DM. All these parameters returned to normal level by insulin therapy. It seems likely that up-regulation of the 5-HT$_{2A}$R may have a role in the regulation of insulin secretion from pancreatic islets. As is known, the increased activity of 5-HT$_{2A}$R in the cerebral cortex and brainstem can increase the sympathetic nerve discharge, thereby increasing the levels of circulating norepinephrine and epinephrine, which leads to inhibition of insulin release from the pancreas. In addition to insulin regulation, an increase in affinity and the number of 5-HT$_{2A}$Rs has a role in pathogenesis of depression and cognitive deficit in DM.

In our view, being a compensatory response of the brain to lower levels of 5-HT and its precursors, the increase of the number of 5-HTRs is also a reaction to the weakening of signal transduction through these receptors. The latter may be associated with a decreased expression or the functions of signal proteins, the components of 5-HT-regulated signaling pathways. It was shown that one week after STZ treatment the flat body posture induced by 5-HT$_{1A}$R agonist 8-hydroxy-2-(dipropylamino)tetralin hydrobromide (8-OH-DPAT) and head twitching induced by 5-HT$_{2A}$R agonist 2,5-dimethoxy-4-iodoamphetamine hydrochloride (DOI) were markedly reduced in the diabetic rats compared with control animals, which indicates that STZ-induced DM profoundly affects the sensitivity to drugs acting at 5-HT$_{1A}$- and 5-HT$_{2A}$Rs (J.X. Li & France, 2008). Insulin treatment during one week restored 8-OH-DPAT and DOI-induced behavioral effects. We found no alteration of the sensitivity of AC signaling system in the brain of STZ rats to selective agonists of 5-HT$_6$R coupled with G$_s$ proteins, while the sensitivity of this system to agonists of 5-HT$_{1A}$R and 5-HT$_{1B}$R coupled with G$_i$ proteins was significantly decreased (Shpakov et al., 2007a). We consider the weakening of 5-HT$_1$R-mediated signaling to be associated with decreased expression and activity of G$_i$ proteins because, as mentioned above, a decrease in activity of the other G$_i$ protein-coupled cascades regulated by somatostatin and DA was also detected in the brain in DM. Note that in the diabetic brain the signaling pathways involving G$_s$ proteins were either unchanged or changed very little (Shpakov et al., 2007b). The impairment of response of the diabetic brain to 5-HT was made evident in the recent clinic study where citalopram, a selective 5-HT reuptake inhibitor, was used in the treatment of patients with DM2. It was shown that citalopram is less effective in diabetic patients compared with healthy individuals (Trento et al., 2010). The appropriate control of glucose and insulin plasma level in patients with DM2 makes it possible to increase the efficiency of citalopram treatment and the response of the hypothalamic-pituitary-adrenal axis to this drug, and to improve the clinical as well as cognitive and emotional variables.

Dysfunctions of the serotonergic system of the brain can be the result of DM, but on the other hand, they can be the cause of DM. The attenuation of 5-HT signaling in the brain induces hyperphagia and other disturbances of feeding behavior, which, in turn, leads to the obesity and DM2 (Heisler et al., 2002). The cause of this is in that the central 5-HT activates, via 5-$HT_{2C}$Rs expressed on POMC neurons, signaling pathways regulated by melanocortin and its analogs via $MC_4R/MC_3R$ located on the same neurons in the arcuate nucleus of the hypothalamus (Zhou et al., 2007; Nonogaki et al., 2008). It follows, these neurons are a potential target for 5-$HT_{2C}$R agonists because they receive direct input from 5-HT dorsal raphe nucleus neurons and project to the regions associated with energy regulation. 5-$HT_{2C}$R agonists significantly improved glucose tolerance and reduced plasma insulin in animals with obesity and DM2. 5-$HT_{2C}$R agonist-induced improvements in glucose homeostasis occurred at concentrations of agonist that had no effect on feeding behavior, energy expenditure, locomotor activity, body weight, and fat mass (Zhou et al., 2007). These data are supported by the results of genetic studies. It was revealed in the murine knockout studies that only deletion of the gene encoding the 5-$HT_{2C}$ receptor produces insulin resistance and DM2 with antecedent hyperphagia and obesity, which demonstrates that 5-$HT_{2C}$Rs are critical for energy homeostasis (Bonasera & Tecott, 2000). It was found that three loci of single nucleotide substitution ($G \rightarrow A$ at -995, $C \rightarrow T$ at -759, $G \rightarrow C$ at -697) and $(GT)_n$ dinucleotide repeat polymorphism in the upstream region (promoter) of the 5-$HT_{2C}$R gene are involved in the development of obesity and DM2 in human (Yuan et al., 2000). The haplotypes containing the nucleotide substitutions are associated with higher transcription levels of the gene and thereby with resistance to obesity and DM2.

### 3.3 Glutamate signaling

Glutamate is the major excitatory neurotransmitter in the CNS. It exerts action via ionotropic glutamate receptors (iGluRs) – AMPA and NMDA receptors, and via metabotropic glutamate receptors (mGluRs). mGluRs are predominantly found in pre- and post-synaptic neurons in synapses of the hippocampus, cerebellum and cerebral cortex but are also present in other parts of the brain and in the peripheral tissues. mGluR subtypes are critical in gating the plasticity and memory formation. mGluRs interact with iGluRs, ion channels and membrane-associated enzymes, the generators of second messengers, that modulate the cellular response involved in the processes of differentiation and degeneration of neuronal cells. The activation of mGlu$_1$R and mGlu$_5$R, belonging to group I of mGluRs, enhances phosphoinositide hydrolysis and mobilization of intracellular $Ca^{2+}$ due to stimulation of PLC, induces the activation of $Na^+$ and $K^+$ channels, modulates voltage-dependent $Ca^{2+}$ channels and inhibits glutamate release, all this being of great importance in the regulation of cascades of biochemical reactions resulting in death of neuronal cells (N.E. Schwartz & Alford, 2000). The iGluRs are ligand-gated nonselective cation channels allowing the flow of $K^+$, $Na^+$ and $Ca^{2+}$ in response to glutamate binding. These receptors, like mGluRs, have influence on synaptic plasticity and are of prime importance in excitotoxicity. An increase or a decrease of the number of iGluRs on post-synaptic neurons leads to LTP or LTD of neuronal cell, respectively. The activation of NMDA receptors in post-synaptic neurons increases $Ca^{2+}$ influx, leading to phospholipase $A_2$-mediated arachidonic acid release and neuronal injury by inhibiting the $Na^+$-channels.

Glutamate is essential for synaptic communication in the CNS, but inadequate increase of extracellular glutamate and excessive activation of GluRs causes toxicity in the brain leading to neurodegenerative disorders (Trudeau et al., 2004). Excessive glutamate over-activates the cognate receptors, specifically NMDA receptors, which gives the influx of high level of $Ca^{2+}$ in the post-synaptic cell. In the diabetic brain the glutamate level and the number of

GluRs are significantly increased, which is the main cause of neurodegenerative changes in DM (N. Li et al., 1999; Tomiyama et al., 2005; Joseph et al., 2008; Anu et al., 2010) (Fig. 3).

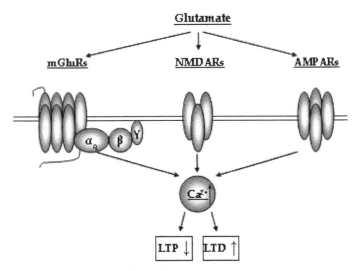

Fig. 3. Signaling pathways responsible for glutamate toxicity

Abbreviations: mGluRs, metabotropic glutamate receptors; NMDARs and AMPARs, ionotropic glutamate receptors of NMDA and AMPA types; $\alpha_q\beta\gamma$, heterotrimeric $G_q$-protein; LTP and LTD, long-term potentiation and long-term depression, respectively.

The synaptic level of glutamate in the brain depends on the high-affinity glutamate transporter GLAST, the major component of synaptic glutamate reuptake system, that plays an important role in the termination of glutamatergic neurotransmission and prevention of excitotoxicity, it also depends on the activity of GluRs regulating synaptic glutamate release (Danbolt, 2001). In nerve terminals specific vesicular transporters GluT1-3 allow incorporation of glutamate into synaptic vesicles. These transporters have an essential role in glutamate recycling and homeostasis in the CNS and the abnormalities of this functioning are responsible for development of neurological disorders (Benarroch, 2010). Synaptic release of endogenous glutamate is mediated with the voltage-dependent N-, L- and P/Q-type $Ca^{2+}$ channels controlling the entry of $Ca^{2+}$ into nerve terminals. In the diabetic brain the content of glutamate transporters and the $\alpha_{1A}$ subunit of P/Q type $Ca^{2+}$ channels are changed. In the cerebellum of STZ rats the expression of the glutamate transporter GLAST gene was decreased, which indicates a decrease of glutamate reuptake (Anu et al., 2010). In the hippocampus a decrease of the level of glutamate transporters was transient, being evident mainly at the early stages of DM. This suggests that after the initial stress induced by DM the hippocampus was somehow able to respond to DM-induced stress, and after two weeks of DM the level of glutamate transporters recovered so that the values remained under control longer. After eight weeks of DM, the levels of glutamate transporters and P/Q-type $Ca^{2+}$ channels did not change but the basal release of glutamate was significantly increased in hippocampal synaptosomes, which may underlie alterations in synaptic transmission at the later stages of DM (Baptista et al., 2011).

In the cerebral synaptosomes from STZ mice the $K^+$- and 4-aminopyridine-evoked $Ca^{2+}$-dependent glutamate release was significantly increased. The treatment of synaptosomes with a combination of $\omega$-agatoxin IVA (a P-type $Ca^{2+}$ channel blocker) and $\omega$-conotoxin GVIA (an N-type $Ca^{2+}$ channel blocker) completely inhibited $K^+$- or 4-aminopyridine-induced increase in glutamate release and prevented glutamate toxicity typical of the diabetic brain (Satoh & Takahashi, 2008). It means that STZ-induced DM enhanced a depolarization-evoked $Ca^{2+}$-dependent glutamate release in cerebral synaptosomes by stimulating $Ca^{2+}$ entry through both P- and N-type $Ca^{2+}$ channels. It was also shown that voltage-dependent $Ca^{2+}$ currents through N-, P- and L-type $Ca^{2+}$ channels were enhanced in dorsal root ganglion neurons of STZ rats and Bio Bred/Worchester diabetic rats, which directly mediated the increase of glutamate exocytosis and induced DM-associated excitotoxicity (Voitenko et al., 2000; Hall et al., 2001). These data allow the selective blockers of the $Ca^{2+}$ channels to be considered possible drugs for the treatment of diabetic patients with neuronal disorders associated with an increased level of synaptic glutamate.

In the cerebral cortex and cerebellum of STZ rats and hypoglycemic diabetic rats the expression of NR1 and NR2B receptor subunits and mGlu5R genes and the number of the receptors were increased (Joseph et al., 2008). The activity of mGlu5R was increased, which led to stimulation of the activity of PLC coupled with mGlu5R via $G_q$ protein and to an increase of the content of intracellular inositol 1,4,5-triphosphate receptors interacting with the second messenger phosphatidyl inositol 1,4,5-triphosphate generated by PLC. The increase of activity of NMDA receptors and the mGlu5R-associated stimulation of PLC activity mediated $Ca^{2+}$ overload in cells causing neuronal cell damage and neurodegeneration in the diabetic brain, affecting as it did the motor learning and memory ability (Anu et al., 2010). In the dorsal horn of the lumbar spinal cord of STZ rats the levels of mRNAs coding several AMPA receptor subunits (GluR1, GluR2, and GluR3), NMDA receptor subunits (NR2A and NR2B), as well as mGlu1R and mGlu5R were also up regulated (Tomiyama et al., 2005). In the deep dorsal horn of STZ rats the level of NMDA receptors with high affinity for glutamate, namely NR1/NR2A or NR1/NR2B receptors, was the highest. Also increased was the number of NMDA and AMPA receptors in the gray matter of the spinal cord of the ob/ob mice responsible for pain, sensory perception and muscle control (N. Li et al., 1999). Thus, the elevated level of specific GluRs/GluR subunits in the spinal cord is a precondition for the pathogenesis of sensory impairment leading to diabetic neuropathy in DM. The use of GluRs antagonists decreasing enhanced activity of these receptors in the diabetic brain significantly ameliorated hyperalgesia and allodynia in experimental DM1 (Malcangio & Tomlinson, 1998; Calcutt & Chaplan, 1997), which suggests that increased excitatory tone in the spinal cord plays an important role in the development of diabetic neuropathy. It should be pointed out that NR2B-selective antagonists are effective in suppressing hyperalgesia in STZ rats with neuropathic pain at doses devoid of negative side effects, which indicates their suitability for control of sensory symptoms induced by DM (Tomiyama et al., 2005). It is worth mentioning that some antagonists of GluRs, e.g. the NMDA receptor antagonists dextromethorphan and amantadine, are used in clinical practice in the treatment of diabetic patients and markedly ameliorate the neuropathic pain in some patients (Nelson et al., 1997; Amin & Sturrock, 2003).

### 3.4 GABA signaling

GABAergic inhibitory function in the cerebral cortex is of great importance in the regulation of excitability and responsiveness of cortical neurons. GABA inhibition is mediated both by

$GABA_A$ receptors, which open membrane chloride channels and stabilize the membrane potential below firing threshold, and $GABA_B$ receptors, which act via G proteins to reduce transmitter release from presynaptic terminals. The inhibitory GABA-releasing interneurons mediate the function of excitatory glutamatergic neurons in the brain regions, which contributes significantly to the control of glutamate content in brain regions and prevents glutamate toxicity induced in the brain of hypo- and hyperglycemic diabetic rats. Disruption of GABAergic inhibition induces seizures leading to neuronal damage and, therefore, the pathophysiology of many seizure disorders is the result of alteration of GABA receptor function (Antony et al., 2010a).

It was shown that the synaptic level of GABA and its release in the diabetic brain are slightly changed or remain unchanged. The extracellular basal level of GABA at dentate gyrus of STZ rats 12 weeks after the induction of DM showed no changes (Reisi et al., 2009). The content of vesicular GABA transporter was significantly decreased in hippocampal synaptosomal membranes in two week DM, although only minor changes in the release of GABA and in the loading capacity of GABA transporters were found (Baptista et al., 2011). This indicates that the alterations of GABA signaling, typical of the diabetic brain, are due to the changes in the level and functional activity of GABA receptors and down-stream signal components of GABA-regulated intracellular cascades.

Actually, the GABA binding and the gene expression of the subunits of $GABA_{A\alpha1}$ and $GABA_B$ receptors were decreased in the cerebral cortex of diabetic rats compared to control animals. In the diabetic hypoglycemic rats having two episodes of insulin-induced hypoglycemia in the course of 10 days GABA binding and expression of GABA receptor subunits were reduced to a greater extent in comparison with diabetic hyper/euglycemic animals. This is the evidence that hypoglycemia amplifies the adverse effects of hyperglycemia on GABAergic system, and the impairments of functions of GABAergic neurons in the diabetic cerebral cortex are intensified in hypoglycemia. The expression of glutamate decarboxylase, the rate-limiting enzyme of GABA synthesis, which is used as a marker of GABAergic activity, was also significantly down regulated in DM and hypoglycemia exacerbated the altered expression (Antony et al., 2010a). The same picture is found in the cerebellum, where GABA receptors are involved in control of coordination and motor learning and, like in the cerebral cortex, play a critical role in neuronal excitability and modulation of synaptic neurotransmission (Luján, 2007). In the cerebellum of STZ rats with hyperglycemia the gene expression of $GABA_{A\alpha1}$ subunit and glutamate decarboxylase was decreased and these molecular alterations were exacerbated by recurrent hypoglycemia (Sherin et al., 2010). The gene expression of CREB, a stimulus-inducible transcription activator implicated in the activation of protein synthesis required for long-term memory and seizure formation, was significantly down regulated in DM and recurrent hypoglycemia. Since CREB up-regulates endogenous $GABA_{A\alpha1}$ transcription, the decreased expression of CREB in the cerebellum of hypoglycemic and hyperglycemic rats led to the attenuation of GABAergic system and, as a result, to excitotoxic damage of neuronal cells (Sherin et al., 2010). It follows that hypo- and hyperglycemia in DM both decrease GABAergic neuroprotective function in the cerebral cortex and cerebellum, which accounts for increased vulnerability of these brain areas to subsequent neuronal damage.

## 3.5 Acetylcholine signaling

In the brain acetylcholine functions either as a  neuromodulator, or as a neutotransmitter, activating via metabotropic muscarinic acetylcholine receptors (MAChRs) a multitude of signaling pathways important for modulating neuronal excitability, synaptic plasticity and feedback regulation of acetylcholine release and, thus, controls the functional, behavioral and pathological states of the CNS (Dani, 2001). Acetylcholine also activates ionotropic nicotinic acetylcholine receptors that form ligand-gated ion channels in the plasma membranes of the neurons and on the postsynaptic side of the neuromuscular junction. The activation of nicotinic receptors in the CNS induces depolarization of the plasma membrane, culminating in an excitatory postsynaptic potential in neuron, the activation of voltage-gated ion channels and the increase of calcium permeability. The changes in the number and activity of the metabotropic and ionotropic acetylcholine receptors have been implicated in the pathophysiology of many diseases of the CNS, including cognitive impairment.

It was shown that in the cerebral cortex, hypothalamus and brainstem of STZ rats the number of $G_q$-coupled $m_1$-MAChRs and the expression of genes encoding $m_1$-MAChR were decreased with an increase in affinity of the receptor to agonists, and the binding parameters of the $m_1$-MAChR were reversed to near control by the treatment with insulin (Gireesh et al., 2008; Peeyush Kumar et al., 2011). In the cerebral cortex of the diabetic and control rats with insulin-induced long-term hypoglycemia the maximal binding of $m_1$-MAChRs and their expression were reduced to a greater extent compared with diabetic animals with hyperglycemia (Sherin et al., 2011). At the same time, in the cerebellum and corpus striatum of both diabetic rats and hypoglycemic diabetic and control rats the binding parameters and gene expression of $m_1$-MAChRs was, on the contrary, increased (Antony et al., 2010b). This indicates that the alterations in the initial steps of $m_1$-MAChR signaling in the diabetic brain are area-specific.

The STZ-induced DM and insulin-induced hypoglycemia both lead to a significant increase of the binding of another $G_q$-coupled $m_3$-MAChR in the cerebral cortex and cerebellum but the extent of changes induced by hypoglycemia was significantly higher compared to DM, which indicates the detrimental effect of recurrent hypoglycemia on cholinergic system in the brain (Antony et al., 2010b; Peeyush Kumar et al., 2011; Sherin et al., 2011). This allows a conclusion that the imbalance in glucose homeostasis affects acetylcholine metabolism and cholinergic muscarinic neurotransmission in the brain, and changes the expression and function of cholinergic receptors. The study of 7-week- and 90-week-old STZ rats showed that in the brainstem of both groups of animals the number of $m_1$-MAChRs was significantly decreased whereas the number of $m_3$-MAChRs greatly increased compared to their respective controls, and the insulin treatment reversed the binding parameters of $m_1$- and $m_3$-MAChRs to near control level (Balakrishnan et al., 2009). In the cerebral cortex of 7-week-old STZ rats the number of $m_1$-MAChRs decreased by 28 %, while the number of $m_3$-MAChRs increased by 30 %. In the cerebral cortex of 90-week-old diabetic rats the number of $m_1$- and $m_3$-MAChRs increased by 43 and 23 %, respectively, and the level of acetylcholine was significantly increased compared to control (Savitha et al., 2010). These alterations of $m_1$- and $m_3$-MAChR expression correlate with cholinergic hypofunction in short-term and prolonged STZ-induced DM. It should be noted that $m_1$- and $m_3$-MAChRs are abundantly expressed in the brain regions involved in cognition, including the cerebral cortex, hippocampus and striatum (Porter et al., 2002).

As a rule, most animal models of obesity and hyperinsulinemia are associated with increased vagal cholinergic activity that is strongly associated with the $m_3$-MAChR expressed in the brain and the peripheral tissues (Gautam et al., 2008). The absence of $m_3$-MAChR protects the animals against experimentally or genetically induced obesity and obesity-associated metabolic deficit and greatly ameliorates the impairments in glucose homeostasis and insulin sensitivity. The $m_3$-MAChR-deficient mice are largely protected against obesity-associated glucose intolerance, insulin resistance, hyperinsulinemia, and hyperglycemia triggered by a high-fat diet, chemical disruption of hypothalamic neurons by gold-thioglucose, and genetic disruption of the leptin gene. These data favor the fact that the $m_3$-MAChR and other subtypes of MAChRs can represent a potential pharmacologic target for the treatment of DM, obesity and associated neurological disorders.

Along with insulin, some substances, vitamin $D_3$ and curcumin in particular, which differ in the chemical nature and the mechanism of action are also capable of restoring the functions of cholinergic system in the diabetic brain. Vitamin $D_3$, as well as insulin, markedly recovers the altered gene expression of $m_1$- and $m_3$-MAChRs in the cerebral cortex and cerebellum of STZ rats and binding parameters of these receptors to near control (P.T. Kumar et al., 2011). Vitamin $D_3$-induced improvement of the cholinergic system and glucose homeostasis in the diabetic brain is due to the influence of vitamin $D_3$ on activity of pancreatic $m_3$-MAChR followed by enhanced synthesis and secretion of insulin and reduction of the neuronal disorders in DM (P.T. Kumar et al., 2011). It was found, in addition, that vitamin $D_3$ restores the disrupted expression of IR in the cerebral cortex of diabetic rats. Curcumin possesses powerful anti-diabetic properties and has the ability to modulate MAChRs thereby ameliorating the impaired cognitive functions in DM (Peeyush Kumar et al., 2011).

Ionotropic nicotine acetylcholine receptors are also involved in the pathogenesis of neurodegenerative processes in DM. Note that the stimulation of nicotinic acetylcholine receptors and MAChRs provokes opposing physiological and behavioral responses, which is due to the existence of multiple nicotinic and muscarinic receptor subtypes and their different anatomical distributions in the CNS. For example, nicotine administration inhibits food intake, increases metabolic rate, and leads to reduced adiposity (M.D. Li et al., 2003), while the activation of $m_3$-MAChRs induces hyperphagia and obesity (Gautam et al., 2008).

$\alpha$7-Nicotinic receptors highly expressed in the course of brain development are implicated in memory, attention and information processing (Picciotto et al., 2000). In the cortex of STZ rats the expression of $\alpha$7-nicotinic receptors was markedly increased. The receptors significantly influenced the activity within the cortex circuitry, and DM-associated deregulation of this activity could contribute to disorders involving the cerebral cortex (Peeyush Kumar et al., 2011). Alongside with the increase in $\alpha$7-nicotinic receptors expression, in the cerebral cortex of diabetic rats were revealed the increased acetylcholine esterase and the decreased choline acetyl transferase mRNA levels, which indicates fast acetylcholine degradation and a subsequent down stimulation of acetylcholine receptors causing undesirable effects on cognitive functions. These changes in the expression of acetylcholine esterase and choline acetyl transferase in DM led to a reduction of cholinergic neurotransmission efficiency due to a decrease in acetylcholine levels in the synaptic cleft, thus contributing to progressive cognitive impairment and other neurological dysfunctions in DM. Insulin therapy and curcumin substantially regularize the increased expression of acetylcholine esterase and choline acetyl transferase, and significantly revert up-regulation of $\alpha$7-nicotinic receptor in the cortex of STZ rats improving the cognitive functions, such as learning and memory.

## 4. Peptide hormones in the diabetic brain

### 4.1 Melanocortin signaling

The DM2 and obesity of humans and animals are strongly associated with variations in a gene encoding $MC_4R$ coupled with AC via $G_s$ proteins (Farooqi et al., 2003) (Fig. 2). $MC_4R$

expression is restricted primarily to the brain, where it is widely expressed. $MC_4R$ agonists α-MSH, a product of POMC, and melanotan II promote a negative energy balance by decreasing the food intake and increasing the CNS activity and energy expenditure, whereas hypothalamic AgRP, $MC_4R$ antagonist, on the contrary, increases food intake (Balthasar et al., 2005). $MC_4R$ pathways also regulate glucose metabolism and insulin sensitivity (Fan et al., 2000; Obici et al., 2001; Nogueiras et al., 2007). Central injection of the $MC_4R$ agonist reduces insulin secretion, while administration of the $MC_4R$ antagonist increases serum insulin levels. Furthermore, elevated plasma insulin level was detected in the young lean $MC_4R$ knockout mice, and impaired insulin tolerance before the onset of detectable hyperphagia or obesity (Fan et al., 2000; Haskell-Luevano et al., 2009). The mice with functionally inactive $MC_4R$ had obesity strikingly reminiscent of the agouti syndrome, which indicates that the disturbances in $MC_4R$ signaling pathways were the primary cause of the agouti obesity. The available data indicate that hypothalamic melanocortin system controls adiposity levels rapidly and perhaps more efficiently than the other CNS signaling pathways (Nogueiras et al., 2007). It should be emphasized that the hypothalamic melanocortin system is regulated by leptin. It must be really so because the conditions associated with low leptin levels, such as fasting or genetic leptin deficiency, provide for decreased hypothalamic POMC mRNA level as well as increased expression of AgRP (Havel et al., 2000). Leptin infusion is followed by an increase in POMC mRNA level as well as in $MC_4R$ mRNA level and inhibits the production of AgRP (Gout et al., 2008).

Despite the lack of data on the relationship between neurodegenerative diseases and the alterations of the hypothalamic melanocotrin system in obesity and DM, a suggestion was made that a decreased activity of this system and increased expression of AgRP are the prime causes of neurodegenerative processes in the diabetic brain. As is known, $MC_4R$-mediated improvement of cognitive functions involves neuroprotective action, regenerative trophic effects, promotion of adaptive plasticity, and suppression of damage pathways triggered by apoptotic and inflammatory factors (Tatro, 2006). The treatment with $Nle^4$,D-$Phe^7$-MSH, a selective $MC_4R$ agonist, reduced postischemic tissue injury and improved the recovery of behavioral functions even when the treatment began as late as 9 hours after ischemia. The neuroprotective effect of $Nle^4$,D-$Phe^7$-MSH was prevented by $MC_4R$ antagonists (Giuliani et al., 2006). The treatment blocked the ischemia-induced impairment of spatial learning and memory for at least 12 days due to the $MC_4R$-mediated reduction of death of hippocampal cells. Because a very high dose of $MC_4R$ agonists actually enhanced learning, it was assumed that their effect is likely to have involved neurotrophic action of melanocortin, including promotion of neurite sprouting and functional recovery from nerve injury. The regulatory effects of α-MSH and selective $MC_4R$ agonists on neuronal plasticity and survival could be mediated by their influence on neuronal signaling pathways regulated by other neurotransmitters. It was shown that $MC_4R$ activation by agonists exerts the inhibitory effect on hypothalamic neurons through inhibition of neuronal firing rate and facilitation of GABA transmission (Nargund et al., 2006). This suggests the central melanocortin system to be responsible for a large number of neurodegenerative processes in the CNS previously associated with the other signaling systems of the brain.

Studying the activity of antibodies against extracellular loops of $MC_3R$ and $MC_4R$ strong evidence was obtained for the involvement of central melanocortin system in DM and obesity. Hofbauer and coworkers immunized the rats with peptides corresponding to the N-terminal extracellular domain $MC_4R$ and to the first and third extracellular loops of $MC_3R$ (Hofbauer et al., 2008; Peter et al., 2010). The antibodies to the N-terminal domain of $MC_4R$

acted as partial agonists and decreased the level of cAMP in cell cultures. In rats injected with peptide corresponding to the N-terminal domain of $MC_4R$, like in the case of blockade of hypothalamic MCRs, the food intake, body weight, plasma insulin and triglycerides levels increased significantly (Hofbauer et al., 2008). Antibodies against peptide derived from the first loop of $MC_3R$ amplified AC stimulating effect of $\alpha$-MSH; contrary to this, antibodies against the peptide derivatives of the third loop of the same receptor reduced the effect of hormone, acting as non-competitive antagonist. In rats injected with peptide derived from the third loop of $MC_3R$, the body weight and blood pressure were increased and motor activity was decreased. In plasma the levels of triglycerides, insulin and leptin were significantly increased compared with control. At the same time, the rats injected with peptide derived from the first loop had no changes of physiological and biochemical parameters (Peter et al., 2010). These data indicate that peptides derived from the MCRs and the antibodies to them directly influence melanocortin signaling pathways and cause changes in brain signaling, their action being receptor- and site-specific, i.e. depends on the antigenic determinants they correspond to, and can either inhibit or enhance signal transduction via the cognate receptor. This is in good agreement with the results obtained with other peptides, the derivatives of extracellular and intracellular regions of G protein-coupled receptors (Shpakov, 2011). Thus, peptides derived from the extracellular loops of MCRs and the other receptors involved in the functioning of the brain are a promising tool in the study of pathogenesis of DM and its CNS complications and give a perspective approach to develop new models of DM and obesity based on antibody-induced deregulation of the central signaling network controlled by hormones of different nature.

### 4.2 Neuropeptide Y signaling

NPY, a 36-amino acid peptide, stimulates feeding and decreases energy expenditure. NPY, one of the most abundant brain peptides in the paraventricular and arcuate nuclei and in the other regions of the hypothalamus is implicated in regulation of the feeding behavior, energy balance, and pituitary secretion. Disruptions in NPY signaling due to high or low abundance of NPY and cognate receptors deregulate the homeostatic milieu to promote hyperinsulinemia, hyperglycemia, fat accrual, and overt DM. In STZ rats the activity of hypothalamic NPY neurons was significantly increased, and induced marked hyperphagia (Sindelar et al., 2002; Kuo et al., 2006). STZ rats between 3 and 14 weeks after induction of DM1 had a significant increase (35–200 %) of NPY concentration in the paraventricular and the ventromedial nuclei and lateral hypothalamic area of hypothalamus, the major appetite-regulating areas sensitive to hyperphagic and polydipsic action of NPY. The concentration of NPY was also increased in the arcuate nucleus and medial preoptic area, the regions involved in modulating hormone secretion. A significant increase of NPY level was found in the hypothalamic sites of diabetic rats 6 months after STZ treatment, and insulin therapy for 3 months completely prevented the STZ-induced increments in NPY levels in all hypothalamic sites (Sahu et al., 1990).

In the rats with DM2 the level of NPY and the activity of arcuate nucleus NPY neurons were also increased, which led to hyperphagia and obesity, and may have contributed to hyperinsulinemia and altered pituitary secretion, and the insulin treatment returned the activity of NPY system (Maekawa et al., 2006). The level of mRNA encoding NPY was increased in cells of the arcuate nucleus of young 11-week-old Goto-Kakizaki rats having hyperphagia associated with leptin resistance. Following i.c.v. injection of the NPY-Y1 receptor antagonist 1229U91, the amount of food intake in Goto-Kakizaki rats was indistinguishable from that in Wistar rats, thus eliminating hyperphagia. Note that in NPY-deficient diabetic mice the mean daily food intake did not change, while in wild diabetic mice it increased two-fold. Alongside, in NPY-deficient mice the level of mRNA encoding POMC was decreased by as little as 11%, but in wild diabetic mice by 65%. Proceeding from these results, the conclusion was made that NPY is required both for an increase of food intake and for a decrease of POMC gene expression in DM (Sindelar et al., 2002).

The NPY signaling system is tightly associated with dopaminergic, melanocortin and leptin systems of the brain. The increased content of hypothalamic NPY plays a major role in attenuating the anorectic response of $D_1/D_2$-DARs agonists in STZ rats (Bina, Cincotta, 2000; Kuo, 2006). Leptin directly restrains the release of NPY and cohorts from the hypothalamic NPY neuronal network, and the complete absence of leptin or hypothalamic leptin receptors induces up-regulation of NPY signaling, which promotes unabated hyperphagia and fat storage (Kalra, 2008). The NPY and melanocortin signaling systems in the arcuate nucleus, where NPY and α-MSH are expressed, act in concert but have opposite functions. Hypothalamic NPY pathways favor anabolic processes and increase the food intake, whereas POMC neurons do the reverse. As a result, in hypothalamus signaling systems both form a complex network integrating hormonal (e.g., insulin and leptin) and metabolic (e.g., glucose) signals of energy homeostasis and initiating the adaptive responses of the diabetic brain (Fioramonti et al., 2007).

### 4.3 Glucagon-like peptide-1 signaling

Glucagon-like peptide-1 (GLP-1), a 30-amino-acid peptide hormone, is responsible for modulating blood glucose concentrations by stimulating glucose-dependent insulin secretion and by activating β-cell proliferation. GLP-1 is effective in restoring first-phase insulin response and lowering hyperglycemia in DM2 (Doyle & Egan, 2007). GLP1 also functions in the brain as a neurotransmitter, has the growth factor-like properties and protects neurons from neurotoxic influence, controlling learning behavior, memory and synaptic plasticity (Hamilton & Holscher, 2009; Hamilton et al., 2011). The action of GLP-1 is realized via GLP-1 receptors that in the brain affect neuronal activity through regulation of intracellular cAMP-dependent pathways, modulation of $Ca^{2+}$ channels, activation of ERK1/ERK2 kinases and other second messenger systems involved in transmitter vesicle release (Gilman et al., 2003) (Fig. 2).

GLP-1 receptor agonists, exendin-4 and Liraglutide, like the inhibitors of GLP-1 degradation (dipeptidylpeptidase IV inhibitors), have been approved for treatment of DM2 (Lovshin & Drucker, 2009; Holst et al., 2011). Note that Liraglutide, analog of human GLP-1 with prolonged half life having a fatty acid palmitoyl group conjugated to the side-chain of $Lys^{26}$ and an $Arg^{34}Ser$ substitution, is now widely used in DM2 therapy (Lovshin, Drucker, 2009). Exendin-4 and Liraglutide injected subcutaneously for 4, 6, or 10 weeks once daily in *ob/ob*, *db/db* and high-fat-diet-fed mice enhanced proliferation rate of progenitor cells by 100–150 % and stimulated differentiation into neurons in the dentate gyrus (Hamilton et al., 2011). The GLP-1 receptor antagonist exendin(9–36) significantly reduced progenitor cell proliferation in these mice. Exendin-4 and Liraglutide enhanced LTP in the brain and once-daily injection of the GLP-1 analog with $Ala^8Val$ substitution enhanced LTP in the brain and reduced the number of amyloid dense-core plaques in mice with insulin resistance and in patients with DM-associated obesity and AD (McClean et al., 2010). These results demonstrate that the

GLP-1 analogs show promise in the treatment of neurodegenerative diseases induced by DM, because they cross the BBB and increase neuroneogenesis. The GLP-1 analogs, such as GLP-1 with the substitution of Ala[8]2-aminobutyric acid, with the increased stability to dipeptidyl peptidase IV elicit the insulinotropic activity and improve the central and peripheral symptoms of DM2 (Green & Flatt, 2007). The dipeptidyl peptidase-stable analogs of GLP-1 stimulate AC activity in neuronal cells and the AC stimulating effect correlates with their neuroprotective properties.

## 5. Conclusion

The data presented in this review suggest that alterations and disturbances occurring in a majority of hormonal signaling systems in the diabetic brain are responsible for the functioning of the CNS, the central regulation of peripheral functions as well as for memory, cognitive processes, emotion, and social behavior. These alterations leading to the DM-associated CNS disorders and centrally induced diseases of the peripheral systems are likely to develop via several mechanisms.

The first mechanism is associated with the appearance of damages in one of the signaling systems that may be caused by alterations in the expression or functional activity of sensory, adaptor or effector protein, a component of this system, and also by a deficit or, on the contrary, an excess of hormonal or hormone-like molecules that specifically regulate the system. The damages may be a result of hyperactivation, weakening or modification of the functions of signal protein due to mutations in the translated region of the gene encoding this protein or in the untranslated regions responsible for gene transcription, or else be induced by gene polymorphism in human DM. The other causes are the gene knockout and the mutations leading to gain, loss or modification of the function of signal proteins in experimental models of DM. The changes in concentration and availability of signal molecules can be ascribed to abnormalities in the systems responsible for their synthesis, transport and degradation. In the case of insulin and IGF-1 that penetrate the BBB, a decrease or increase of their level in plasma induces the corresponding alterations of insulin and IGF-1 levels in the brain, which directly affects the functioning of the signaling pathways regulated by these hormones. DM1 gives rise to peripheral hypoinsulinemia which leads to insulin deficiency in the brain, and DM2 to moderate hyperinsulinemia which leads to an increase of central insulin concentration. The abnormalities in one single signaling system influence the activity of the other signaling cascades coupled with and depending on it and induce changes in their functional activity which is a compensatory response of the brain to the primary local dysfunction of hormonal signaling. If the abnormalities are not eliminated, then the changes of brain signaling will amplify and cause deregulation of a comprehensive neuronal signaling network, which resembles "a domino effect". As a result, the disturbances are systemic and irreversible; they have influence on the signal transduction pathways regulated by insulin, IGF-1, leptin, biogenic amines, glutamate, and neuropeptides.

The second mechanism is based on the systemic response of the hormonal signaling systems in the brain to significant and prolonged changes of cerebral glucose homeostasis, the state of recurrent hypoglycemia and severe long-term hyperglycemia. This causes alterations in the energy balance in the neuronal and glial cells, inducing different compensatory changes in the signal network to allow maintaining the activity of the brain in the case of inadequate glucose concentrations. The short-term fluctuations in cerebral glucose level cause temporary changes in brain signaling, they are reversible and do not significantly affect the physiological functions of the brain, but the long-term alterations of the level and its large amplitude provoke dramatic and irreversible changes and cause the neurodegenerative disorders. For example, a prolonged and untreated DM1 with markedly expressed hyperglycemia as well as DM1 with intensive therapy using high doses of insulin and inadequate control of glucose plasma level, leading to recurrent hypoglycemia, are the major factors causing abnormalities in several signaling systems in parallel including the glutamatergic system responsible for development of glutamate excitotoxicity and CNS disorders.

Until recently, it was generally accepted that abnormalities and alterations in the neurotransmitter systems of the brain and the associated neurodegenerative disorders are the complications of DM and their role in the etiology of this disease is not very important. In the last few years, however, the conception of central genesis of DM has been significantly extended (Cole et al., 2007; de la Monte, 2009). According to this conception, there are cases when the abnormalities in the hormonal signaling systems of the brain will trigger the mechanism leading to insulin resistance or insulin deficiency and, as a result, to the development of DM and its central and peripheral complications. The following factors contribute to DM, a dysfunction in the leptin and the melanocortin systems (leptin and melanocortin model of DM2), and alterations in the $5\text{-HT}_{2C}R$-coupled serotonergic and the $D_2R$-coupled dopaminergic systems (Bonasera & Tecott, 2000; Heisler et al., 2002; Zhou et al., 2007; Hofbauer et al., 2008; Toda et al., 2009; Peter et al., 2010). In the years to come, this list will, no doubt, be extended with the results of study of the forms of DM with central genesis. Some neurodegenerative diseases are considered to be pre-diabetes or specific forms of earlier DM, e.g. AD is referred to as the third type of DM (de la Monte, 2009).

The etiology of DM should be studied in order to find the most optimal strategy for adequate therapy and clinical management of DM and its CNS complications. The neuronal abnormalities precede DM as its causal factors; therefore it seems appropriate to eliminate the changes in the central signaling systems responsible for these abnormalities, and then to use the effective treatment of DM without high doses of insulin causing dangerous hypoglycemic episodes. A high efficiency has been shown in the case of combined use of insulin and IGF-1 and the drugs that improve the function of dopaminergic, serotonergic, melanocortin, GABAergic and glutamatergic systems. The approaches based on restoration of the functioning of a comprehensive signaling network of the brain are a new avenue of the treatment of DM of both central and peripheral genesis. This will allow avoiding many side effects of insulin monotherapy negatively affecting the CNS in diabetic patients.

## 6. Acknowledgment

This work was supported by Grant No. 09-04-00746 from the Russian Foundation of Basic Research and Program of the Russian Academy of Sciences "Fundamental Sciences – Medicine" (2009–2011). We express our thanks to *Inga Menina* for linguistic assistance.

## 7. References

Amin, P. & Sturrock, N.D. (2003). A pilot study of the beneficial effects of amantadine in the treatment of painful diabetic peripheral neuropathy. *Diabetes Medicine,* Vol.20, No2, (August 2002), pp. 114–118, ISSN 0742-3071

Antony, S.; Kumar, T.P.; Kuruvilla, K.P.; George, N. & Paulose, C.S. (2010a). Decreased GABA receptor binding in the cerebral cortex of insulin induced hypoglycemic and streptozotocin induced diabetic rats. *Neurochemical research,* Vol.35, No.10, (June 2010), pp. 1516-1521, ISSN 0364-3190

Antony, S.; Kumar, T.P.; Mathew, J.; Anju, T.R. & Paulose, C. (2010b). Hypoglycemia induced changes in cholinergic receptor expression in the cerebellum of diabetic rats. *Journal of biomedical science,* Vol.17, No.1, (February 2010), pp. 7-15, ISSN 1021-7770

Anu, J.; Peeyush Kumar, T.; Nandhu, M.S. & Paulose, C. (2010). Enhanced NMDAR1, $NMDA_{2B}$ and $mGlu_5$ receptors gene expression in the cerebellum of insulin induced hypoglycaemic and streptozotocin induced diabetic rats. *European journal of pharmacology,* Vol.630, No.1-3, (December 2009), pp. 61-68, ISSN 0014-2999

Balakrishnan, S.; Mathew, J.; Antony, S. & Paulose, C.S. (2009). Muscarinic $M_1$, $M_3$ receptors function in the brainstem of streptozotocin induced diabetic rats: their role in insulin secretion from the pancreatic islets as a function of age. *European journal of pharmacology,* Vol.608, No.1-3, (April 2009), pp.14-22, ISSN 0014-2999

Balthasar, N.; Dalgaard, L.T.; Lee, C.E.; Yu, J.; Funahashi, H.; Williams, T.; Ferreira, M.; Tang, V.; McGovern, R.A,; Kenny, C.D.; Christiansen, L.M.; Edelstein, E.; Choi, B.; Boss, O.; Aschkenasi, C.; Zhang, C.Y.; Mountjoy, K.; Kishi, T.; Elmquist, J.K. & Lowell, B.B. (2005). Divergence of melanocortin pathways in the control of food intake and energy expenditure. *Cell,* Vol.123, No.3, (November 2005), pp. 493–505, ISSN 0092-8674

Baptista, F.I.; Gaspar, J.M.; Cristóvão, A.; Santos, P.F.; Köfalvi, A. & Ambrósio, A.F. (2011). Diabetes induces early transient changes in the content of vesicular transporters and no major effects in neurotransmitter release in hippocampus and retina. *Brain Research,* Vol.1383, (January 2011), pp. 257-269, ISSN 0006-8993

Benarroch, E.E. (2010). Glutamate transporters: diversity, function, and involvement in neurologic disease. *Neurology,* Vol.74, No.3, (January 2010), pp. 259–264, ISSN 0028-3878

Bhattacharya, S.K. & Saraswati, M. (1991). Effect of intracerebroventricularly administered insulin on brain monoamines and acetylcholine in euglycaemic and alloxan-induced hyperglycaemic rats. *Indian journal of experimental biology,* Vol.29, No.12, (December 1991), pp. 1095–1100, ISSN 0019-5189

Biessels, G.J.; Smale, S.; Duis, S.E.; Kamal, A. & Gispen, W.H. (2001). The effect of γ-linolenic acid-α-lipoic acid on functional deficits in the peripheral and central nervous system of streptozotocin-diabetic rats. *Journal of the neurological sciences,* Vol.182, No.2 , (January 2001), pp. 99–106, ISSN 0022-510X

Bina, K.G. & Cincotta, A.H. (2000). Dopaminergic agonists normalize elevated hypothalamic neuropeptide Y and corticotropin-releasing hormone, body weight gain, and hyperglycemia in ob/ob mice. *Neuroendocrinology,* Vol.71, No.1, (January 2000), pp. 68–78, ISSN 0028-3835

Bonasera, S.J. & Tecott, L.H. (2000). Mouse models of serotonin receptor function: toward a genetic dissection of serotonin systems. *Pharmacology & therapeutics,* Vol.88, No.2, (November 2000), pp. 133–142, ISSN 0163-7258

Boura-Halfon, S. & Zick, Y. (2009). Phosphorylation of IRS proteins, insulin action, and insulin resistance. *American journal of physiology. Endocrinology and metabolis,.* Vol.296, No.4, (August 2008), pp. E581–591, ISSN 0193-1849

Boyle, P.J. & Zrebiec, J. (2007). Physiological and behavioral aspects of glycemic control and hypoglycemia in diabetes. *Southern medical journal,* Vol.100, No.2, (February 2007), pp. 175–182, ISSN 0038-4348

Brüning, J.C.; Gautam, D.; Burks, D.J.; Gillette, J.; Schubert, M.; Orban, P.C.; Klein, R.; Krone, W.; Müller-Wieland, D. & Kahn, CR. (2000). Role of brain insulin receptor in control of body weight and reproduction. *Science,* Vol.289, No.5487, (September 2000), pp. 2122-2125, ISSN 0036-8075

Busiguina, S.; Chowen, J.A.; Argente, J. & Torres-Aleman, I. (1996). Specific alterations of the insulin-like growth factor I system in the cerebellum of diabetic rats. *Endocrinology,* Vol.137, No.11, (November 1996), pp. 4980-4987, ISSN 0013-7227

Busiguina, S.; Fernandez, A.M.; Barrios, V.; Clark, R.; Tolbert, D.L.; Berciano, J. & Torres-Aleman, I. (2000). Neurodegeneration is associated to changes in serum insulin-like growth factors. *Neurobiology of disease,* Vol.7, No.6 Pt B, (December 2000), pp. 657-665, ISSN 0969-9961

Calcutt. N.A. & Chaplan, S.R. (1997). Spinal pharmacology of tactile allodynia in diabetic rats, *British journal of pharmacology,* Vol.122, No.7, (December 1997), pp. 1478–1482, ISSN 0007-1188

Clauson, P.G.; Brismar Hall, K.; Linnarsson, R. & Grill, V. (1998). Insulin-like growth factor-I and insulin-like growth factor binding protein-1 in a representative population of type 2 diabetic patients in Sweden. *Scandinavian journal of clinical and laboratory investigation,* Vol.58, No.4, (July 1998), pp. 353-360, ISSN 0036-5513

Clodfelder-Miller, B.J.; Zmijewska, A.A.; Johnson, G.V. & Jope, RS. (2006). Tau is hyperphosphorylated at multiple sites in mouse brain in vivo after streptozotocin-induced insulin deficiency. *Diabetes,* Vol.55, No.12, (December 2006), pp. 3320-3325, ISSN 0012-1797

Cole, A.R.; Astell, A.; Green, C. & Sutherland, C. (2007). Molecular connexions between dementia and diabetes. *Neuroscience and biobehavioral reviews,* Vol.31, No.7, (April 2007.), pp. 1046-1063, ISSN 0149-7634

Danbolt, N.C. (2001). Glutamate uptake. *Progress in neurobiology,* Vol.65, No.1, (May 2001), pp. 1–105, ISSN 0301-0082

Dani, J.A. (2001). Overview of nicotinic receptors and their roles in the central nervous system. *Biological psychiatry,* Vol.49, No.3, (February 2001), pp. 166–174. ISSN 0006-3223

Das, U.N. (2010). Hypothesis: Intensive insulin therapy-induced mortality is due to excessive serotonin autoinhibition and autonomic dysregulation. *World journal of diabetes,* Vol.1, No.4, (September 2010), pp. 101-108, ISSN 1948-9358

de la Monte, S.M. (2009). Insulin resistance and Alzheimer's disease. *BMB reports,* Vol.42, No.8, (August 2009), pp. 475-481, ISSN 1976-6696

D'Ercole, A.J.; Ye, P. & O'Kusky, J.R. (2002). Mutant mouse models of insulin-like growth factor actions in the central nervous system. *Neuropeptides,* Vol.36, No.2-3, (April-June 2002), pp. 209-220, ISSN 0143-4179

Doyle, M.E. & Egan, J.M. (2007). Mechanisms of action of glucagon-like peptide 1 in the pancreas. *Pharmacology & Therapeutics*, Vol.113, No.3, (March 2007), pp. 546–593, ISSN 0163-7258

Fan, W.; Dinulescu, D.M.; Butler, A.A.; Zhou, J.; Marks, D.L. & Cone, R.D. (2000). The central melanocortin system can directly regulate serum insulin levels. *Endocrinology*, Vol.141, No.9, (September 2000), pp. 3072–3079, ISSN 0013-7227

Farooqi, I.S.; Keogh, J.M.; Yeo, G.S.; Lank, E.J.; Cheetham, T. & O'Rahilly, S. (2003) . Clinical spectrum of obesity and mutations in the melanocortin 4 receptor gene. *The New England journal of medicine*, Vol.348, No.12, (March 2003), pp.1085–1095, ISSN 0028-4793

Finkbeiner, S. (2000). CREB couples neurotrophin signals to survival messages. *Neuron*, Vol.25, No.1, (January 2000), pp. 11-14, ISSN 0896-6273

Fioramonti, X.; Contie, S.; Song, Z.; Routh, V.H.; Lorsignol, A. & Penicaud, L. (2007). Characterization of glucosensing neuron subpopulations in the arcuate nucleus: integration in neuropeptide Y and pro-opio melanocortin networks? *Diabetes*, Vol.56, No.6, (May 2007), pp. 1219-1227, ISSN 0012-1797

Garcia, B.G.; Wei, Y.; Moron, J.A.; Lin, R.Z.; Javitch, J.A. & Galli, A. (2005). .Akt is essential for insulin modulation of amphetamine-induced human dopamine transporter cell-surface redistribution. *Molecular pharmacology*, Vol.68, No.1, (July 2005), pp. 102-109, ISSN 0026-895X

Gautam, D.; Jeon, J.; Li, J.H.; Han, S.J.; Hamdan, F.F.; Cui, Y.; Lu, H.; Deng, C.; Gavrilova, O. & Wess, J. (2008). Metabolic roles of the $M_3$ muscarinic acetylcholine receptor studied with $M_3$ receptor mutant mice: a review. *Journal of receptor and signal transduction research*, Vol. 28, No.1-2, pp. 93-108, ISSN 1532-4281

Gelling, R.W.; Morton, G.J.; Morrison, C.D.; Niswender, K.D.; Myers, M.G. Jr.; Rhodes, C.J. & Schwartz, M.W. (2006). Insulin action in the brain contributes to glucose lowering during insulin treatment of diabetes. *Cell metabolism*, Vol.3, No.1, (January 2006), pp. 67–73, ISSN 1550-4131

Gerozissis, K. (2008). Brain insulin, energy and glucose homeostasis; genes, environment and metabolic pathologies. *European journal of pharmacology*, Vol.585, No.1, (May 2008), pp.38-49, ISSN 0014-2999

Gilman, C.P.; Perry, T.; Furukawa, K.; Grieg, N.H.; Egan, J.M. & Mattson, M.P. (2003). Glucagon-like peptide 1 modulates calcium responses to glutamate and membrane depolarization in hippocampal neurons. *Journal of neurochemistry*, Vol.87, No.5 (December 2003), pp. 1137-1144, ISSN 0022-3042

Gireesh, G.; Kaimal, S.B.; Kumar, T.P. & Paulose, C.S. (2008). Decreased muscarinic $M_1$ receptor gene expression in the hypothalamus, brainstem, and pancreatic islets of streptozotocin-induced diabetic rats. *Journal of neuroscience research*, Vol.86, No.4, (March 2008), pp. 947-953, ISSN 0360-4012

Giuliani, D.; Mioni, C.; Altavilla, D.; Leone, S.; Bazzani, C.; Minutoli, L.; Bitto, A.; Cainazzo, M-M.; Marini, H.; Zaffe, D.; Botticelli, A.R.; Pizzala, R.; Savio, M.; Necchi, D.; Schiöth, H.B.; Bertolini, A.; Squadrito, F. & Guarini, S. (2006). Both early and delayed treatment with melanocortin 4 receptor-stimulating melanocortins produces neuroprotection in cerebral ischemia. *Endocrinology*, Vol.147, No.3, (March 2006), pp. 1126–1135, ISSN 0013-7227

Gout, J.; Sarafian, D.; Tirard, J.; Blondet, A.; Vigier, M.; Rajas, F.; Mithieux, G.; Begeot, M. & Naville, D. (2008). Leptin infusion and obesity in mouse cause alterations in the hypothalamic melanocortin system. *Obesity (Silver Spring)*, Vol.16, No.8, (August 2008), pp. 1763-1769, ISSN 1930-7381

Green, B.D. & Flatt, P.R. (2007) Incretin hormone mimetics and analogues in diabetes therapeutics. *Best practice & research. Clinical endocrinology & metabolism*, Vol.21, No.4, (December 2007), pp. 497–516, ISSN 1521-690X

Hall, K.E.; Liu, J.; Sima A.A.F. & Wiley, J.W. (2001). Impaired inhibitory G-protein function contributes to increased calcium currents in rats with diabetic neuropathy, *Journal of neurophysiology*, Vol.86, No.2, (August 2001), pp. 760–770, ISSN 0022-3077

Hamilton, A. & Holscher, C. (2009). Receptors for the insulin-like peptide GLP-1 are expressed on neurons in the CNS. *Neuroreport*, Vol.20, No.13, (August 2009), pp. 1161–1166, ISSN 0959-4965

Hamilton, A.; Patterson, S.; Porter, D.; Gault, V.A. & Holscher, C. (2011). Novel GLP-1 mimetics developed to treat type 2 diabetes promote progenitor cell proliferation in the brain. *Journal of neuroscience research*, Vol.89, No.4, (April 2011), pp. 481-489, ISSN 0360-4012

Haskell-Luevano, C.; Schaub, J.W.; Andreasen, A.; Haskell, K.R.; Moore, M.C.; Koerper, L.M.; Rouzaud, F.; Baker, H.V.; Millard, W.J.; Walter, G.; Litherland, S.A. & Xiang, Z. (2009). Voluntary exercise prevents the obese and diabetic metabolic syndrome of the melanocortin-4 receptor knockout mouse. *The FASEB journal*, Vol.23, No.2, (February 2009), pp. 642-655, ISSN 0892-6638

Havel, P.J.; Hahn, T.M.; Sindelar, D.K.; Baskin, D.G.; Dallman, M.F.; Weigle, D.S. & Schwartz, M.W. (2000). Effects of STZ-induced diabetes and insulin treatment on the hypothalamic melanocortin system and muscle uncoupling protein 3 expression in rats. *Diabetes*, Vol.49, No.2, (February 2000), pp. 44-52, ISSN 0012-1797

Heisler, L.K.; Cowley, M.A.; Tecott, L.H.; Fan, W.; Low, M.J.; Smart, J.L.; Rubinstein, M.; Tatro, J.B.; Marcus, J.N.; Holstege, H.; Lee, C.E.,; Cone, R.D. & Elmquist, J.K. (2002). Activation of central melanocortin pathways by fenfluramine. *Science*, Vol.297, No.5581, (July 2002), pp. 609–611, ISSN 0036-8075

Hegyi, K.; Fulop, K.; Kovacs, K.; Toth, S. & Falus, A. (2004). Leptin-induced signal transduction pathways. *Cell biology international*, Vol.28, No.3, (March 2004), pp. 159-169, ISSN 1065-6995

Herrera, R.; Manjarrez, G. & Hernandez, J. (2005). Inhibition and kinetic changes of brain tryptophan-5-hydroxylase during insulin-dependent diabetes mellitus in the rat. *Nutritional neuroscience*, Vol.8, No.1, (February 2005), pp. 57-62, ISSN 1028-415X

Herrera-Marquez, R.; Hernandez-Rodriguez, J.; Medina-Serrano, J.; Boyzo-Montes de Oca, A. & Manjarrez-Gutierrez, G. (2011). Association of metabolic syndrome with reduced central serotonergic activity. *Metabolic brain disease*, Vol.26, No.1, (March 2011), pp. 29-35, ISSN 0885-7490

Hofbauer, K.G.; Lecourt, A.C. & Peter, J.C. (2008). Antibodies as pharmacologic tools for studies on the regulation of energy balance. *Nutrition*, Vol.24, No.9, (July 2008), pp. 791-797, ISSN 0899-9007

Holst, J.J.; Burcelin, R. & Nathanson, E. (2001). Neuroprotective properties of GLP-1: theoretical and practical applications. *Current medical research and opinion*, Vol.27, No.3, (March 2011), pp. 547-558, ISSN 0300-7995

Hosoi, T.; Hyoda, K.; Okuma, Y.; Nomura, Y. & Ozawa, K. (2007). Inhibitory effect of 4-(2-aminoethyl)-benzenesulfonyl fluoride, a serine protease inhibitor, on PI3K inhibitor-induced CHOP expression. *European journal of pharmacology*, Vol.554, No.1, (January 2007), pp. 8-11, ISSN 0014-2999

Huo, L.; Gamber, K.; Greeley, S.; Silva, J.; Huntoon, N.; Leng, X.H. & Bjørbaek, C. (2009). Leptin-dependent control of glucose balance and locomotor activity by POMC neurons. *Cell metabolism*, Vol.9, No.6, (June 2009), pp. 537-547, ISSN 1550-4131

Irvine, E.E.; Drinkwater, L.; Radwanska, K.; Al-Qassab, H.; Smith, M.A.; O'Brien, M.; Kielar, C.; Choudhury, A.I.; Krauss, S.; Cooper, J.D.; Withers, D.J. & Giese, K.P.(2011). Insulin receptor substrate 2 is a negative regulator of memory formation. *Learning & memory*, Vol.18, No.6, (May 2011), pp. 375-383, ISSN 1072-0502

Iskandar, K.; Cao, Y.; Hayashi, Y.; Nakata, M.; Takano, E.; Yada, T.; Zhang, C.; Ogawa, W.; Oki, M.; Chua, S Jr.; Itoh, H.; Noda, T.; Kasuga, M. & Nakae, J. (2010). PDK-1/FoxO1 pathway in POMC neurons regulates Pomc expression and food intake. *American journal of physiology*, Vol.298, No.4, (January 2010), pp. 787–798, ISSN 0193-1849

Jackson, J. & Paulose, C.S. (1999). Enhancement of [$m$-methoxy $^3$H]MDL100907 binding to 5HT$_{2A}$ receptors in cerebral cortex and brain stem of streptozotocin induced diabetic rats. *Molecular and cellular biochemisty*, Vol.199, No.1-2, (September 1999), pp. 81-85, ISSN 0300-8177

Jolivalt, C.G.; Lee, C.A.; Beiswenger, K.K.; Smith, J.L.; Orlov, M.; Torrance, M.A. & Masliah, E. (2008). Defective insulin signaling pathway and increased glycogen synthase kinase-3 activity in the brain of diabetic mice: parallels with Alzheimer's disease and correction by insulin. *Journal of neuroscience research*, Vol.86, No.15, (November 2008), pp. 3265-3274, ISSN 0360-4012

Joseph, A.; Antony, S. & Paulose, C.S. (2008). Increased glutamate receptor gene expression in the cerebral cortex of insulin induced hypoglycemic and streptozotocin-induced diabetic rats. *Neuroscience*, Vol.156, No.2, (October 2008), pp. 298-304, ISSN 0306-4522

Kalra, S.P. (2008). Disruption in the leptin-NPY link underlies the pandemic of diabetes and metabolic syndrome: new therapeutic approaches. *Nutrition*, Vol.24, No.9, (September 2008), pp. 820-826, ISSN 0899-9007

Kerr, J.L.; Timpe, E.M. & Petkewicz, K.A. (2010). Bromocriptine mesylate for glycemic management in type 2 diabetes mellitus. *Annals of pharmacotherapy*, Vol.44, No.11, (November 2010), pp. 1777-1785, ISSN 1060-0280

Kitamura, T.; Feng, Y.; Kitamura, Y.I.; Chua, S.C. Jr.; Xu, A.W.; Barsh, G.S.; Rossetti, L. & Accili, D. (2006). Forkhead protein FoxO1 mediates Agrp-dependent effects of leptin on food intake. *Nature medicine*, Vol.12, No.5, (April 2006), pp. 534–540, ISSN 1078-8956

Koch, L.; Wunderlich, F.T.; Seibler, J.; Könner, A.C.; Hampel, B.; Irlenbusch, S.; Brabant, G.; Kahn, C.R.; Schwenk, F. & Brüning, J.C. (2008). Central insulin action regulates peripheral glucose and fat metabolism in mice, *The Journal of clinical investigation*, Vol.118, No.6, (May 2008), pp. 2132–2147, ISSN 0021-9738

Kojima, S.; Asakawa, A.; Amitani, H.; Sakoguchi, T.; Ueno, N.; Inui, A. & Kalra, S.P. (2009). Central leptin gene therapy, a substitute for insulin therapy to ameliorate hyperglycemia and hyperphagia, and promote survival in insulin-deficient diabetic mice. *Peptides*, Vol.30, No.5, (January 2009), pp. 962-966, ISSN 0196-9781

Kumar, T.P.; Antony, S.; Gireesh, G.; George, N. & Paulose, C.S. (2010). Curcumin modulates dopaminergic receptor, CREB and phospholipase C gene expression in the cerebral cortex and cerebellum of streptozotocin induced diabetic rats. *Journal of biomedical science*, Vol.17, No.1, (May 2010), pp. 43-53, ISSN 1021-7770

Kumar, P.T.; Antony, S.; Nandhu, M.S.; Sadanandan, J.; Naijil, G. & Paulose, C.S. (2011). Vitamin $D_3$ restores altered cholinergic and insulin receptor expression in the cerebral cortex and muscarinic $M_3$ receptor expression in pancreatic islets of streptozotocin induced diabetic rats. *The Journal of nutritional biochemistry*, Vol.22, No.5, (May 2011), pp. 418-425, ISSN 0955-2863

Kuo, D.Y. (2006). Hypothalamic neuropeptide Y (NPY) and the attenuation of hyperphagia in streptozotocin diabetic rats treated with dopamine D1/D2 agonists. *British journal of pharmacology*, Vol.148, No.5, (July 2006), pp. 640-647, ISSN 0007-1188

Lee, Y.H. & White, M.F. (2004). Insulin receptor substrate proteins and diabetes. *Archives of pharmacal research*, Vol.27, No.4, (April 2004), pp. 361-370, ISSN 0253-6269

Li, X.L.; Aou, S.; Oomura, Y.; Hori, N.; Fukunaga, K. & Hori, T. (2002). Impairment of long-term potentiation and spatial memory in leptin receptor-deficient rodents. *Neuroscience*, Vol.113, No.3, (August 2002), pp. 607–615, ISSN 0306-4522

Li, X.; Wu, X.; Camacho, R.; Schwartz, G.J. & LeRoith, D. (2011). Intracerebroventricular leptin infusion improves glucose homeostasis in lean type 2 diabetic MKR mice via hepatic vagal and non-vagal mechanisms. *PloS one [electronic resource]*, Vol.6, No.2, (February 2011), p. e17058, ISSN 1932-6203

Li, J.X. & France, C.P. (2008). Food restriction and streptozotocin treatment decrease 5-HT1A and 5-HT2A receptor-mediated behavioral effects in rats. *Behavioural pharmacology*, Vol.19, No.4, (July 2008), pp. 292-297, ISSN 0955-8810

Li, M.D.; Kane, J.K. & Konu, O. (2003). Nicotine, body weight and potential implications in the treatment of obesity. *Current topics in medicinal chemistry*, Vol.3, No.8, (August 2003), pp. 899–919, ISSN 1568-0266

Li, N.; Young, M.M.; Bailey, C.J. & Smith, M.E. (1999). NMDA and AMPA glutamate receptor subtypes in the thoracic spinal cord in lean and obese-diabetic *ob/ob* mice. *Brain research*, Vol.849, No.1-2, (December 1999), pp. 34–44, ISSN 0006-8993

Li, Z.G.; Zhang, W. & Sima, A.A. (2007). Alzheimer-like changes in rat models of spontaneous diabetes. *Diabetes*, Vol.56, No.7, (July 2007), pp. 1817-1824, ISSN 0012-1797

Lin, H.V. & Accili, D. (2011). Reconstitution of insulin action in muscle, white adipose tissue, and brain of insulin receptor knock-out mice fails to rescue diabetes. *The Journal of biological chemistry*, Vol.286, No.11, (March 2011), pp. 9797-9804, ISSN 0021-9258

Lin, X.; Taguchi, A.; Park, S.; Kushner, J.A.; Li, F.; Li, Y. & White, M.F. (2004). Dysregulation of insulin receptor substrate 2 in β cells and brain causes obesity and diabetes. *The Journal of clinical investigation*, Vol.114, No.7, (October 2004), pp. 908–916, ISSN 0021-9738

Liu, J.; Wang, W.; Wang, F.; Cai, F.; Hu, Z.L.; Yang, Y.J.; Chen, J. & Chen, J.G. (2009). Phosphatidylinositol-linked novel $D_1$ dopamine receptor facilitates long-term depression in rat hippocampal CA1 synapses. *Neuropharmacology*, Vol.57, No.2, (August 2009), pp. 164-171, ISSN 0028-3908

Liu, Y.; Liu, L.; Lu, S.; Wang, D.; Liu, X.; Xie, L. & Wang, G. (2011). Impaired amyloid β-degrading enzymes in brain of streptozotocin-induced diabetic rats. *Journal of endocrinological investigation*, Vol.34, No.1, (January 2011), pp. 26-31, ISSN 0391-4097

Lozovsky, D.; Saller, C.F. & Kopin, I.J. (1981). Dopamine receptor binding is increased in diabetic rats. *Science*, Vol.214, No.4524, (November 1981), pp. 1031-1033, ISSN 0036-8075

Lovshin, J.A.& Drucker, D.J. (2009). Incretin-based therapies for type 2 diabetes mellitus. *Nature reviews. Endocrinology*, Vol.5, No.5, (May 2009), pp. 262–269, ISSN 1759-5029

Luján R., (2007). Subcellular regulation of metabotropic GABA receptors in the developing cerebellum, *The cerebellum*, Vol.6, No.2, pp. 123–129, ISSN 1473-4222

Luo, J.; Balkin, N.; Stewart, J.; Sarwark, J.; Charrow, J. & Nye, J. (2000). Neural tube defects and the 13q deletion syndrome: evidence for a critical region in 13q33-34. *American journal of medical genetics*, Vol.91, No.3, (March 2000), pp. 227-230, ISSN 0148-7299

Luo, S.; Luo, J. & Cincotta, A.H. (2000). Association of the antidiabetic effects of bromocriptine with a shift in the daily rhythm of monoamine metabolism within the suprachiasmatic nuclei of the Syrian hamster. *Chronobiology international*, Vol.17, No.2, (March 2000), pp. 155-172, ISSN 0742-0528

Lupien, S.B.; Bluhm, E.J. & Ishii, D.N. (2003). Systemic insulin-like growth factor-I administration prevents cognitive impairment in diabetic rats, and brain IGF regulates learning/memory in normal adult rats. *Journal of neuroscience research*, Vol.74, No.4, (November 2003), pp. 512-523, ISSN 0360-4012

Lustman, P.J.; Freedland, K.E.; Griffith, L.S. & Clouse, R.E. (2000). Fluoxetine for depression in diabetes: a randomized double-blind placebo-controlled trial. *Diabetes Care*, Vol.23, No.5, (May 2000), pp. 618–623, ISSN 0149-5992

Lustman, P.J. & Clouse, R.E. (2005). Depression in diabetic patients: the relationship between mood and glycemic control. *Journal of diabetes and its complications*, Vol.19, No.2, (March-April 2005), pp. 113-122, ISSN 1056-8727

Mackenzie, R.G. & Trulson, M.E. (1978). Effects of insulin and streptozotocin-induced diabetes on brain tryptophan and serotonin metabolism in rats. *Journal of neurochemistry*, Vol.30, N0.1, (January 1978), pp. 205–211, ISSN 0022-3042

Maekawa, F.; Fujiwara, K.; Kohno, D.; Kuramochi, M.; Kurita, H. & Yada, T. (2006). Young adult-specific hyperphagia in diabetic Goto-kakizaki rats is associated with leptin resistance and elevation of neuropeptide Y mRNA in the arcuate nucleus. *Journal of neuroendocrinology*, Vol.18, No.10, (October 2006), pp. 748-756, ISSN 0953-8194

Malcangio, M. & Tomlinson, D.R. (1998). A pharmacologic analysis of mechanical hyperalgesia in streptozotocin/diabetic rats. *Pain*, Vol.76, No.1-2, (May 1998), pp. 151–157, ISSN 0304-3959

Manjarrez-Gutierrez, G.; Marquez, R.H.; Mejenes-Alvarez, S.A.; Godinez-Lopez, T. & Hernandez, R.J. (2009). Functional change of the auditory cortex related to brain serotonergic neurotransmission in type 1 diabetic adolescents with and without depression. *World J Biol Psychiatry*, Vol.4, No.10(4 Pt 3), pp. 877-883, ISSN 1562-2975

Marino, J.S.; Xu, Y. & Hill, J.W. (2011). Central insulin and leptin-mediated autonomic control of glucose homeostasis. *Trends in endocrinology and metabolism : TEM*, Vol.22, No.7, (July 2011), pp. 275-285, ISSN 1043-2760

McClean P.L.; Gault, V.A.; Harriott, P. & Hölscher, C. (2010). Glucagon-like peptide-1 analogues enhance synaptic plasticity in the brain: a link between diabetes and Alzheimer's disease. *European journal of pharmacology*, Vol.630, No.1-3, (March 2010), pp. 158-162, ISSN 0014-2999

Morton, G.J.; Gelling, R.W.; Niswender, K.D.; Morrison, C.D.; Rhodes, C.J. & Schwartz, M.W. (2005). Leptin regulates insulin sensitivity via phosphatidylinositol-3-OH kinase signaling in mediobasal hypothalamic neurons, *Cell metabolism*, Vol.2, No.6, (December 2005), pp. 411–420, ISSN 1550-4131

Mutze, J.; Roth, J.; Gersberg, M.; Matsumura, K. & Hubschle, T. (2006). Immunohistocemical evidence of functional leptin receptor expression in neuronal and endothelial cells of the brain. *Neuroscience letters,* Vol..394, No.2, (November 2005), pp. 105-110, ISSN 0304-3940

Nargund, R.P.; Strack, A.M. & Fong, T.M. (2006). Melanocortin-4 receptor (MC4R) agonists for the treatment of obesity. *Journal of medicinal chemistry,* Vol.49, No.14, (July 2006), pp. 4035-4043, ISSN 0022-2623

Nelson, K.A.; Park, K.M.; Robinovitz, E.; Tsigos, C. & Max, M.B. (1997). High-dose oral dextromethorphan versus placebo in painful diabetic neuropathy and postherpetic neuralgia, *Neurology,* Vol.48, No.5, (May 1997), pp. 1212–1218, ISSN 0028-3878

Nogueiras, R.; Wiedmer, P.; Perez-Tilve, D.; Veyrat-Durebex, C.; Keogh, J.M.; Sutton, G.M.; Pfluger, P.T.; Castanada, T.R.; Neschen, S. & Hofmann, S.M. (2007). The central melanocortin system directly controls peripheral lipid metabolism. *The Journal of clinical investigation*, Vol.117, No.11, (November 2007), pp. 3475–3488, ISSN 0021-9738

Nonogaki, K.; Ohba, Y.; Sumii, M.; & Oka, Y. (2008). Serotonin systems upregulate the expression of hypothalamic NUCB2 via 5-HT2C receptors and induce anorexia via a leptin-independent pathway in mice. *Biochemical and biophysical research communications*, Vol.372, No.1, (July 2008), pp. 186-190, ISSN 0006-291X

Obici, S.; Feng, Z.; Karkanias, G.; Baskin, D.G. & Rossetti, L. (2002). Decreasing hypothalamic insulin receptors causes hyperphagia and insulin resistance in rats, *Nature neuroscience*, Vol.5, No.6, (June 2002), pp. 566–572, ISSN 1097-6256

Obici, S.; Feng, Z.; Tan, J.; Liu, L.; Karkanias, G. & Rossetti, L. (2001). Central melanocortin receptors regulate insulin action. *The Journal of clinical investigation*, Vol.108, No.7, (October 2001), pp. 1079–1085, ISSN 0021-9738

Okamoto, H.; Nakae, J.; Kitamura, T.; Park, B.C.; Dragatsis, I. & Accili, D. (2004). Transgenic rescue of insulin receptor-deficient mice. *The Journal of clinical investigation*, Vol.114, No.2, (July 2004), pp. 214-223, ISSN 0021-9738

Okouchi, M.; Okayama, N.; Alexander, J.S. & Aw, T.Y. (2006). NRF2-dependent glutamate-L- cysteine ligase catalytic subunit expression mediates insulin protection against hyperglycemia- induced brain endothelial cell apoptosis. *Current neurovascular research*, Vol.3, No.4, (November 2006), pp. 249-261, ISSN 1567-2026

Peeyush Kumar, T.; Antony, S.; Soman, S.; Kuruvilla, K.P.; George, N. & Paulose, C.S. (2011). Role of curcumin in the prevention of cholinergic mediated cortical dysfunctions in streptozotocin-induced diabetic rats. *Molecular and cellular endocrinology*, Vol.331, No.1, (January 2011), pp. 1-10, ISSN 0303-7207

Peter, J.C.; Zipfel, G.; Lecourt, A.C.; Bekel, A. & Hofbauer, K.G. (2010). Antibodies raised against different extracellular loops of the melanocortin-3 receptor affect energy balance and autonomic function in rats. *Journal of receptor and signal transduction research,* Vol.30, No.6, (December 2010), pp. 444-453, ISSN 1532-4281

Picciotto, M.R,; Caldarone, B.J.; King, S.L. & Zachariou, V. (2000). Nicotinic receptors in the brain. Links between molecular biology and behavior, *Neuropsychopharmacology,* Vol.22, No. 22, (May 2000), pp. 451–465, ISSN 0893-133X

Pijl, H. & Edo, A.M. (2002). Modulation of monoaminergic neural circuits: potential for the treatment of type 2 diabetes mellitus. *Treatments in endocrinology,* Vol.1, No.2, (April 2002), pp. 71-78, ISSN 1175-6349

Pijl, H.; Ohashi, S.; Matsuda, M.; Miyazaki, Y.; Mahankali, A.; Kumar, V.; Pipek, R.; Iozzo, P.; Lancaster, J.L.; Cincotta, A.H. & DeFronzo, R.A..(2000). Bromocriptine: a novel approach to the treatment of type 2 diabetes. *Diabetes care,* Vol.23, No.8, (August 2000), pp. 1154-1161, ISSN 0149-5992

Porter, A.C.; Bymaster, F.P.; DeLapp, N.W.; Yamada, M.; Wess, J.; Hamilton, S.E.; Nathanson, N.M. & Felder, C.C. (2002). $M_1$ muscarinic receptor signaling in mouse hippocampus and cortex. *Brain research,* Vol.944, No.1-2, (July 2002), pp. 82-89, ISSN 0006-8993

Qiu, W.Q. & Folstein, M.F. (2006). Insulin, insulin-degrading enzyme and amyloid-beta peptide in Alzheimer's disease: review and hypothesis. *Neurobiology of aging,* Vol.27, No.2, (February 2006), pp. 190-198, ISSN 0197-4580

Reisi, P.; Alaei, H.; Babri, S.; Sharifi, M.R.; Mohaddes, G. & Soleimannejad, E. (2009). Determination of the extracellular basal levels of glutamate and GABA at dentate gyrus of streptozotocin-induced diabetic rats, *Pathophysiology,* Vol.16, No.1, (June 2009), pp. 63-66, ISSN 0928-4680

Roseberry, A.G.; Painter, T.; Mark, G.P. & Williams, J.T. (2007). Decreased vesicular somatodendritic dopamine stores in leptin-deficient mice. *The Journal of neuroscience,* Vol.27, No.26, (June 2007), pp. 7021-7027, ISSN 0270-6474

Sahu, A.; Sninsky, C.A.; Kalra, P.S. & Kalra, S.P. (1990). Neuropeptide-Y concentration in microdissected hypothalamic regions and *in vitro* release from the medial basal hypothalamus-preoptic area of streptozotocin-diabetic rats with and without insulin substitution therapy. *Endocrinology,* Vol.126, No.1, (January 1990), pp. 192-198, ISSN 0013-7227

Sandrini, M.; Vitale, G.; Vergoni, A.V.; Ottani, A. & Bertolini, A. (1997). Streptozotocin-induced diabetes provokes changes in serotonin concentration and on 5-$HT_{1A}$ and 5-$HT_{2A}$ receptor in rat brain, *Life sciences,* Vol.60, No.16, (March 1997), pp. 1393–1397, ISSN 0024-3205

Satoh, E. & Takahashi, A. (2008). Experimental diabetes enhances Ca2+ mobilization and glutamate exocytosis in cerebral synaptosomes from mice. *Diabetes research and clinical practice,* Vol.81, No.2, (August 2008), pp. e14-e17, ISSN 0168-8227

Savitha, B.; Joseph, B.; Peeyush Kumar, T. & Paulose, C.S. (2010). Acetylcholine and muscarinic receptor function in cerebral cortex of diabetic young and old male Wistar rats and the role of muscarinic receptors in calcium release from pancreatic islets. *Biogerontology,* Vol.11, No.2, (April 2010), pp. 151-166, ISSN 1389-5729

Scheen, A.J. (2010). Central nervous system: a conductor orchestrating metabolic regulations harmed by both hyperglycaemia and hypoglycaemia. *Diabetes & metabolism,* Vol.36, Suppl.3, (October 2010), pp. 31-38, ISSN 1262-3636

Schubert, M.; Brazil, D.P.; Burks, D.J.; Kushner, J.A.; Ye, J.; Flint, C.L.; Farhang-Fallah, J.;
    Dikkes, P.; Warot, X.M.; Rio, C.; Corfas, G. & White, M.F. (2003). Insulin receptor
    substrate-2 deficiency impairs brain growth and promotes tau phosphorylation. *The
    Journal of neuroscience*, Vol.23, No.18, (August 2003), pp. 7084-7092, ISSN 0270-6474
Schubert, M.; Gautam, D.; Surjo, D.; Ueki, K.; Baudler, S.; Schubert, D.; Kondo, T.; Alber, J.;
    Galldiks, N.; Küstermann, E.; Arndt, S.; Jacobs, A.H.; Krone, W.; Kahn, C.R. &
    Brüning, J.C. (2004). Role for neuronal insulin resistance in neurodegenerative
    diseases. *Proceedings of the National Academy of Sciences of the U SA*, Vol.101, No.9,
    (March 2004), pp. 3100-3105, ISSN 0027-8424
Schwartz, N.E. & Alford, S. (2000). Physiological activation of presynaptic metabotropic
    glutamate receptors increases intracellular calcium and glutamate release. *Journal of
    neurophysiology*, Vol.84, No.1, (July 2000), pp. 415-427, ISSN 0022-3077
Schwartz, M.W.; Woods, S.C.; Porte, DJr.; Seeley, R.J. & Baskin, D.G. (2000). Central nervous
    system control of food intake. *Nature*, Vol.404, No.6778, (April 2000), pp. 661-671,
    ISSN 0028-0836
Scranton, R.E.; Gaziano, J.M.; Rutty, D.; Ezrokhi, M. & Cincotta, A. (2007). A randomized,
    double-blind,  placebo-controlled trial to assess safety and tolerability during
    treatment of type 2 diabetes with usual diabetes therapy and either Cycloset or
    placebo. *BMC endocrine disorders [electronic resource]*, Vol.7, No.3 (June 2007), pp. 7,
    ISSN 1472-6823
Serbedzija, P.; Madl, J.E. & Ishii, D.N. (2009). Insulin and IGF-I prevent brain atrophy and
    DNA loss in diabetes. *Brain research*, Vol.1303, (September 2009), pp. 179-194, ISSN
    0006-8993
Shafrir, E. (2010). Contribution of animal models to the research of the causes of diabetes.
    *World journal of diabetes,* Vol.1, No.5, (November 2010), pp. 137-140, ISSN 1948-9358
Shankar, P.N.; Joseph, A. & Paulose, C.S. (2007). Decreased [3H] YM-09151-2 binding to
    dopamine D2  receptors in the hypothalamus, brainstem and pancreatic islets of
    streptozotocin-induced diabetic rats. *European journal of pharmacology*, Vol.557,
    No.2-3, (February 2007), pp. 99–105, ISSN 0014-2999
Sherin, A.; Peeyush, K.T.; Naijil, G.; Chinthu, R. & Paulose, C.S. (2010). Hypoglycemia
    induced behavioural deficit and decreased GABA receptor, CREB expression in the
    cerebellum of streptozotocin induced diabetic rats. *Brain research bulletin*, Vol.83,
    No.6, (November 2010), pp. 360-366, ISSN 0361-9230
Sherin, A.; Peeyush, K.T.; Naijil, G.; Nandhu, M.S.; Jayanarayanan, S.; Jes, P. & Paulose, C.S.
    (2011). The effects of abnormalities of glucose homeostasis on the expression and
    binding of muscarinic receptors in cerebral cortex of rats. *European journal of
    pharmacology*, Vol.65, No.1-3, (January 2011), pp. 128-136, ISSN 0014-2999
Shimizu, H. & Bray, G.A. (1990). Effects of insulin on hypothalamic monoamine metabolism.
    *Brain research*, Vol.510, No.2, (March 1990), pp.251–258, ISSN 0006-8993
Shpakov, A.O. (2011). GPCR-based peptides: structure, mechanisms of action and
    application. *Global Journal of Biochemistry*, Vol.2, No.2, (June 2011), pp. 96–123, ISSN
    2229 – 709X
Shpakov, A.O.; Kuznetsova, L.A.; Plesneva, S.A.; Bondareva, V.M.; Guryanov, I.A.; Vlasov,
    G.P. & Pertseva M.N. (2006). Decrease in functional activity of G-proteins hormone-
    sensitive adenylate cyclase signaling system, during experimental type II diabetes

mellitus. *Bulletin of experimental biology and medicine*, Vol.142, No.6, (December 2006), pp. 685-689, ISSN 0007-4888

Shpakov, A.O.; Kuznetsova, L.A.; Plesneva, S.A.; Gurianov, I.A.; Vlasov, G.P. & Pertseva, M.N. (2007a). The identification of disturbances in hormone-sensitive AC system in rat tissues in types 1 and 2 diabetes mellitus with using functional probes and synthetic peptides. *Tekhnologii zhivykh system*, Vol.4, No.2, (March 2007), pp. 96-108, (in Russian), ISSN 2070-0997

Shpakov, A.O.; Kuznetsova, L.A.; Plesneva, S.A. & Pertseva, M.N. (2007b). The disturbance of the transduction of adenylyl cyclase inhibiting hormonal signal in myocardium and brain of rats with experimental type II diabetes. *Tsitologiia*, Vol.49, No.6, (June 2007), pp. 442-450 (in Russian), ISSN 0041-3771

Signore, A.P.; Zhang, F.; Weng1, Z.; Gao, Y.Q. & Chen, J. (2008). Leptin neuroprotection in the CNS: mechanisms and therapeutic potentials. *Journal of neurochemistry*, Vol.106, No.5, (September 2008), pp. 1977–1990, ISSN 0022-3042

Sindelar, D.K.; Mystkowski, P.; Marsh, D.J.; Palmiter, R.D. & Schwartz, M.W. (2002). Attenuation of diabetic hyperphagia in neuropeptide Y--deficient mice. *Diabetes*, Vol.51, No.3, (March 2002), pp. 778–783, ISSN 0012-1797

Tatro, J.B. (2006). Melanocortins defend their territory: multifaceted neuroprotection in cerebral ischemia. *Endocrinology*, Vol.147, No.3, (March 2006), pp. 1122-1125, ISSN 0013-7227

Toda, C.; Shiuchi, T.; Lee, S.; Yamato-Esaki, M.; Fujino, Y.; Suzuki, A.; Okamoto, S. & Minokoshi, Y. (2009). Distinct effects of leptin and a melanocortin receptor agonist injected into medial hypothalamic nuclei on glucose uptake in peripheral tissues. *Diabetes*, Vol.58, No.12, (December 2009), pp. 2757-2765, ISSN 0012-1797

Tomiyama, M.; Furusawa, K.; Kamijo, M.; Kimura, T.; Matsunaga, M. & Baba, M. (2005). Upregulation of mRNAs coding for AMPA and NMDA receptor subunits and metabotropic glutamate receptors in the dorsal horn of the spinal cord in a rat model of diabetes mellitus. *Brain research*, Vol.138, No.1-2, (May 2005), pp. 275–281, ISSN 0169-328X

Trento, M.; Kucich, C.; Tibaldi, P.; Gennari, S.; Tedesco, S.; Balbo, M.; Arvat, E.; Cavallo, F.; Ghigo, E. & Porta, M. (2010). A study of central serotoninergic activity in healthy subjects and patients with Type 2 diabetes treated by traditional one-to-one care or Group Care. *Journal of endocrinological investigation*, Vol.33, No.9, (October 2010), pp. 624-628, ISSN 0391-4097

Trudeau, F.; Gagnon, S. & Massicotte, G. (2004). Hippocampal synaptic plasticity and glutamate receptor regulation: influences of diabetes mellitus. *European journal of pharmacology*, Vol.490, No.1–3, (April 2004), pp. 177–186, ISSN 0014-2999

Van der Heide, L.P.; Kamal, A.; Artola, A.; Gispen, W.H. & Ramakers, G.M. (2005). Insulin modulates hippocampal activity-dependent synaptic plasticity in N-methyl-D-aspartate receptor and phosphatidyl-inositol-3-kinase-dependent manner. *Journal of neurochemistry*, Vol.94, No.4, (August 2005), pp. 1158-1166, ISSN 0022-3042

Van Tilburg, M.A.; McCaskill, C.C.; Lane, J.D.; Edwards, C.L.; Bethel, A.; Feinglos, M.N. & Surwit, R.S. (2001). Depressed mood is a factor in glycemic control in type 1 diabetes. *Psychosomatic medicine*, Vol.63, No.4, (July-August 2001), pp. 551–555, ISSN 0033-3174

Voitenko, N.V.; Kruglikov, I.A.; Kostyuk, E.P. & Kostyuk, P.G. (2000). Effect of STZ-induced diabetes on the activity of calcium channels in rat dorsal horn neurons. *Neuroscience*, Vol.95, No.2, (February 2000), pp. 519–524, ISSN 0306-4522

Wang, M.Y.; Chen, L.; Clark, G.O.; Lee, Y.; Stevens, R.D.; Ilkayeva, O.R.; Wenner, B.R.; Bain, J.R.; Charron, M.J.; Newgard, C.B. & Unger, R.H. (2010). Leptin therapy in insulin-deficient type I diabetes. *Proceedings of the National Academy of Sciences USA*, Vol.107, No.11, (March 2010), pp. 4813-48199, ISSN 0027-8424

Weng, Z.; Signore, A.P.; Gao, Y.; Wang, S.; Zhang, F.; Hastings, T.; Yin, X.M. & Chen, J. (2007). Leptin protects against 6-hydroxydopamine-induced dopaminergic cell death via mitogen-activated protein kinase signaling. *The Journal of biological chemistry*, Vol.282, No.47, (September 2007), pp. 34479-34491, ISSN 0021-9258

Wredling, R.A.; Theorell, P.G.; Roll, H.M.; Lins, P.E. & Adamson, U.K. (1992). Psychosocial state of patients with IDDM prone to recurrent episodes of severe hypoglycemia, *Diabetes care*, Vol.15, No.4, (April 1992), pp. 518–521, ISSN 0149-5992

Yamato, T.; Misumi, Y.; Yamasaki, S.; Kino, M. & Aomine, M. (2004). Diabetes mellitus decreases hippocampal release of neurotransmitters: an in vivo microdialysis study of awake, freely moving rats. *Diabetes, nutrition & metabolism*, Vol.17, No.3, (June 2004), pp. 128–136, ISSN 0394-3402

Yuan, X.; Yamada, K.; Ishiyama-Shigemoto, S.; Koyama, W. & Nonaka, K. (2000). Identification of polymorphic loci in the promoter region of the serotonin 5-HT2C receptor gene and their association with obesity and type II diabetes. *Diabetologia*, Vol.43, No.3, (March 2000), pp. 373-376, ISSN 0012-186X

Zhou, L.; Sutton, G.M.; Rochford, J.J.; Semple, R.K.; Lam, D.D.; Oksanen, L.J.; Thornton-Jones, Z.D.; Clifton, P.G.; Yueh, C.Y.; Evans, M.L.; McCrimmon, R.J.; Elmquist, J.K.; Butler, A.A. & Heisler, L.K. (2007). Serotonin 2C receptor agonists improve type 2 diabetes via melanocortin-4 receptor signaling pathways. *Cell metabolism*, Vol.6, No.5, (November 2007), pp. 398-405, ISSN 1550-4131

Zhu, X.; Perry, G. & Smith, M.A. (2005). Insulin signaling, diabetes mellitus and risk of Alzheimer disease. *Journal of Alzheimer's disease*, Vol.7, No.1, (February 2005), pp. 81-84, ISSN 1387-2877

# Power of a Metabonomic Approach to Investigate an Unknown Nervous Disease

Céline Domange[1], Alain Paris[2], Henri Schroeder[3] and Nathalie Priymenko[1,4]
*[1]Toulouse Nationale Veterinary School,*
*Alimentation & Botanics, Toulouse*
*[2]INRA - Mét@risk Unit, AgroParisTech, Paris*
*[3]UR AFPA, INRA UC340, Nancy University,*
*Faculty of Sciences & Technologies, Nancy*
*[4]UMR 1331 ToxAlim INRA INP, Toulouse*
*France*

## 1. Introduction

The field of neurological disorders becomes now one of the most important investigation areas in clinical medicine, whatever the toxicological, genetic, degenerative or environmental aetiology they have. Because it involves the main complex organ as target tissue, because also of the intrinsic specificity of the biological network of the nervous system, or the technical difficulty to access such a composite organ, the nervous diseases remain particularly difficult to study. Certainly, the rapid development of transgenic animal models of neurological diseases and the expanding growth of imaging techniques to functionally and non-invasively access some specific brain regions constitute a favourable situation to study the basis and the progression of some nervous diseases. However, the use of such transgenic animals or spontaneous animal models needs that the clinical symptoms are reproducible and that a *prior* knowledge of the aetiopathology of these diseases may exist. These latter conditions are not always available, especially concerning toxicology. In this case, how can both pathophysiology and therapies be investigated? Indeed, classically, when considering a toxicological approach, clinical signs, similar to those ascribed on the target species, need to be reproduced on the animal model. But how to do with disease displaying no known aetiology or with an animal model, on which it is impossible to reproduce, at least partially, some clinical signs of the target species? Furthermore, because of evident ethical reasons added to practical ones, some neurological disorders in humans or in large animals remain scarcely explored. "Omics" approaches seem to be a good alternative in the clinical medical research, enabling to take advantage of the global living system and, simultaneously of the control of the toxicological factor. To illustrate such an original approach, a neurological horse disease, Australian stringhalt, which has been described for several centuries, but for which aetiology is still only partially known, was reassessed using metabonomics in combination with other classical techniques. This has led to show how powerful this method may stand for in clinical medical research and, particularly in neurological studies.

## 2. Current neurological investigations: Advantages and limits of routinely used approaches and techniques

### 2.1 Limits of classical studies

Up to now, the neurological investigations tended to reproduce a human disease using a convenient animal model. However, they laboured to give results. In fact, it may appear surprising to recreate all the metabolic complexity prevailing in the genesis of a given disease and, to work on it, before having any knowledge of the specifically involved metabolic pathways specifically involved. Before considering an animal model as a convenient model of a human disease, it seems more consistent to record and describe all the putative impacts of a controlled *stimulus* on a living system without any *a priori* hypothesis because of our ignorance of the inherent metabolic disruptions involved. Indeed, this may help to efficiently tackle a neurological disease.

### 2.2 Behavioural approaches

The use of animal models of human diseases, on which some behavioural tests are carried out, is fundamental to investigate nervous disorders. The field of psychopharmacology or behavioural pharmacology enables to test and to measure effects of drugs on behaviour. The toxicological studies test the short- or long-term exposure, the acute intoxication or the chronic effects following administration of subclinical doses and the associated effects of chemical compounds or contaminants. Each behavioural manifestation in animal model tends to reflect a specific human behavioural alteration or cognitive effect like depression, anxiety, fear or schizophrenia. This may be susceptible to reveal a disruption in some mean way of neurological transduction involving, for example, dopamine, acetylcholine, amphetamine or catecholamine's impairments. However, this approach has some limits. In case of the lack of any behavioural manifestation in animals, the conclusion isn't that there is a lack of effect but only that there is an impossibility to give an interpretation of this lack of effect because of an inadequate "observation window" as in delayed toxicity of some contaminants for example. Moreover, the putative link between a visible behavioural impairment and a putative mechanistic explanation requires going back to the cerebral metabolism to translate the observed behavioural variance and to confirm the pertinence of metabolic pathways specifically involved. Most of the time, such behavioural approaches are hardly self-sufficient; they need to be completed by other studies such as metabolic, histological, anatomical or immunologic ones.

### 2.3 Imaging techniques

A wide range of imaging techniques provides powerful tools for studying tumours (Cooper et al., 2011), congenital diseases (Toga et al., 2006), metabolic and infectious diseases (Kastrup et al., 2005), development of organisms (Davis et al., 2011) and for realizing preclinical or clinical studies, or for measuring a treatment effect (Song et al., 2011). These techniques can also be used in neurotoxicology (Pogge and Slikker, 2004) or for exploring neurodegenerative or psychiatric disorders (Masdeu, 2011; Stoessl, 2011). The choice of one of these techniques is made according to some awaited answers to a specific anatomical, metabolic or functional information question, some of imaging techniques being able to perform several specific assessments. They are well adapted to describe functions in the frame of non-invasive *in vivo* studies, some being planned with a longitudinal follow-up. Concerning some specific tissues analyses, some compromises have to be done between the spatial or the temporal resolution according to what it has to be focussed on. Among these different techniques, anatomic or functional imaging techniques have to be distinguished. The first ones, tomodensitometry and magnetic resonance imaging or MRI (Griffith et al., 2007) provide highly detailed anatomic information. Their ability to give an access to *in vivo* biological information acquired non-invasively or to define a seemingly normal body composition and its perturbation in response to a pharmacological or a pathological event may facilitate exploration of nervous diseases (Frisoni and Filippi, 2005; Griffith et al., 2007; Tartaglia and Arnold, 2006). In parallel with the description of novel biomarkers coming from transgenic animal models developed for studying neurodegenerative diseases and more efficient therapies, the use of MRI and magnetic resonance spectroscopy (MRS) provide new information for *in vivo* neurochemistry, such as neuronal apoptosis, osmoregulation, energy metabolism, membrane function or signalling disruptions (Choi et al., 2007; Ross and Sachdev, 2004; Ross and Bluml, 2001). Most of clinical researches are based on the metabolites that are detectable using proton spectroscopy (Figure 1), which can quantify them in localized volumes in brain.

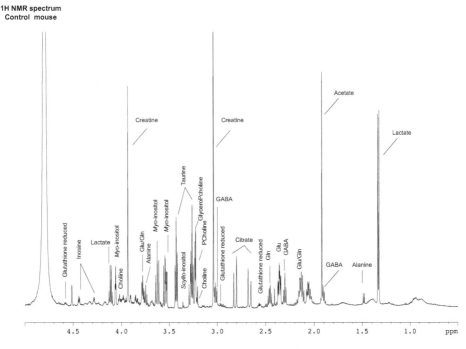

Fig. 1. 600.13 MHz ¹H NMR spectra from aqueous extracts of brain in mouse (control animal) (from Domange, 2008)

Nuclear magnetic resonance (or NMR) methods (MRI or MRS) can be successfully used to reveal neurological markers like N-acetyl-aspartate (a neuronal and axonal marker associated with neuronal viability), *myo*-inositol (a cerebral osmolyte and an astrocytic marker), glutamate and glutamine (the first is a major excitatory neurotransmitter and the second can restore it), creatine (which plays a crucial role in ATP biosynthesis in astrocytes), choline (its increased concentration theoretically means an alteration of myelin) and gamma-amino butyric acid (a main inhibitory neurotransmitter) (Martin, 2007). But MRS can also record intrinsic containing metabolites containing other atoms, as phosphorus, sodium, potassium, carbon, nitrogen and fluorine (this last atom often being a constituent of many drugs). Among the functional imaging techniques, positron emission tomography (PET) is a three-dimensional diagnostic imaging technology used in nuclear medicine that measures physiological function by looking at various functions of the body. It is a non-invasive diagnostic imaging tool enabling to follow some chemical neurotransmitters like dopamine in Parkinson's disease. Whatever the technique used to cover a specific neurological question, most of the time, it often requires laboratory animal and more particularly animal models of given human diseases.

## 2.4 Laboratory animals model contribution

The use of animal models in clinical research is crucial. As models, they usually display the same features and clinical signs as those observed in humans. So, they enable to establish some comparisons and extrapolations with the human physiology, to give access putative metabolic mechanisms involved in the progression of the disease and, hence, to identify biomarkers. A wide range of animal models has been used according to their origin. Animal models can be spontaneous, namely "mutant". Therefore, identification and characterization of novel laboratory animal lines carrying an interesting mutation combined with genotype-driven approaches are useful approaches to investigate some specific mechanistically-related molecules, to give new information about the function of the mammalian nervous system (Banks et al., 2011) or to study how genetic, environmental, toxicological or dietary factors can explain aetiology of a given disease. Animal models can also be created, using surgery, pharmacology or genetic interventions. These models are used to identify aetiological markers of disease or drug target and to test some new therapeutic drugs. The first cases have traditionally been induced by neurotoxins, acting selectively on neurons affected by human diseases. They are particularly useful for the study of the pathogenetic mechanism or to test new therapies for human neurological disorders (psychiatric or motor disorders) like obsessive-compulsive disorder or Parkinson's disease (Nowak et al., 2011). In parallel, the knockout technique, in which a gene is made inoperative leading to animals deficient in one specific gene, enables to evaluate the effects of the depletion of one protein in all the series of biological reactions within an organism and the putative followed consequences (Berman et al., 2011). More recently, the use of transgenic animals, constructed by inserting a human gene downstream into promoter, followed by microinjection in animal, ensures to indicate whether an over- or under-expression of a gene in one or several tissues should be susceptible to promote the pathogenesis and the development of a disease (Liu et al., 2011). The common point of all these animal models is the necessity of having some preliminary knowledge concerning a disease or the deleterious effect of a given xenobiotic. However, this information is not always available. Therefore, researchers have apace become aware of the necessity to access a wider range of knowledge in a living system and not only a specific molecular entity.

## 3. "Omics" approaches and their interest in clinical research

### 3.1 "Omics" approaches presentation

Similarly to imaging techniques, omics-based approaches appeared to be used according to the biological pool they consider (genes, proteins, lipids, metabolites) and the nature of target they have to reach (gene, enzymatic mechanism, biomarker). The full range of metabolites synthesized by a given biological system corresponds to its metabolome. In the same way, the full range of genes is contained in the term genome, the mRNA and the proteins ones, respectively, in the terms transcriptome and proteome (Figure 2). All these systems can be defined according to the level of biological organization, *i.e.* organism, organ, tissue, and cell. Related to these biological levels, omics-based approaches, mainly genomics, transcriptomics, proteomics (Colucci-D'Amato et al., 2011), lipidomics (Li et al., 2007), and metabolomics are terms standing for various global molecular-oriented approaches to better understand the underlying mechanisms, as the physiological regulations and the networks involved on all levels of gene products (mRNA, proteins, metabolites) in their respective systems and, if possible, between different sub-networks. Indeed, the observable property of organisms, *i.e.* their phenotype, is issued from genotype submitted to the concomitantly interactive action of the environment. Most of the time, the association between some of these approaches can be beneficial, enabling to understand the temporal progression of a pathophysiological state or the functioning of metabolic networks (Fiehn, 2001). Interest of these methods is to apply a controlled disruption to a biological system, whatever its nature (genetic, toxicological, pathophysiological, dietary), under some

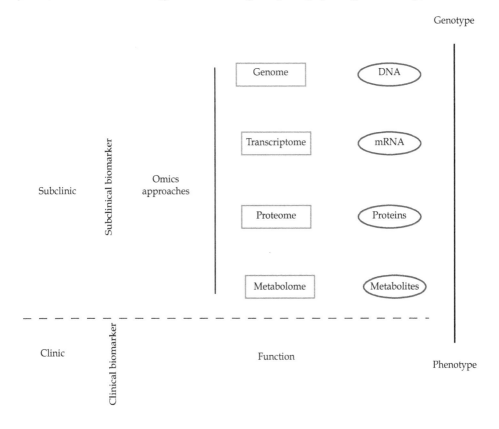

Fig. 2. "Omics" approaches and their different levels of biological living systems investigation

specific conditions (most of the time, the investigation is focused on an animal model), and to consider the subclinical consequences of such a disruptive perturbation. Therefore, "omics" approaches are widely used in biomedical research to make easier the understanding of disease mechanisms and to give access target tissues, to make easier the identification of biomarkers useful for therapeutic and diagnostic development and to predict clinical responses to treatments. The large amount of acquired data is as much an advantage as a hindrance. Indeed, the challenging subtlety is that all this information needs to be explored without any *a priori* hypothesis but by extracting only the interesting data. This fact partially explains why the real capacity of "omics" technologies stays in some instances rather limited because of the necessary requirement of some specific bioinformatics tools to efficiently mine multidimensional data but also the requirement of some specific analytical database to identify the candidate biomarkers at the gene, mRNA, enzyme, protein, or metabolite level. Moreover, transcriptomic studies require high-cost technologies and so, are less used than proteomic ones, which are based on two-dimensional gel-electrophoresis, which is cheaper and can be more easily used in many laboratories. However, analytical techniques related to the detection of large arrays of metabolites seem more robust, the resulting information being often easier to interpret because of the lower number of molecular entities, even though a rigorous identification of new metabolites still remains particularly fussy. According to the aim of studies and considering an increasing level of complexity of the analytical strategy used, investigation of metabolites may require either a metabolic profiling approach, which is focused on a small number of known metabolites (targeted metabolic profiling), or metabolomics including investigation of several classes of compounds (open metabolic profiling) or functional genomics, also called metabolic fingerprinting or metabonomics. This latter one is based on classification of samples according to their biological relevance to the studied disruption event and on identification of the fully informative markers detected at the statistical and functional sides and measured within the analyzed biological matrices.

Therefore, among these omics-based approaches, metabonomics stands for one of the most used holistic methods. Its emergence and its development mainly come from pioneering works of Pr J. Nicholson from the Imperial College of London. Because metabonomics enables to identify and quantify simultaneously low molecular weight compounds (metabolites) using spectroscopic methods such as nuclear magnetic resonance (NMR) or mass spectroscopy (MS), it gives access to a molecular level and may define the quantitative measurement of multiparametric metabolic responses of living system to pathophysiological stimuli. This can bring to the determination of some comprehensive metabolic signatures of biological matrices (Nicholson et al., 1999; Robertson, 2005). Metabonomics approach can be divided into successive steps. After the crucial step concerning the development of the experimental design, the choice of the animal model, the choice of the instrumentation used to quantitatively generate the metabolic information, the choice of samples of interest to be collected during the animal or the human experiment (biofluids such as plasma, urine, cerebral spinal fluid, saliva or faeces, tissues or organs), these biological samples are treated using appropriate analytical techniques. These latter ones enable to establish a metabolic fingerprint through the spectrum recording for every sample. All these fingerprints are summed up into datasets, in which metabolic information is subdivided and identified through coding variables. Each of them stands for either an integration bucket in NMR spectra corresponding to a defined chemical shift, or a relative or an absolute intensity of the ionic current measured at a specific mass to charge ratio in MS. Datasets are then treated using sophisticated statistical tools, *i.e.* multivariate or multidimensional statistical analysis tools, to access the most suitable model able to discriminate the different groups of samples according to the studied factors and to reveal main variables explaining this segregation. These variables can be considered at this step as many putative biomarkers, which need to be fully characterized by convenient structural identification methods. Finally, a detailed map of regulation and interaction between identified metabolites, their disruptions and the putative explanation of the pathophysiological state according to all involved factors may be suggested. Among analytical techniques mainly used in metabolomics, MS spectroscopy coupled to liquid (LC-MS) or gas chromatography (GC-MS) and NMR spectroscopy are the most appropriate ones concerning analysis of biofluids or liquid samples, whereas high resolution magic angle spinning (HR-MAS) NMR and MRS are adapted to solid samples like tissue or to achieve *in vivo* studies, respectively.

### 3.2 An integrated and functional approach

As previously mentioned above, the major constraint the "omics" approaches have to answer to, is to give access to a global pool of information belonging to the living system without focusing on a specific molecular entity. Indeed, one of the main assets of these approaches is the property of data integration necessary to render it as functionally understandable as possible. These features can be revealed through three complementary characteristics, namely *i)* the global nature of living systems underlined by homeostasis, *ii)* the multifactorial nature of diseases with both intrinsic and extrinsic factors, and *iii)* the ability to access multiple biological levels in living systems, and then to compile them to reveal one of the most realistic progressions of a disruption within a complex organism. Let's go into details of these three points. i) Contrary to classical biochemical approaches, which are set out to study only a single or few metabolites or metabolic reactions at the same time, metabolomics provides quantitative data on a wide range of known and unknown metabolites. It enables to visualize an overall pattern comprehensively linked to a set of interactions between metabolites or metabolic pathways and, hence, to an intrinsic homeostasis defined in these specific conditions (Kaddurah-Daouk et al., 2008). Indeed, whatever the stress applied on living systems, some allostatic changes, defined as an adaptive process, lead to short-term corrective changes of the different relevant regulatory systems to maintain a metabolic homeostasis. Concept of homeostasis is fundamental in biology and in clinical medicine to understand pathophysiological processes. The current clinical medicine tends now to come back to a more global view and, at the same time, on a more individualized approach of every patient because each of them differently answers to the environment according to their own homeostatic specificity. Clinical and subclinical signs give personalized information for every subject and, hence, physiological "means" used to adapt for everybody the set of parameters of homeostatic control in response to a disruptive stimulus and so to avoid falling down in a pathological state. The understanding of overall adaptation requires a good knowledge of metabolic pathways and related biochemical networks involved in the efficient control of homeostasis. For example, the knowledge of the glucose metabolism and the different ways by which homeostatic control of the circulating glucose concentration is achieved is crucial in the investigation of the Type 2 diabetes (Fiehn et al., 2010). ii) From global approaches can emerge a more accurate understanding of a given disease considering it is not only a single functional entity which is concerned, that is not only the consequence of a single causative explanation with a single mechanism involved in a single cell type in a given condition. Indeed, most of the pathophysiological disorders are not unique functional events but are resulting from complex interactions. These latter ones involve different concomitant actions in different biological compartments leading to different disruptions, which can be categorized according to the environmental conditions encountered and the inherent variability of subjects. Becoming aware of the importance of the environment and, more particularly, of the multifactorial nature of most of the disruptive events displayed by a living system is among the first pillars of the concept of global approach used in biological research in clinical medicine or in toxicology. iii) Finally, as a microscope could do it, omics-based approaches enable to focus on a specific level of a living system depending on the available analytical techniques used to generate data, but also to statistically integrate data coming from complementary fingerprinting techniques by using canonical analyses.

### 3.3 A metabolomic-based approach to reveal subclinical metabolic disruptions: A powerful tool in investigation of biomarkers

Besides the ability to define and to understand the aetiology of a disease, the discovery of novel biomarkers stands for a fundamental step to characterize and to manage it, especially to spot the homeostatic break down before appearance of the first clinical signs. Biomarkers, which are relevant indicators of disrupted biological processes in a given pathophysiological context, have to disclose features of disease (Moore et al., 2007; Nicholson and Lindon, 2008). The metabonomic approach is particularly interesting to explore subclinical disruptions of a living system before the outset of manifest clinical signs, and to identify biomarkers of disease risk and, if possible, to initiate prevention like in cancer (Roberts et al., 2011), diabetes (Wang et al., 2011), or nervous system illnesses (Kaddurah-Daouk and Krishnan, 2009; Nicholson and Lindon, 2008; Quinones and Kaddurah-Daouk, 2009). The identification of the metabolites requires the use of up-to-date structural databases of metabolites and metabolic pathway resources (Kouskoumvekaki and Panagiotou, 2011). As it has been previously mentioned, the use of complementary approaches stands for a wise way search of biomarkers displayed at different levels, namely biochemical, neuroanatomical, metabolic, genetic and neuropsychological ones, as it can be reported in the case of Alzheimer's disease investigation (Wattamwar and Mathuranath, 2010).

### 3.4 Examples of "omics" approaches in neurological investigation area

Use of metabolomics in neurological studies has been reported in many reviews (Choi et al., 2003; Rudkin and Arnold, 1999). It has been applied to a variety of biological samples for a better understanding of pathogenesis. This approach, because of its integrated and functional nature, stands for a powerful tool to study normal or pathological living systems, especially in central nervous system disorders through the use of specific animal models (Pears et al., 2005). Thus, it allows the identification of biomarkers of such diseases, but also of illness progression or response to therapy. In the drug discovery process, metabolomics brings some biochemical information about drug candidates, their mechanism of action and their therapeutic potential. In the field of neurosciences, the use of metabolomic approach can generate some questionings. Contrary to other organs in mammals, brain is isolated from the rest of organism by the blood-brain barrier, with consequences on the passage of some metabolites. Therefore, a metabolic fingerprint of brain predicted from a blood or urine metabolomic analysis is not prone to reflect the real state of the subject, contrary to data coming from other organs like liver and kidney. Nevertheless, some first encouraging studies on neurological disorders performed using metabolomics have confirmed the interest of application of this approach in the field of neuroscience (Griffin and Salek, 2007). Analysis of blood or urine gives access to putative cerebral disruptions and can help to successfully reveal some biomarkers, as in the case of the manganese neurotoxicity, which is a significant public health concern (Dorman et al., 2008). So, because it reflects the presence of both extrinsic and intrinsic disruptive factors, metabonomics can define accurate biomarkers in neurology. Moreover, some specific metabolic pathways or some biological disruptions can be particularly interesting to study, because of their central or ubiquitous role in many pathological states. One example is the oxidative stress, leading to neuronal death, a mechanism that is found in early stages but also in secondary manifestations of many neurodegenerative states like Alzheimer's, Parkinson's and Huntington's diseases, amyotrophic lateral sclerosis, and neuroinflammatory disorders (Sayre et al., 2008). Because of the pivotal role of a metabolite in many biological functions, a

better understanding of some metabolic pathways like the biosynthesis of the amino acid L-serine can be interesting to investigate (Tabatabaie et al., 2010). Metabolic profiles acquired on human or animal biofluids like urine, cerebrospinal fluid (Lutz et al., 2007b), plasma, serum or tissue extracts, using either NMR or MS techniques, can give some precious information concerning neurological disorders (Sinclair et al., 2009). For example, ultra performance liquid chromatography/mass spectroscopy (UPLC/MS) metabolic profiles from serum collected on cerebral infarction patients have been analyzed using a metabonomic approach (Jiang et al., 2011). Quantitative analysis of human cerebrospinal fluid using NMR spectroscopy has been performed in multiple sclerosis (Lutz et al., 2007a), to identify biomarkers in the early stages of the amyotrophic lateral sclerosis (Blasco et al., 2010). Plasmatic metabolic disruptions between healthy and old persons with Alzheimer's disease were investigated using UPLC/MS-based metabonomic approach (Li et al., 2010). CRND8 transgenic mouse, model of this disease, enabled to analyze brain extracts using $^1$H NMR spectroscopy (Salek et al., 2010). The interest of brain extracts coming from an animal model has been also illustrated to investigate epilepsy, for which the pharmacologically-induced animal model was obtained using pentylenetetrazole, a drug that induces seizures (Carmody and Brennan, 2010). Plasma from an experimental animal model of the spinal cord injury (Blasco et al., 2010) has been analyzed by $^1$H NMR to get fingerprint profiles of this pathology (Jiang et al., 2010). Other cerebral alterations like brain tumors (Tate et al., 1996; Tate et al., 1998), schizophrenia and meningitis (Holmes et al., 2006; Lutz et al., 2007a) have also been investigated.

Beyond the use of a unique "omics" approach, it seems that it is all the more interesting and powerful to call for several complementary approaches and to tend to integrate so-generated data to yield a more comprehensive understanding of many diseases. In this way, Caudle et al. have used "omics" to characterize and identify some biomarkers of Parkinson's disease (Caudle et al., 2010). As an example, the following part illustrates the power of such a use, in a rodent model, of a neuro-intoxication caused in the horse by a plant, *Hypochoeris radicata* (L.). Indeed, because of the lack of knowledge about a neurological disease described only in the horse, we have tempted to use a laboratory animal model of this intoxication by applying metabonomics combined to imaging or behavioural experiments to reveal, in brain, candidate biomarkers of this pathology.

## 4. Example of a metabonomic approach of a neurological horse disease, the Australian stringhalt or how to address a toxicological issue on a seemingly non-target species without referring to a known toxic molecule

### 4.1 Problem for studying such an animal disease

Australian stringhalt is the name of a horse disease described since the middle of the 19th century in Australia (Robertson-Smith et al., 1985). It is defined as a syndrome characterized by an abnormal gait and an involuntary hyperflexion of both hind limbs during movement (Figure 3).

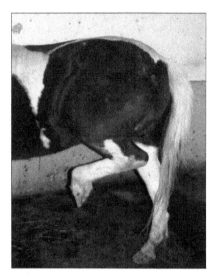

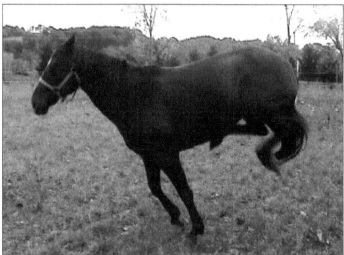

Fig. 3. Horses displaying clinical signs of Australian stringhalt (grade IV on the left, grade V on the right) (from (Collignon, 2007))

Since this time, several other outbreaks had been reported in many countries such as New Zealand (Cahill et al., 1985; Cahill et al., 1986; Cahill and Goulden, 1992), Chile (Araya et al., 1998), United States (Gay et al., 1993; Huntington et al., 1989; Robertson-Smith et al., 1985; Slocombe et al., 1992), Italy (Torre, 2005), Brasil (Araujo), more recently in France (Domange et al., 2010; Gouy et al., 2005) and were suspected in Japan (Takahashi et al., 2002). According to most of the authors, a plant of the Asteraceae family (formerly Compositeae family), *Hypochoeris radicata* L. also named cat's ear, flatweed or capeweed was suspected to be responsible for this disease (Araujo et al., 2008; Gardner et al., 2005; Gay et al., 1993; Gouy et al., 2005). This rosette-forming herb with a yellow terminal flower has a deep taproot, giving it resistance to drought. This explains a growth achieved preferentially on poor-quality pastures after a prolonged dry period, mainly in late summer and early autumn. Such climatic conditions, associated with the aggressiveness and the dominance of *Hypochoeris radicata* L. on other species, enable it to colonize pastures and to become the major plant available as herbivore feeding. These favouring factors, in aggravation for many years because of the global change in climatic conditions, appeared particularly marked in 2003 in France, after a blistering and dry summer, leading to an epizooty with a few tens of recorded intoxicated horses (Domange et al., 2010; Gouy et al., 2005). These latter's showed a wide range of symptoms but mainly dominated by several severity degrees from grade I to grade V, (Huntington et al., 1989) with an involuntary exaggerated hyperflexion of hind limbs and a delayed extension of hocks during forward movement. A marked atrophy of the hind limbs musculature, especially in the distal muscles, is often associated with this gait in the most affected animals. Most of the time, this amyotrophy is related to neurological lesions of the hind limbs with a proximal-to-distal gradient in the intensity, *i.e.* a loss of fibres, a decrease of the number of large myelinated nerve fibres, in agreement with the supposed pathogenesis described as a distal axonopathy (Cahill et al., 1986; Domange et al., 2010). However, in spite of these rare epidemiological and pathological data, the link between this horse disease and the toxicity of *Hypochoeris radicata* (HR) has been poorly investigated in spite of a recent study, which tended to reproduce the disease on animals after a 50-day HR treatment (9.8 kg HR/animal/day) (Araujo et al., 2008). The lack of investigation of such a disease is further partially explained by the critical approach of the nervous system, especially the peripheral nervous system and by the only target species. Besides, we need to consider ethical and financial issues. Moreover, as Araujo and colleagues underlined, the plant material is susceptible to differ in toxicity depending on several factors, one being the geographical location (Araujo et al., 2008).

## 4.2 Concept of orthology and interest in metabonomics

Most of the time, investigating a disease often requires a convenient laboratory animal model enabling to reproduce clinical symptoms, to access pharmacological data, to reveal some biomarkers of the disease and, in the best cases, to suggest some therapeutic treatments. Because of the nervous nature of Australian stringhalt, the fact that this illness was only described in target species, and the difficulties to link the supposed plant (more particularly if a specific secondary metabolite present in the plant would be involved) to the pathogenesis, the assessment of such an induced intoxication using a "classical" neurological approach seemed not efficient enough to reveal valuable biomarkers. Data obtained until recently remained too scarce. The "omics" approach, more particularly metabonomics, appears to be the most suitable mean to obtain some pertinent information about the target organs and candidate metabolic biomarkers by using an *a priori* "metabolically competent" animal model. The orthologous hypothesis considered in the case of an induction of a metabolic disruption in a rodent animal model of another animal species, here horse species, is crucial in characterizing a set of candidate metabolic biomarkers. Even though clinical signs may strikingly differ between the two species, some metabolic similarities may exist between their metabolic networks, particularly in their ability to be similarly disrupted by one or few toxicants. Among these latter's, plant secondary metabolites, for which nothing is known at the chemical and pharmacological sides, can be studied.

### 4.3 Use of complementary approaches: [1]H NMR-based metabonomics, MRI and behavioural tests
### 4.3.1 Metabolic fingerprints on biofluids and tissue extracts

Using the orthologous metabolic disruption assumption existing between two species, horse and mouse in the present case, metabonomics was used to investigate at the metabolic side this orphan neurological disease, Australian stringhalt. The purpose was to combine it with MRI as published elsewhere (Griffith et al., 2007) and with behavioural tests to improve the functional understanding of the metabolic data. Based on the orthologous hypothesis previously mentioned, the mouse was chosen as a "metabolically competent" laboratory animal model of horse intoxicated by HR, even though this rodent model of exposure to HR does not display any observable clinical sign. In a first time, metabonomic studies using male and female C57BL/6J mice fed for 21 days a diet containing 3 or 9% HR had been performed (Domange et al., 2008). [1]H NMR spectroscopy analyses have been done on weekly collected urine samples but also on tissue extracts prepared from liver and brain tissues collected at 0, 8, 15 and 21 days of treatment, after sacrifice of a subpopulation of the animals included in the experimental design. Urine and liver analyses were performed to detect the putative systemic disruption after the HR ingestion, and the brain analysis to access the nervous system disruption. All [1]H NMR spectra were acquired at 300 K on a Bruker DRX-600 Avance NMR spectrometer operating at 600.13 MHz for [1]H resonance frequency, using a cryoprobe and the 1D "Improved Watergate" sequence for suppression of water resonance. Multidimensional statistical analyses of fingerprint data were achieved on log-transformed variables. After removing redundant variables, linear discriminant analyses and partial least-squares regression-based discriminant analyses (PLS-DA) were performed on NMR data to maximize the groups' separation on a factorial map. Projection of these groups on every factorial axis enables to associate canonical [1]H NMR variables to the axis construction revealing thus the respective influence of the different factors of interest (gender, intoxication duration, toxicant dose). Therefore, the main part of the metabolic information related to urine [1]H NMR data and enabling the discrimination between the different groups of animals can be summed up in a factorial map (Figure 4). On this map, appears the temporal evolution between day 0 and day 21 of the metabolism of animals. This latter depends significantly on the gender of mice, through the 1st axis (this factor contains the main part of the variance explained by the statistical model used) and on the diet factor, through the second axis, covering from the bottom part of the factorial map diets without HR (named "control") to the middle part, diets with 3% HR (named "3%HR"), then to the top part, diets with 9% HR (named "9%HR"). By searching the first variables involved in the second axis construction, we reached the main metabolites, the concentration of which was influenced by a HR-induced metabolic disruption (Domange et al., 2008).

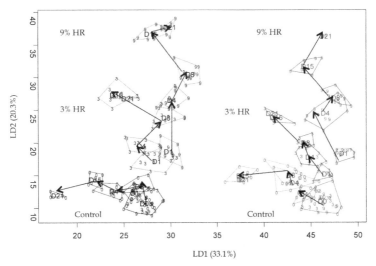

Fig. 4. LDA performed on 150 metabolic variables selected from fingerprints obtained by ¹H NMR performed at 600.13 MHz on 332 urinary samples (from Domange et al., 2008). The dummy variable selected is the « group » factor. A 61.5% amount of the total metabolic information is projected on the factorial plan LD1 x LD2. Arrows stand for metabolic trajectories throughout the study followed by every group fed either a control or a 3 or 9% HR diet. Barycenters give the dates of urine collection and correspond to the duration of HR intoxication (d8, day 8; d15, day 15; d21, day 21)

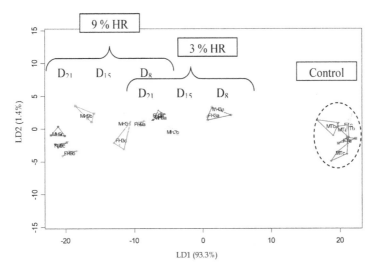

Fig. 5. LDA performed on 20 variables filtered from 600.13 MHz ¹H NMR data of brain aqueous extracts from male and female mice according to groups and in agreement with the two first components (from Domange, 2008). Barycenters give the date of brain collection and correspond to the duration of HR intoxication (d8, day 8; d15, day 15; d21, day 21)

In a same way, the main part of metabolic information contained in ¹H NMR data characterizing liver and brain hydrosoluble extracts and enabling the discrimination between the different groups of animals during the experiment could be summed up into a more complex factorial map (Figure 5). Firstly, is displayed the temporal evolution of the brain metabolism of mice orally exposed or not to HR, which holds almost all the part of the variance explained by the statistical model with, respectively from the right to the left side, a projection of the cerebral metabolisms of control animals, then the 3%HR-treated mice, and finally, the 9%HR-treated ones (Domange, 2008). The factor "time" is clearly revealed through every HR treatment with, respectively, from the right to the left side, an emphasis of the disrupted metabolism in a given direction all along the experiment duration. Given the fact that the two matrices of ¹H NMR fingerprinting data obtained on hydrosoluble brain and liver extracts were issued from the same individuals, a global correlation using a canonical analysis (PLS2 here) have been performed between them. A significant correlation between the two first PLS2 components has been revealed (Figure 6), in which, the gender factor is orthogonally projected to the diet one. Concerning the projection of variables involved in the variance calculation, *i.e.* the information explaining this construction, on the same plot, we can show that liver and brain ¹H NMR fingerprint data display close

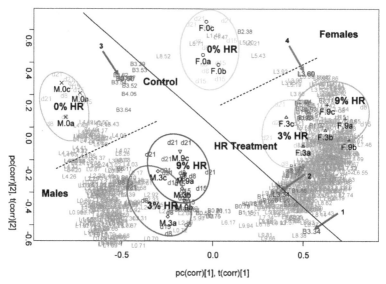

Fig. 6. Resulting biplot performed on the two first PLS2 components calculated between the hydrosoluble liver and brain extracts (from (Domange et al., 2008). Only the projection of the variables with contribution is above 0.5 is displayed (in grey for brain variables, in pink for the liver ones). Most of the variables containing the variance explained by the statistical model is spread according to the gender factor for the liver and according to the diet concerning the brain. The brain variable named B3.34 (arrow numbered 1) and the corresponding liver variable named L3.34 (arrow numbered 2) stand for the *scyllo*-inositol, detected at δ = 3.34 ppm. The brain variable named B3.60 (arrow numbered 3) and the corresponding liver variable named L3.60 (arrow numbered 4) stand for the *myo*-inositol detected at δ = 3.60 ppm

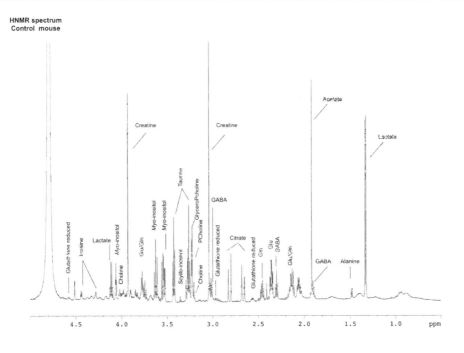

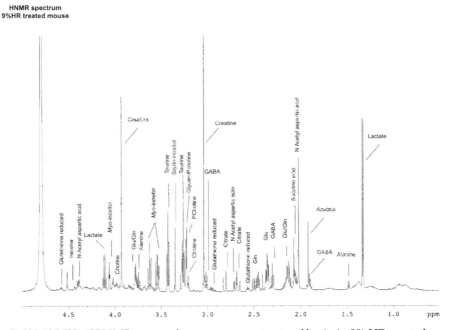

Fig. 7. 600.13 MHz ¹H NMR spectra from aqueous extracts of brain in 9% HR-treated mouse and control mouse (from Domange, 2008)

information. Among the main variables involved in the segregation of the groups of animals, *i.e.* which are related to the HR-treatment factor, and whatever the biological matrix analysed, the first identified variables correspond to the chemical shifts of the *scyllo*-inositol ($\delta = 3.35$ or 3.36 ppm in urine and in liver extract fingerprints, $\delta = 3.34$ ppm in cerebral and liver fingerprints), which are positively correlated to HR-treatment, when the *myo*-inositol ones ($\delta = 3.60$ ppm) are negatively correlated to HR-treatment (Figures 7 and 8). Moreover, the comparison between [1]H-NMR metabolic fingerprints in control and HR-fed laboratory animals revealed a dose-dependent increase of the ratio *scyllo*-inositol/*myo*-inositol in urine, plasma, and hydrosoluble extracts of liver and brain of the HR-treated animals, enabling us to reveal some putative candidate metabolic biomarker(s) even though no aetiological factor was characterized, and no requirement of the target species was performed in this toxicological exploration.

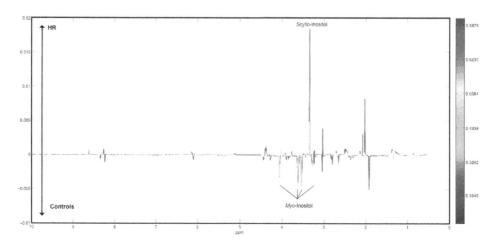

Fig. 8. Loading plot from O-PLS models performed from the aqueous extracts of brain in 9% HR-treated mice

### 4.3.2 Magnetic resonance imaging

To get access *in situ* to some potent cerebral metabolic changes thanks to a second spectroscopic technique, [1]H NMR localized spectroscopy, six male mice given a 9% HR diet and six control mice were used for *in vivo* metabolite quantification. All experiments were performed at 9.4 T on a Bruker Avance DRX 400 microimaging system with a wide-bore vertical magnet and a Micro 2.5 gradient system (Bruker Ettlingen, Germany). Because a preliminary experiment performed on a spectroscopic volume of interest (VOI) positioned in the cortex of mice was inconclusive, spectra have been performed from [1]H NMR data acquired by *in vivo* MRI using a VOI positioned in the thalamus of control and 9% HR-treated male mice (Figure 9.a). In this region, only the 9% HR-treated mice displayed a significant although minor signal found at $\delta = 3.34$ ppm corresponding to *scyllo*-inositol (Figure 9.b). A one-way ANOVA performed for every other identified variables quantified at the same time from raw integrated spectra coming from *in vivo* MRI enables us to give significant results only for *scyllo*-inositol (p = 0.0013). As it could be described above, and as one of the interests of metabonomic approach is to combine data generated by different techniques to get more powerful biomarkers, a PLS2-based canonical regression between the set of brain metabolites issued by *in vivo* MRI and the ¹H NMR fingerprints of hydrosoluble brain extracts performed on the same animals has been obtained after correction of the two data sets by an OSC-PLS-driven correction procedure. The canonical analysis obtained by the PLS2 analysis between these two corrected data sets showed that the ¹H NMR variable called B3.34, namely *scyllo*-inositol, was projected in the region where scores of HR-treated animals were also projected (Figure 9.c). Moreover, the relative contents of $N$-acetyl-aspartate (NAA), lactate and choline were increased ($p < 10^{-5}$, $p = 0.02$ and $p = 0.03$, respectively) whereas the glutamine one was decreased ($p = 0.04$) in response to the 9% HR treatment. MRI studies were also conducted in poisoned living mice and corroborated the abnormal higher presence of *scyllo*-inositol in the thalamus of poisoned animals. Even this result was unable to explain the exact pathophysiological mechanism involved and the outset of the illness, it confirmed that *scyllo*-inositol was a biomarker of interest in the central nervous system, particularly when it is related to some brain metabolic disturbances (Griffith et al., 2007; Jenkins et al., 1993; Viola et al., 2004). The increase in NAA, which has been previously revealed following MRI and ¹H NMR spectroscopy of hydrosoluble brain extracts was suggested to be linked to the enhanced locomotor activity observed in 9% HR-treated mice. Besides, NAA has been reported in epileptic seizures cases (Akimitsu et al., 2000).

This accumulation of NAA has also been shown in a rat model of the Canavan's disease, suggesting that NAA increase in brain should be linked to neuroexcitation and neurodegeneration (Kitada et al., 2000).

### 4.3.3 Behavioural testing

The two previous exploratory studies led us to consider in more details the role of inositols in the development of the Australian stringhalt. The location of such metabolic disturbances, the current knowledge of the metabolism and the pathways involved, such as neurotransmission, signalling system and regulation of many cellular functions, depending on the balance between *scyllo* and *myo* inositol needed to be rounded out by a complementary functional assessment as a large extent behavioural testing of HR-treated animals can provide it. Indeed, the administration of inositol (*myo*-inositol) is used as a therapeutic molecule in depression (Einat et al., 1999), panic disorder, obsessive-compulsive disorder (Cohen et al., 1997; Levine, 1997). It partially explains an enhanced locomotion (Kofman et al., 1998) and may be linked to a putative anxiolytic effect (Kofman et al., 2000) with possible involvement of serotoninergic (5-HT₂) receptors (Einat et al., 2001). Therefore, to investigate the functional consequences of such previous disrupted metabolic events, various behavioural aspects of C57BL/6J mice orally exposed to 9% HR for 3 weeks were performed in parallel with the ¹H NMR metabolomic exploration of the brain. Several behavioural tests related to locomotor activity (open-field test), motor coordination (Locotronic® apparatus, Wespoc test), learning and memory [Y maze, (Hughes, 2004), Figure 10.a and Morris water maze], anxiety [elevated plus maze, (Rodgers and Johnson, 1995), hole board (do-Rego et al., 2006; Takeda et al., 1998), Figure 10.b], and depression forced swimming test or test of Porsolt (Porsolt et al., 1977; Porsolt et al., 1979), social interaction (resident/intruder model), and addiction (place preference test) were carried out (Domange et al., submitted).

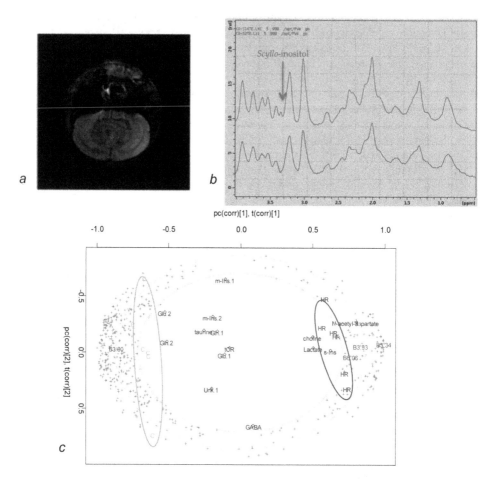

Fig. 9. a) MRI performed at 9.4 T on a Bruker Avance DRX 400 microimaging system positioned in the thalamus region with an *in vivo* parallel metabolite quantification using [1]H NMR localized spectroscopy (VOI, 12 mm[3]). b) Spectrum comparison between the sum of six [1]H NMR spectra acquired on control male mice and the sum of six [1]H NMR spectra acquired on 9%HR-treated male mice with the presence of *scyllo*-inositol (chemical shift detected at $\delta = 3.34$ ppm). c) PLS2 between MRI quantitative data and [1]H NMR data. A loading projection is given for metabonomic variables having a norm above 0.5 (pale blue circle) or above 0.75 (pale green circle). The purple and the dark-blue ellipses, respectively, correspond to the scores of control and 9% HR-treated mice. Among the main MRI loadings having a positive correlation with HR treatment are *scyllo*-inositol (*s*-Ins), *N*-acetyl-aspartate, lactate and choline. For MRI variables having a negative correlation with HR treatment are glutamate (Glu.2, second chemical shift) and glutamine (Gln.2, second chemical shift). Uninformative MRI loadings: *myo*-inositol (*m*-Ins), glutamate, first chemical shift (Glu.1), glutamine, first chemical shift (Gln.1), GABA, taurine and unknown 1 are projected in the centre of the biplot (from Domange et al., 2008)

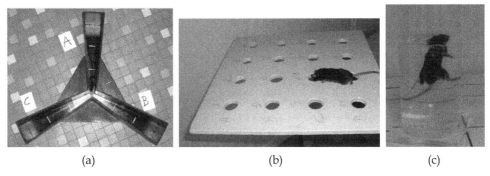

|       |       |       |
|:-----:|:-----:|:-----:|
|  (a)  |  (b)  |  (c)  |

Fig. 10. Examples of behavioural tests used in mice: a) Y-maze or Y-maze spontaneous alternation that estimates the immediate working memory performance. b) Hole board test that evaluates the exploratory rate and the anxiety level. c) Forced swimming test defined to visualize a depression state (from Domange et al., submitted)

Although the lack of motor coordination impairment is commonly observed in the sick horses, 9% HR-treated mice displayed a motor hyperactivity, which is reflected by the decrease of immobility time in the forced swimming test, and the increased numbers of head dipping in the hole board test, of arms visited in Y-maze and of the number of entries in the upper quarter of the maze in the Morris water maze (Domange et al., submitted). This increased activity of treated mice, which is clearly observable at the end of tests, could be linked to a decrease in the resignation state or an enhanced motivation. Moreover, the 9% HR-contaminated mice seem to be addicted to the plant as indicated by results obtained in the place preference test. A regularized canonical analyses performed using mixOmics, an R package (Le Cao et al., 2009) to establish a canonical link between the two multidimensional data sets, *i.e.* the one containing the ¹H NMR fingerprints of hydrosoluble brain extracts and the one corresponding to the behavioural data set, which comprises nearly 100 variables, has revealed a clear relationship between some behavioural impairment variables (the motor hyperactivity and the addiction for the plant) and the main metabolic disruptions, *i.e.* the increase in *scyllo*-inositol in the brain of HR-treated mice and the relative decrease in *myo*-inositol. These results underlie the interest of such a dual and combined approach to characterize the functional end-points of a pathophysiological model of the horse Australian stringhalt in a seemingly metabolically orthologous murine species.

## 5. Conclusion

In this chapter, we underlined the interest of "omics" approaches and their recent introduction in the field of neuro-toxicological research. Indeed, metabonomics can especially be considered as a potentially powerful mean to explore the subclinical disruptions of an organism before the outset of clinical signs, and would particularly be useful in discovery markers of disease risk. This approach would help to prevent some risks in spite of the difficulty to detect some minor metabolites or molecules in tiny doses or mixtures, with the ability to access and explore some isolated and intricate tissues (like brain) *via* the general metabolism (urine, plasma) and to link statistically these subclinical metabolic changes with complementary data coming from other phenotyping approaches and across multiple physiological levels. Besides, these combined techniques have been applied in some toxico-environmental assessments possibly aetiologically linked to some neuro-physiological diseases. Thus, coupling metabolomic and behavioural studies may help to functionally describe neurotoxicity resulting from ingestion of milk of lactating goats fed a hay contaminated with various persistent organic pollutants (POPs) like Polycyclic Aromatic Hydrocarbons (PAHs), PolyChloroDibenzo-p-Dioxins (PCDDs), PolyChloroDibenzoFurans (PCDFs) and PolyChloroBiphenyls (PCBs) (Schroeder et al., in preparation). Nevertheless, these "omics" technologies required new specific bioinformatics tools to mine multifactorial data and, in the case of metabolomics, some well-documented analytical databases to structurally characterize metabolites revealed as candidate biomarkers. Therefore, further progress needs to be obtained to improve at the statistical side these integration strategies and to reduce some still existing drawbacks. Nonetheless, such techniques have also the outstanding capacity to give some interpretation of the results in a larger biological perspective, given that this holistic approach stands for an emerging level of knowledge in clinical medical research.

## 6. Acknowledgment

We gratefully acknowledge the excellent technical support and the contribution in the animal experimentation of Florence Blas Y Estrada and Raymond Gazel (INRA Toulouse, INP, UMR1331 ToxAlim) during metabonomic studies, Amidou Traoré, Guy Biélicki and Cécile Keller (INRA Clermont-Ferrand/Theix, QuaPA STIM, F-63122 St Genès Champanelle) during MRI experiments and Nicolas Violle and Julie Peiffer (UR AFPA, INRA UC340, Nancy University) during behavioural tests.

## 7. References

Akimitsu, T., Kurisu, K., Hanaya, R., Iida, K., Kiura, Y., Arita, K., Matsubayashi, H., Ishihara, K., Kitada, K., Serikawa, T., Sasa, M., 2000. Epileptic seizures induced by N-acetyl-L-aspartate in rats: in vivo and in vitro studies. *Brain Research*. Vol.861, pp. 143-150.

Araujo, J.A., Curcio, B., Alda, J., Medeiros, R.M., Riet-Correa, F., 2008. Stringhalt in Brazilian horses caused by Hypochaeris radicata. *Toxicon*. Vol.52, pp. 190-193.

Araya, O., Krause, A., Solis de Ovando, M., 1998. Outbreaks of stringhalt in southern Chile. *The Veterinary Record*. Vol.142, pp 462-463.

Banks, G.T., Haas, M.A., Line, S., Shepherd, H.L., Alqatari, M., Stewart, S., Rishal, I., Philpott, A., Kalmar, B., Kuta, A., Groves, M., Parkinson, N., Acevedo-Arozena, A., Brandner, S., Bannerman, D., Greensmith, L., Hafezparast, M., Koltzenburg, M., Deacon, R., Fainzilber, M., Fisher, E.M., 2011. Behavioral and other phenotypes in a cytoplasmic Dynein light intermediate chain 1 mutant mouse. *Journal of Neurosciences*. Vol.31, pp. 5483-5494.

Berman, A.E., Chan, W.Y., Brennan, A.M., Reyes, R.C., Adler, B.L., Suh, S.W., Kauppinen, T.M., Edling, Y., Swanson, R.A., 2011. N-acetylcysteine prevents loss of dopaminergic neurons in the EAAC1-/- mouse. *Annals of Neurology*. Vol.69, pp. 509-520.

Blasco, H., Corcia, P., Moreau, C., Veau, S., Fournier, C., Vourc'h, P., Emond, P., Gordon, P., Pradat, P.F., Praline, J., Devos, D., Nadal-Desbarats, L., Andres, C.R., 2010. 1H-

NMR-based metabolomic profiling of CSF in early amyotrophic lateral sclerosis. *PLoS One*. Vol.5, e13223.

Cahill, J.I., Goulden, B.E., Pearce, H.G., 1985. A review and some observations on stringhalt. *New Zealand Veterinarian Journal*. Vol.33, pp. 101-104.

Cahill, J.I., Goulden, B.E., Jolly, R.D., 1986. Stringhalt in horses: a distal axonopathy. *Neuropathology Applied Neurobiolology*. Vol.12, pp 459-475.

Cahill, J.I., Goulden, B.E., 1992. Stringhalt--current thoughts on aetiology and pathogenesis. *Equine Veterinary Journal*. Vol.24, pp. 161-162.

Carmody, S., Brennan, L., 2010. Effects of pentylenetetrazole-induced seizures on metabolomic profiles of rat brain. *Neurochemistry International*. Vol.56, pp. 340-344.

Caudle, W.M., Bammler, T.K., Lin, Y., Pan, S., Zhang, J., 2010. Using 'omics' to define pathogenesis and biomarkers of Parkinson's disease. *Expert Review of Neurotherapeutics*. Vol.10, pp. 925-942.

Choi, I.Y., Lee, S.P., Guilfoyle, D.N., Helpern, J.A., 2003. In vivo NMR studies of neurodegenerative diseases in transgenic and rodent models. *Neurochemical Research*. Vol.28, pp. 987-1001.

Choi, J.K., Dedeoglu, A., Jenkins, B.G., 2007. Application of MRS to mouse models of neurodegenerative illness. *NMR in Biomedicine*. Vol.20, pp. 216-237.

Cohen, H., Kotler, M., Kaplan, Z., Matar, M.A., Kofman, O., Belmaker, R.H., 1997. Inositol has behavioral effects with adaptation after chronic administration. *Journal of Neural Transmission*. Vol.104, pp. 299-305.

Collignon, G., 2007. Contribution à l'étude épidémiologique de l'enzootie de harper australien en France depuis 2003 chez le cheval. Veterinary Thesis of University of Toulouse.

Colucci-D'Amato, L., Farina, A., Vissers, J.P., Chambery, A., 2011. Quantitative neuroproteomics: classical and novel tools for studying neural differentiation and function. *Stem Cell Reviews*. Vol.7, pp. 77-93.

Cooper, K.L., Meng, Y., Harnan, S., Ward, S.E., Fitzgerald, P., Papaioannou, D., Wyld, L., Ingram, C., Wilkinson, I.D., Lorenz, E., 2011. Positron emission tomography (PET) and magnetic resonance imaging (MRI) for the assessment of axillary lymph node metastases in early breast cancer: systematic review and economic evaluation. *Health Technology Assessment*. Vol.15, pp. iii-iv, 1-134.

Davis, E.P., Buss, C., Muftuler, L.T., Head, K., Hasso, A., Wing, D.A., Hobel, C., Sandman, C.A., 2011. Children's Brain Development Benefits from Longer Gestation. *Frontiers in Psychology*. Vol.2, p. 1.

do-Rego, J.C., Viana, A.F., Le Maitre, E., Deniel, A., Rates, S.M., Leroux-Nicollet, I., Costentin, J., 2006. Comparisons between anxiety tests for selection of anxious and non anxious mice. *Behavioural Brain Research*. Vol.169, pp. 282-288.

Domange, C., 2008. Etude des disruptions métaboliques provoquées chez le modèle murin par l'ingestion d'Hypochoeris radicata (L.), plante toxique pour l'espèce équine. Validation de l'approche métabonomique par des études comportementales et par imagerie cérébrale. Thesis of University of Toulouse.

Domange, C., Canlet, C., Traore, A., Bielicki, G., Keller, C., Paris, A., Priymenko, N., 2008. Orthologous metabonomic qualification of a rodent model combined with magnetic resonance imaging for an integrated evaluation of the toxicity of Hypochoeris radicata. *Chemical Research in Toxicology*. Vol.21, pp. 2082-2096.

Domange, C., Casteignau, A., Collignon, G., Pumarola, M., Priymenko, N., 2010. Longitudinal study of Australian stringhalt cases in France. *Journal of Animal Physiology and Animal Nutrition (Berl)*. Vol.94, pp. 712-720.

Dorman, D.C., Struve, M.F., Norris, A., Higgins, A.J., 2008. Metabolomic analyses of body fluids after subchronic manganese inhalation in rhesus monkeys. *Toxicological Sciences*. Vol.106, pp. 46-54.

Einat, H., Clenet, F., Shaldubina, A., Belmaker, R.H., Bourin, M., 2001. The antidepressant activity of inositol in the forced swim test involves 5-HT(2) receptors. *Behavioural Brain Research*. Vol.118, pp. 77-83.

Einat, H., Karbovski, H., Korik, J., Tsalah, D., Belmaker, R.H., (1999). Inositol reduces depressive-like behaviors in two different animal models of depression. *Psychopharmacology (Berl)*. Vol.144, pp. 158-162.

Fiehn, O., 2001. Combining genomics, metabolome analysis, and biochemical modelling to understand metabolic networks. *Comparative and Functional Genomics*. Vol.2, pp. 155-168.

Fiehn, O., Garvey, W.T., Newman, J.W., Lok, K.H., Hoppel, C.L., Adams, S.H., 2010. Plasma metabolomic profiles reflective of glucose homeostasis in non-diabetic and type 2 diabetic obese African-American women. *PLoS One*. Vol.5, e15234.

Frisoni, G.B., Filippi, M., 2005. Multiple sclerosis and Alzheimer disease through the looking glass of MR imaging. *AJNR American Journal of Neuroradiology*. Vol.26, pp. 2488-2491.

Gardner, S.Y., Cook, A.G., Jortner, B.S., Troan, B.V., Sharp, N.J.H., Campbell, N.B., Brownie, C.F., 2005. Stringhalt associated with a pasture infested with Hypochoeris radicata. *Equine Veterinary Education*. Vol.17, pp. 118-122.

Gay, C.C., Fransen, S., Richards, J., Holler, S., 1993. Hypochoeris-associated stringhalt in North America. *Equine Veterinary Journal*. Vol.25, pp. 456-457.

Gouy, I., Leblond, A., Egron-Morand, G., Cadore, J.L., 2005. Etude de cas de harper australien après sa recrudescence dans la région lyonnaise. *Pratique Vétérinaire Equine*. Vol.37, pp. 53-60.

Griffin, J.L., Salek, R.M., 2007. Metabolomic applications to neuroscience: more challenges than chances? *Expert Review of Proteomics*. Vol.4, pp. 435-437.

Griffith, H.R., den Hollander, J.A., Stewart, C.C., Evanochko, W.T., Buchthal, S.D., Harrell, L.E., Zamrini, E.Y., Brockington, J.C., Marson, D.C., 2007. Elevated brain scyllo-inositol concentrations in patients with Alzheimer's disease. NMR in Biomedicine. Vol.20, pp. 709-716.

Holmes, E., Tsang, T.M., Tabrizi, S.J., 2006. The application of NMR-based metabonomics in neurological disorders. *NeuroRx*. Vol.3, pp. 358-372.

Hughes, R.N., 2004. The value of spontaneous alternation behavior (SAB) as a test of retention in pharmacological investigations of memory. *Neuroscience and Biobehavioral Reviews*. Vol.28, pp. 497-505.

Huntington, P.J., Jeffcott, L.B., Friend, S.C., Luff, A.R., Finkelstein, D.I., Flynn, R.J., 1989. Australian Stringhalt--epidemiological, clinical and neurological investigations. *Equine Veterinary Journal*. Vol.21, pp 266-273.

Jenkins, B.G., Koroshetz, W.J., Beal, M.F., Rosen, B.R., 1993. Evidence for impairment of energy metabolism in vivo in Huntington's disease using localized 1H NMR spectroscopy. *Neurology*. Vol.43, pp. 2689-2695.

Jiang, H., Peng, J., Zhou, Z.Y., Duan, Y., Chen, W., Cai, B., Yang, H., Zhang, W., 2010. Establishing (1)H nuclear magnetic resonance based metabonomics fingerprinting profile for spinal cord injury: a pilot study. *Chinese Medical Journal (Engl)*. Vol.123, pp. 2315-2319.

Jiang, Z., Sun, J., Liang, Q., Cai, Y., Li, S., Huang, Y., Wang, Y., Luo, G., 2011. A metabonomic approach applied to predict patients with cerebral infarction. *Talanta*. Vol.84, pp. 298-304.

Kaddurah-Daouk, R., Kristal, B.S., Weinshilboum, R.M., 2008. Metabolomics: a global biochemical approach to drug response and disease. Annu Rev Pharmacol Toxicol. 48, 653-83.

Kaddurah-Daouk, R., Krishnan, K.R., 2009. Metabolomics: a global biochemical approach to the study of central nervous system diseases. *Neuropsychopharmacology*. Vol.34, pp. 173-186.

Kastrup, O., Wanke, I., Maschke, M., 2005. Neuroimaging of infections. *NeuroRx*. Vol.2, pp. 324-332.

Kitada, K., Akimitsu, T., Shigematsu, Y., Kondo, A., Maihara, T., Yokoi, N., Kuramoto, T., Sasa, M., Serikawa, T., 2000. Accumulation of N-acetyl-L-aspartate in the brain of the tremor rat, a mutant exhibiting absence-like seizure and spongiform degeneration in the central nervous system. *Journal of Neurochemistry*. Vol.74, pp. 2512-2519.

Kofman, O., Agam, G., Shapiro, J., Spencer, A., 1998. Chronic dietary inositol enhances locomotor activity and brain inositol levels in rats. *Psychopharmacology (Berl)*. Vol.139, pp. 239-242.

Kofman, O., Einat, H., Cohen, H., Tenne, H., Shoshana, C., 2000. The anxiolytic effect of chronic inositol depends on the baseline level of anxiety. *Journal of Neural Transmission*. Vol.107, pp. 241-253.

Kouskoumvekaki, I., Panagiotou, G., 2011. Navigating the human metabolome for biomarker identification and design of pharmaceutical molecules. *Journal of Biomedicine and Biotechnology*. Vol.2011, ID 525497.

Le Cao, K.A., Gonzalez, I., Dejean, S., 2009. integrOmics: an R package to unravel relationships between two omics datasets. *Bioinformatics*. Vol.25, pp. 2855-2856.

Levine, J., 1997. Controlled trials of inositol in psychiatry. *European Neuropsychopharmacology*. Vol.7, pp. 147-155.

Li, J., Cui, Z., Zhao, S., Sidman, R.L., 2007. Unique glycerophospholipid signature in retinal stem cells correlates with enzymatic functions of diverse long-chain acyl-CoA synthetases. *Stem Cells*. Vol.25, pp. 2864-2873.

Li, N.J., Liu, W.T., Li, W., Li, S.Q., Chen, X.H., Bi, K.S., He, P., 2010. Plasma metabolic profiling of Alzheimer's disease by liquid chromatography/mass spectrometry. *Clinical Biochemistry*. Vol.43, pp. 992-997.

Liu, J., Wang, H., Zhang, L., Xu, Y., Deng, W., Zhu, H., Qin, C., 2011. S100B transgenic mice develop features of Parkinson's disease. *Archives of Medical Research*. Vol.42, pp. 1-7.

Lutz, N.W., Viola, A., Malikova, I., Confort-Gouny, S., Audoin, B., Ranjeva, J.P., Pelletier, J., Cozzone, P.J., 2007a. Inflammatory multiple-sclerosis plaques generate characteristic metabolic profiles in cerebrospinal fluid. *PLoS One*. Vol.2, e595.

Lutz, N.W., Viola, A., Malikova, I., Confort-Gouny, S., Ranjeva, J.P., Pelletier, J., Cozzone, P.J., 2007b. A branched-chain organic acid linked to multiple sclerosis: first identification by NMR spectroscopy of CSF. *Biochemical and Biophysical Research Communications*. Vol.354, pp. 160-164.

Martin, W.R., 2007. MR spectroscopy in neurodegenerative disease. *Molecular Imaging and Biology*. Vol.9, pp. 196-203.

Masdeu, J.C., 2011. Neuroimaging in psychiatric disorders. *Neurotherapeutics*. Vol.8, pp. 93-102.

Moore, R.E., Kirwan, J., Doherty, M.K., Whitfield, P.D., 2007. Biomarker discovery in animal health and disease: the application of post-genomic technologies. *Biomarker Insights*. Vol.2, pp. 185-196.

Nicholson, J.K., Lindon, J.C., Holmes, E., 1999. 'Metabonomics': understanding the metabolic responses of living systems to pathophysiological stimuli via multivariate statistical analysis of biological NMR spectroscopic data. *Xenobiotica*. Vol.29, pp. 1181-1189.

Nicholson, J.K., Lindon, J.C., 2008. Systems biology: Metabonomics. *Nature*. Vol.455, pp. 1054-1056.

Nowak, K., Mix, E., Gimsa, J., Strauss, U., Sriperumbudur, K.K., Benecke, R., Gimsa, U., 2011. Optimizing a rodent model of Parkinson's disease for exploring the effects and mechanisms of deep brain stimulation. *Parkinson's Disease*. Vol.2011, 414682.

Pears, M.R., Cooper, J.D., Mitchison, H.M., Mortishire-Smith, R.J., Pearce, D.A., Griffin, J.L., 2005. High resolution 1H NMR-based metabolomics indicates a neurotransmitter cycling deficit in cerebral tissue from a mouse model of Batten disease. *The Journal of Biological Chemistry*. Vol.280, pp. 42508-42514.

Pogge, A., Slikker, W., Jr., 2004. Neuroimaging: new approaches for neurotoxicology. *Neurotoxicology*. Vol.25, pp. 525-531.

Porsolt, R.D., Bertin, A., Jalfre, M., 1977. Behavioral despair in mice: a primary screening test for antidepressants. *Archives internationales de pharmacodynamie et de thérapie*. Vol.229, pp. 327-336.

Porsolt, R.D., Bertin, A., Blavet, N., Deniel, M., Jalfre, M., 1979. Immobility induced by forced swimming in rats: effects of agents which modify central catecholamine and serotonin activity. *European Journal of Pharmacology*. Vol.57, pp. 201-210.

Quinones, M.P., Kaddurah-Daouk, R., 2009. Metabolomics tools for identifying biomarkers for neuropsychiatric diseases. *Neurobiology of Disease*. Vol.35, pp. 165-176.

Roberts, M.J., Schirra, H.J., Lavin, M.F., Gardiner, R.A., 2011. Metabolomics: a novel approach to early and noninvasive prostate cancer detection. *Korean Journal of Urology*. Vol.52, pp. 79-89.

Robertson, D.G., 2005. Metabonomics in toxicology: a review. *Toxicological Sciences*. Vol.85, pp. 809-822.

Robertson-Smith, R.G., Jeffcott, L.B., Friend, S.C., Badcoe, L.M., 1985. An unusual incidence of neurological disease affecting horses during a drought. *Australian Veterinary Journal*. Vol.62, pp. 6-12.

Rodgers, R.J., Johnson, N.J., 1995. Factor analysis of spatiotemporal and ethological measures in the murine elevated plus-maze test of anxiety. *Pharmacology Biochemistry and Behavior*. Vol.52, pp. 297-303.

Ross, A.J., Sachdev, P.S., 2004. Magnetic resonance spectroscopy in cognitive research. *Brain Research Brain Research Reviews*. Vol.44, pp. 83-102.

Ross, B., Bluml, S., 2001. Magnetic resonance spectroscopy of the human brain. *The Anatomical Record*. Vol.265, pp. 54-84.

Rudkin, T.M., Arnold, D.L., 1999. Proton magnetic resonance spectroscopy for the diagnosis and management of cerebral disorders. *Archives of Neurology*. Vol.56, pp. 919-926.

Salek, R.M., Xia, J., Innes, A., Sweatman, B.C., Adalbert, R., Randle, S., McGowan, E., Emson, P.C., Griffin, J.L., 2010. A metabolomic study of the CRND8 transgenic mouse model of Alzheimer's disease. *Neurochemistry International*. Vol.56, pp. 937-947.

Sayre, L.M., Perry, G., Smith, M.A., 2008. Oxidative stress and neurotoxicity. *Chemical Research in Toxicology*. Vol.21, pp. 172-188.

Sinclair, A.J., Viant, M.R., Ball, A.K., Burdon, M.A., Walker, E.A., Stewart, P.M., Rauz, S., Young, S.P., 2009. NMR-based metabolomic analysis of cerebrospinal fluid and serum in neurological diseases--a diagnostic tool? *NMR in Biomedicine*. Vol.23, pp. 123-132.

Slocombe, R.F., Huntington, P.J., Friend, S.C., Jeffcott, L.B., Luff, A.R., Finkelstein, D.K., 1992. Pathological aspects of Australian Stringhalt. *Equine Veterinary Journal*. Vol.24, pp. 174-183.

Song, I.H., Hermann, K., Haibel, H., Althoff, C.E., Listing, J., Burmester, G., Krause, A., Bohl-Buhler, M., Freundlich, B., Rudwaleit, M., Sieper, J., 2011. Effects of etanercept versus sulfasalazine in early axial spondyloarthritis on active inflammatory lesions as detected by whole-body MRI (ESTHER): a 48-week randomised controlled trial. *Annals of the Rheumatic Diseases*. Vol.70, pp. 590-596.

Stoessl, A.J., 2011. Neuroimaging in Parkinson's disease. *Neurotherapeutics*. Vol.8, pp. 72-81.

Tabatabaie, L., Klomp, L.W., Berger, R., de Koning, T.J., 2010. L-serine synthesis in the central nervous system: a review on serine deficiency disorders. *Molecular Genetics and Metabolism*. Vol.99, pp. 256-262.

Takahashi, T., Kitamura, M., Endo, Y., Eto, D., Aoki, O., Kusunose, R., Yoshihara, T., Kai, M., 2002. An outbreak of stringhalt resembling australian stringhalt in Japan. *Journal of Equine Science*. Vol.13, pp. 93-100.

Takeda, H., Tsuji, M., Matsumiya, T., 1998. Changes in head-dipping behavior in the hole-board test reflect the anxiogenic and/or anxiolytic state in mice. *European Journal of Pharmacology*. Vol.350, pp. 21-29.

Tartaglia, M.C., Arnold, D.L., 2006. The role of MRS and fMRI in multiple sclerosis. *Advances in Neurology*. Vol.98, pp. 185-202.

Tate, A.R., Crabb, S., Griffiths, J.R., Howells, S.L., Mazucco, R.A., Rodrigues, L.M., Watson, D., 1996. Lipid metabolite peaks in pattern recognition analysis of tumour in vivo MR spectra. *Anticancer Research*. Vol.16, pp. 1575-1579.

Tate, A.R., Griffiths, J.R., Martinez-Perez, I., Moreno, A., Barba, I., Cabanas, M.E., Watson, D., Alonso, J., Bartumeus, F., Isamat, F., Ferrer, I., Vila, F., Ferrer, E., Capdevila, A., Arus, C., 1998. Towards a method for automated classification of 1H MRS spectra from brain tumours. *NMR Biomedicine*. Vol.11, pp. 177-191.

Toga, A.W., Thompson, P.M., Sowell, E.R., 2006. Mapping brain maturation. *Trends in Neurosciences*. Vol.29, pp. 148-159.

Torre, F., 2005. Clinical diagnosis and results of surgical treatment of 13 cases of acquired bilateral stringhalt (1991--2003). *Equine Veterinarian Journal*. Vol.37, pp 181-183.

Viola, A., Nicoli, F., Denis, B., Confort-Gouny, S., Le Fur, Y., Ranjeva, J.P., Viout, P., Cozzone, P.J., 2004. High cerebral scyllo-inositol: a new marker of brain metabolism disturbances induced by chronic alcoholism. *Magnetic resonance materials in physics, biology, and medicine MAGMA*. Vol.17, pp. 47-61.

Wang, T.J., Larson, M.G., Vasan, R.S., Cheng, S., Rhee, E.P., McCabe, E., Lewis, G.D., Fox, C.S., Jacques, P.F., Fernandez, C., O'Donnell, C.J., Carr, S.A., Mootha, V.K., Florez, J.C., Souza, A., Melander, O., Clish, C.B., Gerszten, R.E., 2011. Metabolite profiles and the risk of developing diabetes. *Nature Medicine.* Vol.17, pp. 448-453.

Wattamwar, P.R., Mathuranath, P.S., 2010. An overview of biomarkers in Alzheimer's disease. *Annals of Indian Academy of Neurology.* Vol.13, S116-123.

# 3

# Can VEGF-B Be Used to Treat Neurodegenerative Diseases?

Xuri Li, Anil Kumar, Chunsik Lee, Zhongshu Tang,
Yang Li, Pachiappan Arjunan, Xu Hou and Fan Zhang
*National Eye Institute, National Institutes of Health, Rockville, Maryland*
*United States of America*

## 1. Introduction

Studies on vascular endothelial growth factor B (VEGF-B) during the past decade or so have shown that VEGF-B appears to be a mysterious molecule with obscure, if not controversial, functions. When VEGF-B was initially discovered (Grimmond et al., 1996; Olofsson et al., 1996a), it was naturally believed to be an angiogenic factor, due to its high sequence homology and similar receptor binding pattern to VEGF, the prototypic angiogenic molecule. Much of our research effort was focused on this speculated angiogenic activity of VEGF-B for a long time. However, studies into this aspect, most of the time, turned out to be disappointing because of the negative findings. Unlike VEGF-A, VEGF-B did not seem to play a significant role in inducing blood vessel growth or vascular permeability, etc (Li et al., 2009). In addition, VEGF-B deficiency in mice did not seem to matter greatly, since VEGF-B-null mice appeared largely healthy (Aase et al., 2001; Bellomo et al., 2000; Louzier et al., 2003; Reichelt et al., 2003), in contrast to the early embryonic lethality of VEGF-A null mice (Carmeliet et al., 1996; Ferrara et al., 1996). Based on the negative findings, we had once suspected that VEGF-B might be a redundant molecule. In recent years, VEGF-B has been shown to be a potent neuroprotective factor and an apoptosis inhibitor (Li et al., 2009; Li et al., 2008b; Poesen et al., 2008; Sun et al., 2004; Sun et al., 2006), opening up a new research avenue in VEGF-B biology.

Thus far, there are five members within the VEGF family, VEGF-A, VEGF-B, PlGF, VEGF-C and VEGF-D (Li and Eriksson, 2001; Lohela et al., 2009). As a prototypic angiogenic factor, VEGF-A has a potent and "universal" angiogenic effect under most physiological and pathological conditions (Carmeliet & Jain, 2000; Ferrara & Kerbel, 2005; Folkman, 2007). The placenta growth factor (PlGF) is required for pathological angiogenesis (Luttun et al., 2002). However, when PlGF-1 is produced in the same population of cells with VEGF-A, it can also act as a natural antagonist of VEGF-A (Cao, 2009; Eriksson et al., 2002). VEGF-C and VEGF-D are important players in lymphangiogenesis (Alitalo et al., 2005; Lohela et al., 2009). Remarkably, the biological function of VEGF-B has remained less studied. VEGF-B displays a high degree of sequence homology to VEGF-A and PlGF, and also binds to the tyrosine kinase VEGF receptor-1 (VEGFR-1) and neuropilin-1 (NP-1), like VEGF-A and PlGF (Olofsson et al., 1998; Olofsson et al., 1996a). VEGF-B is abundantly expressed in most tissues and organs (Aase et al., 1999; Li et al., 2001; Olofsson et al., 1996a). However, VEGF-B under most conditions appeared to be "redundant" or "inert" with no obvious function. The *in vivo* role of VEGF-B therefore remained enigmatic for a long time. In this review, we summarize the recent advances on VEGF-B biology, with a particular interest in its neuroprotective/survival effect on neuronal and vascular cells (Claesson-Welsh, 2008; Karpanen et al., 2008; Lahteenvuo et al., 2009; Li et al., 2008a; Li et al., 2008b; Poesen et al., 2008; Zhang et al., 2009), and further discuss the therapeutic potential of VEGF-B in treating different types of neurodegenerative diseases.

## 2. VEGF-B is a neuronal protective factor

VEGF-B is highly expressed in different types of neural tissues, such as the brain (Li et al., 2001; Sun et al., 2004), retina (Li et al., 2008b), spinal cord (Poesen et al., 2008), etc.

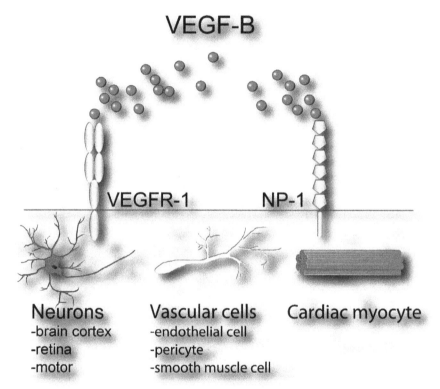

Fig. 1. Pleiotropic protective/survival effect of VEGF-B on multiple cell types. Both *in vitro* data derived from cultured neurons and *in vivo* work using different types of animal models have shown that VEGF-B is a critical protective/survival factor for different types of neurons, including cortical, retinal, and spinal cord motor neurons. In addition, VEGF-B is also a potent protective/survival factor for different types of vascular cells, including vascular endothelial cells, smooth muscle cells and pericytes. Moreover, VEGF-B has also been reported to be a protective factor for cardiac myocytes

We and others have shown that VEGF-B is a potent protective/survival factor for different types of neurons, including brain cortical neurons (Li et al., 2008b; Sun et al., 2004), retinal neurons (Li et al., 2008b), and motor neurons in the spinal cord (Poesen et al., 2008). *In vitro,* VEGF-B protein treatment dose-dependently increased the survival of cultured primary brain cortex neurons (Li et al., 2008b; Sun et al., 2004). *In vivo,* VEGF-B treatment inhibited apoptosis of brain cortical neurons and reduced stroke volume in a middle cerebral artery ligation-induced brain stroke model (Li et al., 2008b). In the retina, we have shown that VEGF-B treatment protected different types of retinal neurons from apoptosis under different pathological conditions. In an optic nerve crush injury model, VEGF-B treatment increased the survival of retinal ganglion cells. In a NMDA-induced retinal neuron apoptosis model, VEGF-B treatment protected retinal neurons in the ganglion cell layer, inner nuclear layer, and outer nuclear layer (Li et al., 2008b). Moreover, Poesen, K *et al* recently showed that VEGF-B treatment protected cultured primary motor neurons from apoptosis (Poesen et al., 2008). Indeed, the neuroprotective effect of VEGF-B was further confirmed using mice in which VEGF-B was genetically deleted. VEGF-B deficiency led to more severe strokes in an experimental stroke model, and exacerbated retinal ganglion cell death in an optic nerve crush injury model (Li et al., 2008b). Moreover, VEGF-B deficient mice developed a more severe form of motor neuron degeneration when intercrossed with the mutant SOD1 mice, whereas VEGF-B intracerebroventricular injection prolonged the survival of mutant SOD1 rats (Poesen et al., 2008). Taken together, both *in vitro* data derived from cultured neurons and *in vivo* work obtained using different animal models showed that VEGF-B is a critical survival factor for different types of neurons (Fig. 1).

### 3. VEGF-B is a vascular survival factor

VEGF-B and its receptors are expressed by different types of vascular cells (Aase et al., 1999; Li et al., 2008a; Zhang et al., 2009). We recently found that VEGF-B is a potent survival factor for multiple types of vascular cells, including vascular endothelial cells (EC), pericytes (PC), and smooth muscle cells (SMC) (Li et al., 2009; Zhang et al., 2009). *In vitro,* in both cultured primary vascular cells and established vascular cell lines, VEGF-B treatment increased the survival of not only ECs, but also that of PCs and SMCs (Zhang et al., 2009). In contrast, VEGF-B inhibition by shRNA treatment led to apoptosis in the ECs and PCs. Moreover, increased apoptosis was found in VEGF-B deficient ECs and SMCs isolated from VEGF-B null mice, when the cells were cultured in serum-free medium or under $H_2O_2$-induced oxidative stress (Zhang et al., 2009). *In vivo,* VEGF-B deficiency led to poorer blood vessel survival in the cornea after withdrawal of the implanted growth factors, fewer surviving hyaloid vessels in postnatal mouse eyes, and greater oxygen-induced retinal blood vessel degeneration in neonatal mice (Zhang et al., 2009). Thus, both gain- and loss-of-function analyses showed that VEGF-B is required for the survival of multiple types of vascular cells, especially, under pathological conditions (Fig. 1).

### 4. VEGF-B promotes energy metabolism

The human brain weighs only about 2% of the total body weight. However, it consumes about 20% of the total energy produced in the body, demonstrating the importance of energy metabolism to the neural systems. Indeed, numerous reports have shown that energy deficit is involved in various neurodegenerative disorders, such as Alzheimer's disease (AD) (Beal, 2007), Huntington's Disease (HD) (Browne and Beal, 2004), Parkinson's disease (PD) (Elstner et al., 2011) and Amyotrophic lateral sclerosis (ALS) (D'Alessandro et al., 2011). In addition, dysregulation of lipid pathways has been implicated in AD (Di Paolo and Kim, 2011). These findings thus warrant investigating and developing therapeutic reagents that can regulate neuronal bioenergetic pathways. Recently, VEGF-B has been shown to be involved in energy metabolism, where it facilitates fatty acid uptake from circulation and transfer to metabolically active tissues (Hagberg et al., 2010). We have also seen that VEGF-B upregulated the expression of a number of key enzymes that are involved in lipid and glucose metabolism in cultured cells (our own unpublished data). Based on the above findings, VEGF-B might be an important molecule that could be used to regulate neuronal bioenergetic pathways. Further studies are needed to verify this.

## 5. VEGF-B does not induce blood vessel permeability

It is known that all the other VEGF family members, VEGF-A (Dvorak et al., 1995), PlGF (Carmeliet et al., 2001), VEGF-C (Joukov et al., 1997), VEGF-D (Rissanen et al., 2003) and VEGF-E (Ogawa et al., 1998), induce blood vessel permeability. However, numerous studies using different models and approaches, such as VEGF-B deficient and transgenic mice, recombinant protein or gene transfer, have shown that VEGF-B does not affect blood vessel permeability (Aase et al., 2001; Mould et al., 2005; Reichelt et al., 2003) (Fig. 2). Intradermal injection of VEGF-A$_{165}$, VEGF-A$_{121}$, and VEGF-C in mice ears increased vascular permeability, while VEGF-B administration had no such effect (Brkovic & Sirois, 2007). VEGF-B$_{167}$ recombinant protein injection into mouse brain or eye did not induce blood vessel permeability (Li et al., 2008b). In preserved lung grafts, VEGF-A and VEGF-C, but not VEGF-B mediate increased vascular permeability (Abraham et al., 2002). Indeed, when overexpressed in the lung by adenoviral gene transfer, VEGF-B had no effect on blood vessel permeability (Louzier et al., 2003). Adenoviruses expressing VEGF-A and VEGF-D delivered into rabbit hind limb skeletal muscles induced vascular permeability, while adenovirus encoding VEGF-B did not affect blood vessel permeability when administered into skeletal muscles (Rissanen et al., 2003). Thus, data derived from different model systems showed that VEGF-B is the only member of the VEGF family that does not have a significant role in inducing blood vessel permeability

## 6. Minimum side effect of VEGF-B and its negligible role in angiogenesis

Due to its high sequence homology and similar receptor binding patterns to VEGF-A (Li and Eriksson, 2001; Nash et al., 2006), VEGF-B was initially believed to be an angiogenic factor. However, studies along this line using VEGF-B deficient and transgenic mice and gene transfer approaches have, most of the time, led to negative findings (Fig. 2).
VEGF-A or VEGF-C deficiency caused embryonic lethality in mice (Carmeliet et al., 1996; Ferrara et al., 1996; Karkkainen et al., 2004). VEGF-B deficient mice, however, are largely healthy with normal physiological angiogenesis (Aase et al., 2001; Bellomo et al., 2000; Louzier et al., 2003; Reichelt et al., 2003). PlGF deficient mice display impaired pathological angiogenesis (Carmeliet et al., 2001; Luttun et al., 2002). VEGF-B deficiency, however, does not affect pathological angiogenesis in most organs studied, such as the wounded skin, hypoxic lung, ischemic retina and limb (Li et al., 2008a). Even though one study reported a role of VEGF-B in pathological (inflammatory) angiogenesis using arthritis models (Mould et al., 2003), we did not observe such an effect in our study (unpublished observation). In contrast to VEGF-A and PlGF, VEGF-B is not required for neovessel formation in

proliferative retinopathy (Reichelt et al., 2003) or blood vessel remodeling in pulmonary hypertension (Louzier et al., 2003).

Transgenic expression of all the other VEGF family members, such as VEGF-A (Detmar et al., 1998; Larcher et al., 1998; Xia et al., 2003), PlGF (Odorisio et al., 2002), VEGF-C (Jeltsch et al., 1997), VEGF-D (Karkkainen et al., 2009) or VEGF-E (Kiba et al., 2003) induced either angiogenesis or lymphangiogenesis. VEGF-B is the only member of the VEGF family, transgenic overexpression of which in different organs did not induce angiogenesis or lymphangiogenesis (Karpanen et al., 2008; Mould et al., 2005). VEGF-B overexpression in cardiac myocytes under the alpha-myosin heavy chain promoter did not induce angiogenesis in the heart (Karpanen et al., 2008). Instead, blood vessel density was decreased in the hearts overexpressing VEGF-B (Karpanen et al., 2008). In addition, VEGF-B

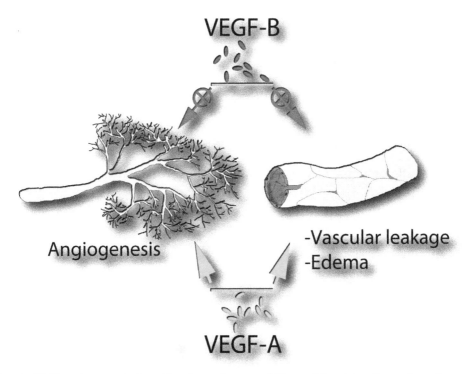

Fig. 2. VEGF-B does not induce blood vessel permeability and is minimally angiogenic. Adenoviral gene transfer of the other VEGF family members, such as VEGF-A, VEGF-C and VEGF-D, into rabbit hindlimb skeletal muscles induced strong angiogenesis, vascular permeability, or lymphangiogenesis (Rissanen et al., 2003). VEGF-B adenoviral gene transfer, however, did not induce angiogenesis or lymphangiogenesis in the same model system (Rissanen et al., 2003). Similarly, adenoviral gene transfer of VEGF-A and VEGF-D to rabbit carotid arteries induced robust adventitial angiogenesis, whereas VEGF-B adenoviral gene transfer failed to do so (Bhardwaj et al., 2003, 2005). Another study also showed that VEGF-B$_{167}$ gene delivery to the mouse skin or ischemic limb did not induce blood vessel growth (Li et al., 2008a)

transgenic expression in endothelial cells under Tie2 promoter did not induce angiogenesis in different types of organs (liver, heart, kidney, etc) (Mould et al., 2005), and VEGF-B transgenic expression in the skin under keratin-14 promoter only marginal potentiated angiogenesis (Karpanen et al., 2008).

Studies using VEGF-B protein treatment also showed a minimum side effect of VEGF-B and a negligible role in angiogenesis. VEGF-B$_{167}$ recombinant protein injection into adult mouse eyes at a dose effective for retinal neuron survival did not induce ocular angiogenesis (Li et al., 2008b). Poesen, K., *et al* has also shown that intracerebroventricular injection of the VEGF-B$_{186}$ recombinant protein did not cause any blood vessel growth or blood-brain barrier leakage (Poesen et al., 2008).

VEGF-B is most abundantly expressed in the heart (Li et al., 2001; Olofsson et al., 1996a). Using a cardiac ischemia model, we found that VEGF-B has a restricted role in the revascularization of ischemic myocardium (Claesson-Welsh, 2008; Li et al., 2008a). Indeed, this observation was also reported by another study demonstrating that in pigs and rabbits, VEGF-B$_{186}$ gene transfer induced myocardium-specific angiogenesis and arteriogenesis (Lahteenvuo et al., 2009). Thus, ours and others' work have shown that in most organs, VEGF-B is dispensable for blood vessel growth in development, normal physiology, and many pathological conditions but with a selective angiogenic activity in the ischemic heart. Taken together, compared with the other VEGF family members, VEGF-B appears to have a unique safety profile that is highly desirable as a potential therapeutic reagent to treat human diseases.

## 7. Therapeutic potential of VEGF-B in treating neurodegenerative diseases

Currently, for most neurodegenerative diseases, there are no effective treatments. Although novel remedies such as gene or cell therapies are being explored intensively, few have proved to be clinically beneficial. Neurodegenerative diseases often involve complex multi-etiological aspects. Neuronal apoptosis is a central characteristic of neurodegenerative diseases. In addition, blood vessel degeneration in the relevant neural system is often seen in many of the neurodegenerative disorders. Therefore, therapeutic reagents targeting one pathway only will most likely not be sufficient to cure the disease. Reagents that can improve multiple pathological aspects are more desirable. Based on our recent findings that VEGF-B is a potent protective/survival factor for both the neuronal and vascular systems, which are two critical components in most neurodegenerative disorders, we hypothesize that VEGF-B may have therapeutic implications in treating various types of neurodegenerative diseases, such as Alzheimer's disease (AD), Parkinson's disease (PD), Huntington's disease (HD), amyotrophic lateral sclerosis (ALS) stroke, retinitis pigmentosa (RP), glaucoma, diabetic retinopathy (DR) and atrophic age-related macular degeneration (AMD). Below, we discuss the therapeutic potential of VEGF-B in relation to these pathologies.

### 7.1 Alzheimer's Disease

Alzheimer's Disease (AD) is a major contributor to dementia in the elderly, and affects about 2% of the population in developed countries. The total number of AD patients is estimated to increase significantly in the near future due to the growing aging population (Mattson, 2004). In AD patients, plaques containing the beta-amyloid protein deposit extracellularly, and neurofibrillary tangles of hyperphosphorylated tau protein accumulate intracellularly in the brain, leading to the degeneration of synapses and neurons, and eventually the loss of memory and cognitive ability (Mattson, 2004). Both genetic and environmental factors contribute to the development of AD. Several drugs are currently available for AD treatment, such as tacrine, donepezil, rivastigmine tartrate and galantamine hydrobromide. These drugs can sometimes relieve the symptoms of early stage AD patients. However, they cannot stop or reverse the progression of the illness, and the effects of these drugs are often inconsistent and diminished over time. Therefore, more effective treatments are still needed. Many new reagents have been tested in preclinical or clinical studies, such as intravenous immunoglobulin (Relkin et al., 2008), γ-secretase inhibitors (Siemers et al., 2006; Wilcock et al., 2008), blockers of the receptor for advanced glycation end product (Chen et al., 2007), Dimebon (Doody et al., 2008), etc. However, their therapeutic efficacies are yet to be proven. It is noteworthy that in recent years, AD has been considered more as a vascular, rather than a neural disease based on clinical imaging, epidemiological, pharmacotherapy and histopathological evidence (Chow et al., 2007; de la Torre, 2002; de la Torre, 2004; Kalaria and Hedera, 1995). Indeed, vascular degeneration has been observed in different experimental Alzheimer's disease models (Girouard and Iadecola, 2006; Wu et al., 2005),(Hsu et al., 2007). In addition, it has been known that the functional relationships among neuronal, glial, and vascular cells within the so-called neurovascular unit is compromised in Alzheimer's disease (Salmina, 2009). Thus, mounting evidence indicates that vascular abnormalities, such as capillary degeneration, are important factors that can initiate Alzheimer's disease. Due to the potent survival effect of VEGF-B on both neuronal and vascular cells, VEGF-B may have a therapeutic potential in the prevention and treatment of Alzheimer's disease. Further studies are needed to verify this.

### 7.2 Parkinson's Disease

Parkinson's Disease (PD) is the second most prevalent neurodegenerative disease following AD. PD is characterized by the age-related progressive loss of dopaminergic neurotransmission in the basal ganglia (Nutt and Wooten, 2005). The etiology of PD is complicated and involves multiple factors and mechanisms. PD patients suffer from severe motor symptoms, including uncontrollable resting tremor, bradykinesia, rigidity and postural imbalance. Current treatment for PD can only attenuate the symptoms. There is no effective drug that can stop the neuronal death in PD patients. Levodopa, in combination with a peripheral dopa decarboxylase inhibitor, is the most effective therapy thus far (Lees et al., 2009). However, levodopa motor and nonmotor complications are challenging issues to overcome clinically (Jankovic, 2005). Dopamine agonists and monoamine oxidase-B inhibitors can reduce the symptoms either as a monotherapy or in combination with levodopa (Jankovic, 2006). However, even though the symptoms may be controlled after the administration of these drugs, at least following the initial treatment, the death of the dopaminergic neurons persists and the disease continues to progress.

Neuroprotection is at the forefront of PD research, and many neuroprotective reagents have been investigated (Bonuccelli and Del Dotto, 2006; Djaldetti and Melamed, 2002). The glial cell derived neurotrophic factor (GDNF) has been shown to enhance the survival of midbrain dopaminergic neurons *in vitro* and rescued degenerating neurons *in vivo* (Love et al., 2005). However, a multicenter clinical trial showed no clinical benefit (Lang et al., 2006), and GDNF antibody development was observed in some PD patients (Sherer et al., 2006).

Indeed, in a rat α-synuclein PD model, overexpression of GDNF failed to exert effective neuroprotection (Decressac et al., 2011). The vascular endothelial growth factor–A (VEGF-A) has been shown to induce neuroprotection in a PD model of the 6-hydroxydopamine (6-OHDA) lesioned rats (Yasuhara et al., 2004). However unwarranted side effect of VEGF-A proved to be detrimental to the brain, since VEGF-A also induced edema and undesired angiogenesis in the brain (Yasuhara et al., 2005). In addition, it has also been reported that VEGF-A induces astrogliosis, microgliosis and disrupts the blood-brain barrier (Rite et al., 2007). Thus, new and better neuroprotective reagents are still needed.

Apart from neuronal death, normal contact between nigral neurons and capillaries is often impaired in the brains of PD patients. Capillary basement membrane thickening and collagen accumulation are often seen in PD patients, suggesting that capillary dysfunction may play an important role in PD development (Farkas et al., 2000; Faucheux et al., 1999). Indeed, it is believed that markers of cerebrovascular disease may predict the development of different types of dementia, including PD (Staekenborg et al., 2009). Recent work has shown that VEGF-B expression was upregulated by neurodegenerative challenges in the midbrain, and exogenous application of VEGF-B has a neuroprotective effect in a culture model of PD (Falk et al., 2009). In another study, VEGF-B$_{186}$ was used to test its neuroprotective effect in a PD model since it is more diffusable and hardly binds to extracellular matrix than VEGF-B$_{167}$ (Olofsson et al., 1996b; Poesen et al., 2008). In this study, a single dose of VEGF-B$_{186}$ (3µg/rat) rescued dopaminergic neurons from death in the caudal sub region of substantia nigra in rats (Falk et al., 2011). Thus, as a potent neuronal and vascular protective factor, VEGF-B may have therapeutic implications in PD treatment. Future investigations are needed to investigate into this.

### 7.3 Amyotrophic lateral sclerosis

Amyotrophic lateral sclerosis (ALS) is a devastating adult-onset neurodegenerative disorder characterized by progressive loss of motoneurons in the primary motor cortex, corticospinal tracts, brainstem and spinal cord, leading to muscular paralysis and eventually death (Wijesekera and Leigh, 2009). The pathogenesis of familial ALS is unclear. Sporadic ALS is believed to be related to superoxide dismutase (SOD) 1 mutation in about 20-30% of the patients (Yamamoto et al., 2008). Although many drug candidates have been tested, such as antioxidants, neurotrophic factors, anti-apoptotic, anti-inflammatory and anti-aggregation reagents, the only drug currently available for ALS patients is Riluzole, a glutamate antagonist (Traynor et al., 2006; Yamamoto et al., 2008). Recently, it is believed that vascular defect may be a critical contributor to the pathogenesis of ALS. In the amyotrophic lateral sclerosis-linked SOD1 mutant mice, vascular endothelial damage accumulates before motor neuron degeneration and plays a central role in ALS initiation (Segura et al., 2009). The therapeutic promise of VEGF-B in ALS treatment has been shown by Poesen et al. VEGF-B$_{186}$ protected cultured primary motor neurons against degeneration (Poesen et al., 2008). *In vivo*, VEGF-B treatment protected motor neurons from degeneration in several experimental ALS models (Poesen et al., 2008). In the future, it will be exciting to see whether this effect of VEGF-B holds true in ALS patients.

### 7.4 Stroke

Ischemic stroke due to sudden loss of blood supply in the brain is a leading cause of morbidity and mortality in the United States. Currently, there is no satisfying therapy for stroke patients despite extensive effort on identifying better interventions. Since early 1990s, neuroprotection as a potential therapeutic strategy for stroke treatment has received much attention (Ginsberg, 2008). During the past decade or so, about 160 clinical trials on neuroprotection for ischemic stroke treatment have been conducted (Ginsberg, 2008). However, no effective neuroprotective drug has been identified. The potential therapeutic value of VEGF-B for stroke treatment has been supported by several studies. It has been shown that VEGF-B is a potent survival factor for cortical neurons. VEGF-B deficiency in mouse increased stroke volume by about 40% in an experimental stroke model, and led to more severe neurologic impairment (Sun et al., 2004). Indeed, VEGF-B protein treatment protected cultured cerebral cortical neurons from hypoxic injury, demonstrating a direct survival effect of VEGF-B on neurons (Sun et al., 2004). Furthermore, intraventricular administration of VEGF-B decreased stroke volume (Li et al., 2008b) and restored neurogenesis to normal level in VEGF-B deficient mice (Sun et al., 2006). Mechanistically, we have shown that VEGF-B exerts its neuronal survival effect by inhibiting the expression of many proapoptotic BH3-only protein genes (Li et al., 2008b). In summary, both *in vitro* and *in vivo* data from several groups have suggested a therapeutic potential of VEGF-B in stroke treatment and warrant further studies to investigate into this.

### 7.5 Huntington's Disease

Huntington's Disease (HD) is a hereditary autosomal dominant neurodegenerative disorder characterized by the selective degeneration of striatal projection neurons that are responsible for choreic movements, resulting in progressive movement disorder, cognitive decline and psychiatric disturbances. Over the course of HD, the mutated huntingtin protein leads to intracellular dysfunctions and neuronal death in the striatum, selected layers of the cerebral cortex, as well as other brain regions (Gil and Rego, 2008). Currently, no effective therapy exists for HD. Pharmacological treatment may ameliorate hyperkinesis and psychiatric symptoms, but neuropsychological deficits and dementia remain untreatable. The apoptotic cascade is believed to be a possible cause of neurodegeneration in HD (Pattison et al., 2006). The therapeutic potential of some neuroprotective reagents in HD treatment, such as GDNF, coenzyme Q10, minocycline and unsaturated fatty acids, has been investigated (Alberch et al., 2002; Bonelli and Hofmann, 2007). Since VEGF-B is a potent apoptosis inhibitor (Li et al., 2008b), it will be interesting to test whether VEGF-B could slow down, if not stop, neuronal degeneration in HD.

### 7.6 Retinal degenerative diseases

Retinal degenerative diseases are a group of disorders involving degeneration of the retina. Progressive loss of retinal neurons is a common characteristic of such disorders and the major reason for vision impair or loss. Further, blood vessel deterioration is often seen in many of the retinal degenerative diseases. Unfortunately, thus far, there is no efficacious treatment for most of the retinal degenerative diseases.

### 7.6.1 Retinitis pigmentosa (RP)

Retinitis pigmentosa (RP) is a heterogeneous retinal dystrophy characterized by the progressive loss of photoreceptors and subsequent degeneration of retinal pigmented epithelial (RPE) cells (Hartong et al., 2006). RP is the leading cause of blindness in inherited retinal degeneration-associated diseases world-wide. The first symptom of RP is often night blindness, followed by the gradual loss of peripheral visual field, and ultimately blindness. Apart from the photoreceptor dystrophy, retinal arterioles are attenuated in RP, leading to poor oxygenation of rods and cones and increased apoptosis in the neural retina. It is known that about 45 genes/loci are involved in this pathology. Due to the large number of genes and mutations implicated, correcting the defective genes/mutations represents an overwhelming challenge. The current available therapies are vitamin supplement and sunlight protection, which can only slow down the degenerative process (Hamel, 2006). There is no treatment that can stop the progress of the disease or restore vision in RP patients. Since VEGF-B can protect both neuronal and vascular cells from apoptosis, VEGF-B administration may preserve both the photoreceptors and blood vessels in RP. Future studies are needed to verify this.

### 7.6.2 Glaucoma

Glaucoma is the most prevalent form of adult optic neuropathies affecting approximately 2% of the population over the age of 40 (Levin, 2005; Marcic et al., 2003). Glaucoma is characterized by the increased apoptosis of retinal ganglion cells, loss of optic nerve fibers, and, if uncontrolled, impair or loss of vision (Weinreb, 2005). Apoptosis of retinal ganglion cells is believed to be an early event in glaucoma (Cheung et al., 2008). The number of glaucoma patients is significantly increasing because of the growing ageing population and other factors (Morley and Murdoch, 2006). Currently, there is no general treatment effective for all glaucoma patients. Recent years have seen increasing evidence showing that glaucoma is, to a large extent, a neurodegenerative disease similar to other neurodegenerative disorders in the central nervous system, such as Alzheimer's disease (Cheung et al., 2008). Traditionally, lowering the intraocular pressure (IOP) has been a major therapeutic goal in glaucoma treatment. However, such therapeutic approaches have not been effective in preventing many patients from progressive vision loss. Thus, the fact that retinal ganglion cells (RGC) continue to die in some glaucoma patients with normal or even lower IOP has changed the research focus to neuroprotection for glaucoma treatment in recent years. Therefore, neuroprotective reagents used to treat other neurodegenerative diseases have been under considerable investigation for glaucoma treatment, and neuroprotection in glaucoma treatment has gained more and more attention. However, the number of effective neuroprotective reagents is limited. We have recently revealed that VEGF-B is expressed in normal retinal ganglion cells (Li et al., 2008b). Importantly, the expression of VEGF-B is up-regulated after optic nerve crush injury in the retina (Li et al., 2008b), suggesting a role of VEGF-B in retinal ganglion cell function. Indeed, VEGF-B inhibits the expression of many apoptotic genes in the retina and protected retinal ganglion cells from axotomy-induced apoptosis (Li et al., 2008b). These data have provided evidence that VEGF-B may be a promising drug candidate for glaucoma treatment as a neuroprotective factor. Further studies are warranted to investigate this.

### 7.6.3 Diabetic retinopathy

Diabetic retinopathy (DR) is a common complication of diabetes. About 50-75% of diabetic patients develop DR. In the United States, DR is the leading cause of legal blindness in the 20 to 74 year-old population (Imai et al., 2009). Conventionally, DR is believed mainly to be a microvascular disease. However, it is now considered to be also a neurodegenerative disease involving functional and structural defects of different types of neurons in the retina (Imai et al., 2009). Indeed, neuronal apoptosis has been found to be an early event in a rat model of diabetes (Barber et al., 1998). Four months after the onset of diabetes, there were only about 50% of total neurons left in the retinae of the rats (Barber et al., 1998), and the number of retinal ganglion cells (RGC) and the thickness of the inner retina layer were significantly reduced (Barber et al., 1998). In diabetic patients, increased apoptosis was also observed in the retina (Imai et al., 2009). Moreover, significant nerve fibre loss in the superior segment of the retina was observed in type 1 diabetic patients, suggesting RGC loss (Kern and Barber, 2008; Lopes de Faria et al., 2002). In addition, thinning of the inner retinal layer was observed in early stage of type 1 diabetic patients (van Dijk et al., 2009). It is reported that the mitochondria- and caspase-dependent cell-death pathways are involved in the neuronal degeneration in diabetic retinopathy (Oshitari et al., 2008). The potential role of VEGF-B in diabetic retinopathy has not been investigated thus far. However, given that VEGF-B is a potent apoptosis inhibitor and has a strong protective effect on both retinal ganglion cells and different types of vascular cells, it is reasonable to speculate that VEGF-B could be used to rescue the chronic retinal degeneration in DR. However, further investigation and research into this aspect are still needed.

### 7.6.4 Atrophic AMD

Age-related macular degeneration (AMD) is the most common cause of blindness in developed countries. Atrophic (dry) AMD is a late-onset, multifactorial, slowly progressing retinal neurodegenerative disease caused by the degeneration of retinal pigment epithelium (RPE) that lies beneath the photoreceptor cells in the retina. Although RPE is a central element in the pathogenesis of age-related macular degeneration, RPE dysfunction results in the secondary death of macular rods and cones due to abnormal metabolic support from the RPE, eventually leading to irreversible vision loss (de Jong, 2006). Drusen formation, oxidative stress, accumulation of lipofuscin, local inflammation and reactive gliosis are believed to be involved in the pathogenesis of atrophic AMD (Petrukhin, 2007). Currently, there is no effective treatment for atrophic AMD. There are reports showing that antioxidants supplement can provide protection against age-related macular degeneration. A high dietary intake of beta carotene, vitamin C, vitamin E, and zinc may reduce the risk of AMD in elderly people substantially (Johnson, 2009; van Leeuwen et al., 2005). Compared with the other types of retinal degenerative diseases, neuroprotection as a potential therapeutic strategy has been less studied in atrophic AMD. Our recent findings showed that VEGF-B is a potent apoptosis inhibitor. Moreover, the anti-apoptotic property of VEGF-B is likely a general effect on many different types of cells, including RPE cells (Li et al., 2009; Li et al., 2008b; Zhang et al., 2009). VEGF-B therefore might potentially be used to enhance RPE survival for AMD treatment.

## 8. Conclusion

In summary, despite the complex etiology of different types of neurodegenerative diseases, one common characteristic of them is the apoptotic neuronal death. In addition, degeneration of the blood vessels is often seen in many of the neurodegenerative diseases. Thus, combination therapy acting on both aspects is highly desirable. We and others have recently shown that VEGF-B appears to be a multi-functional molecule with a potent protective/survival effect on both the neuronal and vascular systems. Importantly, the protective/survival effect of VEGF-B is accompanied by a unique and rare safety profile, since VEGF-B under most conditions appears to be inert, but acts only when there is a pathological challenge. Thus, VEGF-B may have important therapeutic values in treating different types of neurodegenerative diseases by preserving both the endangered neurons and blood vessels, and, possibly, other cell types as well.

## 9. Acknowledgment

This research was supported in part by the Macular Degeneration Research, a program of the American Health Assistance Foundation, and the Intramural Research Program of the NIH, National Eye Institute.

## 10. References

Aase, K.; Lymboussaki, A.; Kaipainen, A.; Olofsson, B.; Alitalo, K. & Eriksson, U. (1999). Localization of VEGF-B in the mouse embryo suggests a paracrine role of the growth factor in the developing vasculature. *Developmental Dynamics*. 215:12-25.

Aase, K.; von Euler, G.; Li, X.; Ponten, A.; Thoren, P.; Cao, R.; Cao, Y.; Olofsson, B.; Gebre-Medhin, S.; Pekny, M.; Alitalo, K.; Betsholtz, C. & Eriksson, U. (2001). Vascular Endothelial Growth Factor-B-Deficient Mice Display an Atrial Conduction Defect. *Circulation*. 104:358-364.

Abraham, D.; Taghavi, S.; Riml, P.; Paulus, P.; Hofmann, M.; Baumann, C.; Kocher, A.; Klepetko, W. & Aharinejad, S. (2002). VEGF-A and -C but not -B mediate increased vascular permeability in preserved lung grafts. *Transplantation*. 73:1703-1706.

Alberch, J.; Perez-Navarro, E. &. Canals, J.M. (2002). Neuroprotection by neurotrophins and GDNF family members in the excitotoxic model of Huntington's disease. *Brain Res Bull*. 57:817-822.

Alitalo, K.; Tammela, T. & Petrova, T.V. (2005). Lymphangiogenesis in development and human disease. *Nature*. 438:946-953.

Barber, A.J.; Lieth, E.; Khin, S.A.; Antonetti, D.A.; Buchanan, A.G. & Gardner, T.W. (1998). Neural apoptosis in the retina during experimental and human diabetes. Early onset and effect of insulin. *J Clin Invest*. 102:783-791.

Beal, M.F. (2007). Mitochondria and neurodegeneration. *Novartis Found Symp*. 287:183-92; discussion 192-196.

Bellomo, D.; Headrick, J.P.; Silins, G.U.; Paterson, C.A.; Thomas, P.S.; Gartside, M.; Mould, A.; Cahill, M.M.; Tonks, I.D. ; Grimmond, S.M.; Townson, S.; Wells, C.; Little, M.; Cummings, M.C.; Hayward N.K. & Kay, G.F. (2000). Mice lacking the vascular endothelial growth factor-B gene (Vegfb) have smaller hearts, dysfunctional coronary vasculature, and impaired recovery from cardiac ischemia. *Circulation Research*. 86:E29-E35.

Bhardwaj, S.; Roy, H.; Gruchala, M.; Viita, H.; Kholova, I.; Kokina, I.; Achen, M.G.; Stacker, S.A.; Hedman, M.; Alitalo, K. & Yla-Herttuala, S. (2003). Angiogenic responses of vascular endothelial growth factors in periadventitial tissue. *Hum Gene Ther*. 14:1451-1462.

Bhardwaj, S.; Roy, H.; Heikura, T. & Yla-Herttuala, S. (2005). VEGF-A, VEGF-D and VEGF-D induced intimal hyperplasia in carotid arteries. *Eur J Clin Invest.* 35:669-676.

Bonelli, R.M. & Hofmann, P. (2007). A systematic review of the treatment studies in Huntington's disease since 1990. *Expert Opin Pharmacother.* 8:141-153.

Bonuccelli, U. & Del Dotto, P. (2006). New pharmacologic horizons in the treatment of Parkinson disease. *Neurology.* 67:S30-38.

Brkovic, A. & Sirois, M.G. (2007). Vascular permeability induced by VEGF family members in vivo: Role of endogenous PAF and NO synthesis. *J Cell Biochem.* 100:727-737.

Browne, S.E. & Beal, M.F. (2004). The energetics of Huntington's disease. *Neurochem Res.* 29:531-546.

Cao, Y. (2009). Positive and negative modulation of angiogenesis by VEGFR1 ligands. *Sci Signal.* 2:re1.

Carmeliet, P.; Ferreira, V.; Breier, G.; Pollefeyt, S.; Kieckens, L.; Gertsenstein, M.; Fahrig, M.; Vandenhoeck, A.; Harpal, K.; Eberhardt, C.; Declercq, C.; Pawling, J.; Moons, L.; Collen, D.; Risau, W. & Nagy, A. (1996). Abnormal blood vessel development and lethality in embryos lacking a single VEGF allele. *Nature.* 380:435-439.

Carmeliet, P. & Jain, R.K. (2000). Angiogenesis in cancer and other diseases. *Nature.* 407:249-257.

Carmeliet, P.; Moons, L.; Luttun, A.; Vincenti, V.; Compernolle, V.; De Mol, M.; Wu, Y.; Bono, F.; Devy, L.; Beck, H.; Scholz, D.; Acker, T.; DiPalma, T.; Dewerchin, M.; Noel, A.; Stalmans, I.; Barra, A.; Blacher, S.; Vandendriessche, T.; Ponten, A.; Eriksson, U.; Plate, K.H.; Foidart, J.M.; Schaper, W.;. Charnock-Jones, D.S.; Hicklin, D.J.; Herbert, J.M.; Collen, D. & Persico, M.G. (2001). Synergism between vascular endothelial growth factor and placental growth factor contributes to angiogenesis and plasma extravasation in pathological conditions. *Nat Med.* 7:575-583.

Chen, X.; Walker, D.G.; Schmidt, A.M.; Arancio, O.; Lue, L.F. & Yan, S.D. (2007). RAGE: a potential target for Abeta-mediated cellular perturbation in Alzheimer's disease. *Curr Mol Med.* 7:735-742.

Cheung, W.; Guo, L. & Cordeiro, M.F. (2008). Neuroprotection in glaucoma: drug-based approaches. *Optom Vis Sci.* 85:406-416.

Chow, N.; Bell, R.D.; Deane, R.; Streb, J.W.; Chen, J.; Brooks, A.; Van Nostrand, W.; Miano, J.M. & Zlokovic, B.V. (2007). Serum response factor and myocardin mediate arterial hypercontractility and cerebral blood flow dysregulation in Alzheimer's phenotype. *Proc Natl Acad Sci U S A.* 104:823-828.

Claesson-Welsh, L. (2008). VEGF-B taken to our hearts: specific effect of VEGF-B in myocardial ischemia. *Arterioscler Thromb Vasc Biol.* 28:1575-1576.

D'Alessandro, G.; Calcagno, E.; Tartari, S.; Rizzardini, M.; Invernizzi, R.W. & Cantoni, L. (2011). Glutamate and glutathione interplay in a motor neuronal model of amyotrophic lateral sclerosis reveals altered energy metabolism. *Neurobiol Dis.* 43:346-355.

de Jong, P.T. (2006). Age-related macular degeneration. *N Engl J Med.* 355:1474-1485.

de la Torre, J.C. (2002). Alzheimer disease as a vascular disorder: nosological evidence. *Stroke.* 33:1152-1162.

de la Torre, J.C. (2004). Is Alzheimer's disease a neurodegenerative or a vascular disorder? Data, dogma, and dialectics. *Lancet Neurol.* 3:184-190.

Decressac, M.; Ulusoy, A.; Mattsson, B.; Georgievska, B.; Romero-Ramos, M.; Kirik, D. & Bjorklund, A. (2011). GDNF fails to exert neuroprotection in a rat {alpha}-synuclein model of Parkinson's disease. *Brain*. [Epub ahead of print]

Detmar, M.; Brown, L.F.; Schon, M.P.; Elicker, B.M.; Velasco, P.; Richard, L.; Fukumura, D.; Monsky, W.; Claffey, K.P. & Jain, R.K. (1998). Increased microvascular density and enhanced leukocyte rolling and adhesion in the skin of VEGF transgenic mice. *J Invest Dermatol*. 111:1-6.

Di Paolo, G. & Kim, T.W. (2011). Linking lipids to Alzheimer's disease: cholesterol and beyond. *Nat Rev Neurosci*. 12:284-296.

Djaldetti, R. & Melamed, E. (2002). New drugs in the future treatment of Parkinson's disease. *J Neurol*. 249 Suppl 2:II30-35.

Doody, R.S.; Gavrilova, S.I.; Sano, M.; Thomas, R.G.; Aisen, P.S.; Bachurin, S.O.; Seely, L. & Hung, D. (2008). Effect of dimebon on cognition, activities of daily living, behaviour, and global function in patients with mild-to-moderate Alzheimer's disease: a randomised, double-blind, placebo-controlled study. *Lancet*. 372:207-215.

Dvorak, H.F.; Brown, L.F.; Detmar, M. & Dvorak, A.M. (1995). Vascular permeability factor/vascular endothelial growth factor, microvascular hyperpermeability, and angiogenesis. *Am J Pathol*. 146:1029-1039.

Elstner, M.; Morris, C.M.; Heim, K.; Bender, A.; Mehta, D.; Jaros, E.; Klopstock, T.; Meitinger, T.; Turnbull, D.M. & Prokisch, H. (2011). Expression analysis of dopaminergic neurons in Parkinson's disease and aging links transcriptional dysregulation of energy metabolism to cell death. *Acta Neuropathol*. 122:75-86.

Eriksson, A.; Cao, R.; Pawliuk, R.; Berg, S.M.; Tsang, M.; Zhou, D.; Fleet, C.; Tritsaris, K.; Dissing, S.; Leboulch, P.& Cao, Y. (2002). Placenta Growth Factor-1 antagonizes VEGF-induced angiogenesis and tumor growth by the formation of functionally inactive PlGF-1/VEGF heterodimers. *Cancer Cell*. 1:99-108.

Falk, T.; Yue, X.; Zhang, S.; McCourt, A.D.; Yee, B.J.; Gonzalez, R.T. & Sherman S.J. (2011). Vascular endothelial growth factor-B is neuroprotective in an in vivo rat model of Parkinson's disease. *Neurosci Lett*. 496:43-47.

Falk, T.; Zhang, S. & Sherman, S.J. (2009). Vascular endothelial growth factor B (VEGF-B) is up-regulated and exogenous VEGF-B is neuroprotective in a culture model of Parkinson's disease. *Mol Neurodegener*. 4:49.

Farkas, E.; De Jong, G.I.; de Vos, R.A.; Jansen Steur, E.N. & Luiten, P.G. (2000). Pathological features of cerebral cortical capillaries are doubled in Alzheimer's disease and Parkinson's disease. *Acta Neuropathol*. 100:395-402.

Faucheux, B.A.; Bonnet, A.M.; Agid Y. & Hirsch, E.C. (1999). Blood vessels change in the mesencephalon of patients with Parkinson's disease. *Lancet*. 353:981-982.

Ferrara, N.; Carver-Moore, K.; Chen, H.; Dowd, M.; Lu, L.; O'Shea, K.S.; Powell-Braxton, L.; Hillan, K.J. & Moore, M.W. (1996). Heterozygous embryonic lethality induced by targeted inactivation of the VEGF gene. *Nature*. 380:439-442.

Ferrara, N. & Kerbel, R.S. (2005). Angiogenesis as a therapeutic target. *Nature*. 438:967-974.

Folkman, J. 2007. Angiogenesis: an organizing principle for drug discovery? *Nat Rev Drug Discov*. 6:273-286.

Gil, J.M. & Rego, A.C. (2008). Mechanisms of neurodegeneration in Huntington's disease. *Eur J Neurosci*. 27:2803-2820.

Ginsberg, M.D. (2008). Neuroprotection for ischemic stroke: past, present and future. *Neuropharmacology.* 55:363-389.

Girouard, H. & Iadecola, C. (2006). Neurovascular coupling in the normal brain and in hypertension, stroke, and Alzheimer disease. *J Appl Physiol.* 100:328-335.

Grimmond, S.; Lagercrantz, J.; Drinkwater, C.; Silins, G.; Townson, S.; Pollock, P.; Gotley, D.; Carson, E.; Rakar, S.; Nordenskjold, M.; Ward, L.; Hayward, N. & Weber, G. (1996). Cloning and characterization of a novel human gene related to vascular endothelial growth factor. *Genome Res.* 6:124-131.

Hagberg, C.E.; Falkevall, A.; Wang, X.; Larsson, E.; Huusko, J.; Nilsson, I.; van Meeteren, L.A.; Samen, E.; Lu, L.; Vanwildemeersch, M.; Klar, J.; Genove, G.; Pietras, K.; Stone-Elander, S.; Claesson-Welsh, L.; Yla-Herttuala, S.; Lindahl, P. & Eriksson, U. (2010). Vascular endothelial growth factor B controls endothelial fatty acid uptake. *Nature.* 464:917-921.

Hamel, C. (2006). Retinitis pigmentosa. *Orphanet J Rare Dis.* 1:40.

Hartong, D.T.; Berson, E.L. & Dryja, T.P. (2006). Retinitis pigmentosa. *Lancet.* 368:1795-809.

Hsu, M.J.; Hsu, C.Y.; Chen, B.C.; Chen, M.C.; Ou, G. & Lin, C.H. (2007). Apoptosis signal-regulating kinase 1 in amyloid beta peptide-induced cerebral endothelial cell apoptosis. *J Neurosci.* 27:5719-5729.

Imai, H.; Singh, R.S.; Fort, P.E. & Gardner, T.W. (2009). Neuroprotection for diabetic retinopathy. *Dev Ophthalmol.* 44:56-68.

Jankovic, J. (2005). Motor fluctuations and dyskinesias in Parkinson's disease: clinical manifestations. *Mov Disord.* 20 Suppl 11:S11-16.

Jankovic, J. (2006). An update on the treatment of Parkinson's disease. *Mt Sinai J Med.* 73:682-689.

Jeltsch, M.; Kaipainen, A.; Joukov, V.; Meng, X.; Lakso, M.; Rauvala, H.; Swartz, M.; Fukumura, D.; Jain, R.K. & Alitalo, K. (1997). Hyperplasia of lymphatic vessels in VEGF-C transgenic mice. *Science.* 276:1423-1425.

Johnson, E.J. (2010). Age-related macular degeneration and antioxidant vitamins: recent findings. *Curr Opin Clin Nutr Metab Care.* 13(1):28-33.

Joukov, V.; Sorsa, T.; Kumar, V.; Jeltsch, M.; Claesson-Welsh, L.; Cao, Y.; Saksela, O.; Kalkkinen, N. & Alitalo, K. (1997). Proteolytic processing regulates receptor specificity and activity of VEGF-C. *Embo J.* 16:3898-3911.

Kalaria, R.N. & Hedera, P. (1995). Differential degeneration of the cerebral microvasculature in Alzheimer's disease. *Neuroreport.* 6:477-480.

Karkkainen, A.M.; Kotimaa, A.; Huusko, J.; Kholova, I.; Heinonen, S.E.; Stefanska, A.; Dijkstra, M.H.; Purhonen, H.; Hamalainen, E.; Makinen, P.I.; Turunen, M.P. & Yla-Herttuala, S. (2009). Vascular endothelial growth factor-D transgenic mice show enhanced blood capillary density, improved postischemic muscle regeneration, and increased susceptibility to tumor formation. *Blood.* 113:4468-4475.

Karkkainen, M.J.; Haiko, P.; Sainio, K.; Partanen, J.; Taipale, J.; Petrova, T.V.; Jeltsch, M.; Jackson, D.G.; Talikka, M.; Rauvala, H.; Betsholtz, C. & Alitalo, K. (2004). Vascular endothelial growth factor C is required for sprouting of the first lymphatic vessels from embryonic veins. *Nat Immunol.* 5:74-80.

Karpanen, T.; Bry, M.; Ollila, H.M.; Seppanen-Laakso, T.; Liimatta, E.; Leskinen, H.; Kivela, R.; Helkamaa, T.; Merentie, M.; Jeltsch, M.; Paavonen, K.; Andersson, L.C.;

Mervaala E.; Hassinen, I.E.; Yla-Herttuala, S.; Oresic, M. & Alitalo, K. (2008). Overexpression of vascular endothelial growth factor-B in mouse heart alters cardiac lipid metabolism and induces myocardial hypertrophy. *Circ Res*. 103:1018-1026.

Kern, T.S. & Barber, A.J. (2008). Retinal ganglion cells in diabetes. *J Physiol*. 586:4401-8.

Kiba, A.; Sagara, H.; Hara, T. & Shibuya, M. (2003). VEGFR-2-specific ligand VEGF-E induces non-edematous hyper-vascularization in mice. *Biochem Biophys Res Commun*. 301:371-7.

Lahteenvuo, J.E.; Lahteenvuo, M.T.; Kivela, A.; Rosenlew, C.; Falkevall, A.; Klar, J.; Heikura, T.; Rissanen, T.T.; Vahakangas, E.; Korpisalo, P.; Enholm, B.; Carmeliet, P.; Alitalo K.; Eriksson, U & Yla-Herttuala, S. (2009). Vascular endothelial growth factor-B induces myocardium-specific angiogenesis and arteriogenesis via vascular endothelial growth factor receptor-1- and neuropilin receptor-1-dependent mechanisms. *Circulation*. 119:845-856.

Lang, A.E.; Gill, S.; Patel, N.K.; Lozano, A.; Nutt, J.G.; Penn, R.; Brooks, D.J.; Hotton, G.; Moro, E.; Heywood, P.; Brodsky, M.A.; Burchiel, K.; Kelly, P.; Dalvi, A.; Scott, B.; Stacy, M.; Turner, D.;. Wooten, V.G.; Elias, W.J.; Laws, E.R.; Dhawan, V.; Stoessl, A.J.; Matcham, J.; Coffey, R.J. & Traub, M. (2006). Randomized controlled trial of intraputamenal glial cell line-derived neurotrophic factor infusion in Parkinson disease. *Ann Neurol*. 59:459-466.

Larcher, F.; Murillas, R.; Bolontrade, M.; Conti, C.J. & Jorcano, J.L. (1998). VEGF/VPF overexpression in skin of transgenic mice induces angiogenesis, vascular hyperpermeability and accelerated tumor development. *Oncogene*. 17:303-311.

Lees, A.J.; Hardy, J. & Revesz, T. (2009). Parkinson's disease. *Lancet*. 373:2055-2066.

Levin, L.A. (2005). Neuroprotection and regeneration in glaucoma. *Ophthalmol Clin North Am*. 18:585-596, vii.

Li, X.; Aase, K.; Li, H.; von Euler, G.& Eriksson, U. (2001). Isoform-specific expression of VEGF-B in normal tissues and tumors. *Growth Factors*. 19:49-59.

Li, X. & Eriksson, U. (2001). Novel VEGF family members: VEGF-B, VEGF-C and VEGF-D. *Int J Biochem Cell Biol*. 33:421-426.

Li, X.; Lee, C.; Tang, Z.; Zhang, F.; Arjunan, P.; Li, Y.; Hou, X.; Kumar, A. & L. Dong. (2009). VEGF-B: a survival, or an angiogenic factor? *Cell Adh Migr*. 3:322-327.

Li, X.; Tjwa, M.; Van Hove, I.; Enholm, B.; Neven, E.; Paavonen, K.; Jeltsch, M.; Juan, T.D.; Sievers, R.E.; Chorianopoulos, E.; Wada, H.; Vanwildemeersch, M.; Noel, A.; Foidart, J.M.; Springer, M.L.; von Degenfeld, G.; Dewerchin, M.; Blau, H.M.; Alitalo, K.; Eriksson, U.; Carmeliet, P. & Moons, L. (2008a). Reevaluation of the role of VEGF-B suggests a restricted role in the revascularization of the ischemic myocardium. *Arterioscler Thromb Vasc Biol*. 28:1614-1620.

Li, Y.; Zhang, F.; Nagai, N.; Tang, Z.; Zhang, S.; Scotney, P.; Lennartsson, J.; Zhu, C.; Qu, Y.; Fang, C.; Hua, J.; Matsuo, O.; Fong, G.H.; Ding, H.; Cao, Y.; Becker, K.G.; Nash, A.; Heldin, C.H.& Li, X. (2008b). VEGF-B inhibits apoptosis via VEGFR-1-mediated suppression of the expression of BH3-only protein genes in mice and rats. *J Clin Invest*. 118:913-923.

Lohela, M.; Bry, M.; Tammela, T. & Alitalo, K. (2009). VEGFs and receptors involved in angiogenesis versus lymphangiogenesis. *Curr Opin Cell Biol*. 21:154-165.

Lopes de Faria, J.M.; Russ, H. & Costa, V.P. (2002). Retinal nerve fibre layer loss in patients with type 1 diabetes mellitus without retinopathy. *Br J Ophthalmol.* 86:725-728.

Louzier, V.; Raffestin, B.; Leroux, A.; Branellec, D.; Caillaud, J.M.; Levame, M.; Eddahibi, S. & Adnot, S. (2003). Role of VEGF-B in the lung during development of chronic hypoxic pulmonary hypertension. *Am J Physiol Lung Cell Mol Physiol.* 284:L926-L937.

Love, S.; Plaha, P.; Patel, N.K.; Hotton, G.R.; Brooks, D.J. & Gill, S.S. (2005). Glial cell line-derived neurotrophic factor induces neuronal sprouting in human brain. *Nat Med.* 11:703-704.

Luttun, A.; Tjwa, M.; Moons, L.; Wu, Y.; Angelillo-Scherrer, A.; Liao, F.; Nagy, J.A.; Hooper, A.; Priller, J.; De Klerck, B.; Compernolle, V.; Daci, E.; Bohlen, P.; Dewerchin, M.; Herbert, J.M.; Fava, R.; Matthys, P.; Carmeliet, G.; Collen, D.; Dvorak, H.F.; Hicklin, D.J. & Carmeliet, P. (2002). Revascularization of ischemic tissues by PlGF treatment, and inhibition of tumor angiogenesis, arthritis and atherosclerosis by anti-Flt1. *Nat Med.* 1:1.

Marcic, T.S.; Belyea, D.A. & Katz, B. (2003). Neuroprotection in glaucoma: a model for neuroprotection in optic neuropathies. *Curr Opin Ophthalmol.* 14:353-356.

Mattson, M.P. (2004). Pathways towards and away from Alzheimer's disease. *Nature.* 430:631-639.

Morley, A.M. & Murdoch, I. (2006). The future of glaucoma clinics. *Br J Ophthalmol.* 90:640-645.

Mould, A.W.; Greco, S.A.; Cahill, M.M.; Tonks, I.D.; Bellomo, D.; Patterson, C.; Zournazi, A.; Nash, A.; Scotney, P.; Hayward, N.K. & Kay, G.F. (2005). Transgenic overexpression of vascular endothelial growth factor-B isoforms by endothelial cells potentiates postnatal vessel growth in vivo and in vitro. *Circ Res.* 97:e60-70.

Mould, A.W.; Tonks, I.D.; Cahill, M.M.; Pettit, A.R.; Thomas, R.; Hayward, N.K. & Kay, G.F. (2003). Vegfb gene knockout mice display reduced pathology and synovial angiogenesis in both antigen-induced and collagen-induced models of arthritis. *Arthritis Rheum.* 48:2660-2669.

Nash, A.D.; Baca, M.; Wright, C. & Scotney, P.D. (2006). The biology of vascular endothelial growth factor-B (VEGF-B). *Pulm Pharmacol Ther.* 19:61-69.

Nutt, J.G. & Wooten, G.F. (2005). Clinical practice. Diagnosis and initial management of Parkinson's disease. *N Engl J Med.* 353:1021-1027.

Odorisio, T.; Schietroma, C.; Zaccaria, M.L.; Cianfarani, F.; Tiveron, C.; Tatangelo, L.; Failla, C.M. & Zambruno, G. (2002). Mice overexpressing placenta growth factor exhibit increased vascularization and vessel permeability. *J Cell Sci.* 115:2559-2567.

Ogawa, S.; Oku, A.; Sawano, A.; Yamaguchi, S.; Yazaki, Y. & Shibuya, M. (1998). A novel type of vascular endothelial growth factor, VEGF-E (NZ-7 VEGF), preferentially utilizes KDR/Flk-1 receptor and carries a potent mitotic activity without heparin-binding domain. *J Biol Chem.* 273:31273-1282.

Olofsson, B.; Korpelainen, E.; Pepper, M.S.; Mandriota, S.J.; Aase, K.; Kumar, V.; Gunji, Y.; Jeltsch, M.M.; Shibuya, M.; Alitalo, K. & Eriksson, U. (1998). Vascular endothelial growth factor B (VEGF-B) binds to VEGF receptor-1 and regulates plasminogen activator activity in endothelial cells. *Proc Natl Acad Sci U S A.* 95:11709-11714.

Olofsson, B.; Pajusola, K.; Kaipainen, A.; von Euler, G.; Joukov, V.; Saksela, O.; Orpana, A.; Pettersson, R.F.; Alitalo, K. & Eriksson, U. (1996a). Vascular endothelial growth factor B, a novel growth factor for endothelial cells. *Proc Natl Acad Sci U S A*. 93:2576-2581.

Olofsson, B.; Pajusola, K.; von Euler, G.; Chilov, D.; Alitalo, K. & Eriksson, U. (1996b). Genomic organization of the mouse and human genes for vascular endothelial growth factor B (VEGF-B) and characterization of a second splice isoform. *J Biol Chem*. 271:19310-19317.

Oshitari, T.; Yamamoto, S.; Hata, N. & Roy. S. (2008). Mitochondria- and caspase-dependent cell death pathway involved in neuronal degeneration in diabetic retinopathy. *Br J Ophthalmol*. 92:552-556.

Pattison, L.R.; Kotter, M.R.; Fraga, D. & Bonelli, R.M. (2006). Apoptotic cascades as possible targets for inhibiting cell death in Huntington's disease. *J Neurol*. 253:1137-1142.

Petrukhin, K. (2007). New therapeutic targets in atrophic age-related macular degeneration. *Expert Opin Ther Targets*. 11:625-639.

Poesen, K.; Lambrechts, D.; Van Damme, P.; Dhondt, J.; Bender, F.; Frank, N.; Bogaert, E.; Claes, B.; Heylen, L.; Verheyen, A.; Raes, K.; Tjwa, M.; Eriksson, U.; Shibuya, M.; Nuydens, R.; Van Den Bosch, L.; Meert, T.; D'Hooge, R.; Sendtner, M.; Robberecht, W. & Carmeliet, P. (2008). Novel role for vascular endothelial growth factor (VEGF) receptor-1 and its Ligand VEGF-B in motor neuron degeneration. *J Neurosci*. 28:10451-10459.

Reichelt, M.; Shi, S.; Hayes, M.; Kay, G.; Batch, J.; Gole, G.A. & Browning, J. (2003). Vascular endothelial growth factor-B and retinal vascular development in the mouse. *Clin Experiment Ophthalmol*. 31:61-65.

Relkin, N.R.; Szabo, P.; Adamiak, B.; Burgut, T.; Monthe, C.; Lent, R.W.; Younkin, S.; Younkin, L.; Schiff, R. & Weksler, M.E. (2008). 18-Month study of intravenous immunoglobulin for treatment of mild Alzheimer disease. *Neurobiol Aging*. 30(11):1728-1736.

Rissanen, T.T.; Markkanen, J.E.; Gruchala, M.; Heikura, T.; Puranen, A.; Kettunen, M.I.; Kholova, I.; Kauppinen, R.A.; Achen, M.G.; Stacker, S.A.; Alitalo, K. & Yla-Herttuala, S. (2003). VEGF-D is the strongest angiogenic and lymphangiogenic effector among VEGFs delivered into skeletal muscle via adenoviruses. *Circ Res*. 92:1098-1106.

Rite, I..; Machado, A.; Cano, J. & Vener,. J.L. (2007). Blood-brain barrier disruption induces in vivo degeneration of nigral dopaminergic neurons. *J Neurochem*. 101:1567-1582.

Salmina, A.B. (2009). Neuron-glia interactions as therapeutic targets in neurodegeneration. *J Alzheimers Dis*. 16:485-502.

Segura, I., De Smet, F.; Hohensinner, P.J.; Almodovar, C.R. & Carmeliet, P. (2009). The neurovascular link in health and disease: an update. *Trends Mol Med*. 15:439-451.

Sherer, T.B.; Fiske, B.K.; Svendsen, C.N.; Lang, A.E. & Langston, J.W. (2006). Crossroads in GDNF therapy for Parkinson's disease. *Mov Disord*. 21:136-141.

Siemers, E.R.; Quinn, J.F.; Kaye, J.; Farlow, M.R.; Porsteinsson, A.; Tariot, P.; Zoulnouni, P.; Galvin, J.E.; Holtzman, D.M.; Knopman, D.S.; Satterwhite, J.; Gonzales, C.; Dean,

R.A. & May, P.C. (2006). Effects of a gamma-secretase inhibitor in a randomized study of patients with Alzheimer disease. *Neurology*. 66:602-604.

Staekenborg, S.S.; Koedam, E.L.; Henneman, W.J.; Stokman, P.; Barkhof, F.; Scheltens, P. & van der Flier, W.M. (2009). Progression of mild cognitive impairment to dementia: contribution of cerebrovascular disease compared with medial temporal lobe atrophy. *Stroke*. 40:1269-1274.

Sun, Y.; Jin, K.; Childs, J.T.; Xie, L.; Mao, X.O. & Greenberg, D.A. (2004). Increased severity of cerebral ischemic injury in vascular endothelial growth factor-B-deficient mice. *J Cereb Blood Flow Metab*. 24:1146-1152.

Sun, Y.; Jin, K.; Childs, J.T.; Xie, L.; Mao, X.O. & Greenberg, D.A. (2006). Vascular endothelial growth factor-B (VEGFB) stimulates neurogenesis: evidence from knockout mice and growth factor administration. *Dev Biol*. 289:329-335.

Traynor, B.J.; Bruijn, L.; Conwit, R.; Beal, F.; O'Neill, G.; Fagan, S.C. & Cudkowicz, M.E. (2006). Neuroprotective agents for clinical trials in ALS: a systematic assessment. *Neurology*. 67:20-27.

van Dijk, H.W.; Kok, P.H.; Garvin, M.; Sonka, M.; Devries, J.H.; Michels, R.P.; van Velthoven, M.E.; Schlingemann, R.O.; Verbraak, F.D. & Abramoff, M.D. (2009). Selective loss of inner retinal layer thickness in type 1 diabetic patients with minimal diabetic retinopathy. *Invest Ophthalmol Vis Sci*. 50:3404-3409.

van Leeuwen, R.; Boekhoorn, S.; Vingerling, J.R.; Witteman, J.C.; Klaver, C.C.; Hofman, A. & de Jong, P.T. (2005). Dietary intake of antioxidants and risk of age-related macular degeneration. *Jama*. 294:3101-107.

Weinreb, R.N. (2005). Clinical trials of neuroprotective agents in glaucoma. *Retina*. 25:S78-S79.

Wijesekera, L.C. & Leigh, P.N. (2009). Amyotrophic lateral sclerosis. *Orphanet J Rare Dis*. 4:3.

Wilcock, G.K.; Black, S.E.; Hendrix, S.B.; Zavitz, K.H.; Swabb, E.A. & Laughlin, M.A. (2008). Efficacy and safety of tarenflurbil in mild to moderate Alzheimer's disease: a randomised phase II trial. *Lancet Neurol*. 7:483-493.

Wu, Z.; Guo, H.; Chow, N.; Sallstrom, J.; Bell, R.D.; Deane, R.; Brooks, A.I.; Kanagala, S.; Rubio, A.; Sagare, A.; Liu, D.; Li, F.; Armstrong, D.; Gasiewicz, T.; Zidovetzki, R.; Song, X.; Hofman, F. & Zlokovic, B.V. (2005). Role of the MEOX2 homeobox gene in neurovascular dysfunction in Alzheimer disease. *Nat Med*. 11:959-965.

Xia, Y.P.; Li, B.; Hylton, D.; Detmar, M.; Yancopoulos, G.D. & Rudge, J.S. (2003). Transgenic delivery of VEGF to mouse skin leads to an inflammatory condition resembling human psoriasis. *Blood*. 102:161-168.

Yamamoto, M.; Tanaka, F.; Tatsumi, H. & Sobue, G. (2008). A strategy for developing effective amyotropic lateral sclerosis pharmacotherapy: from clinical trials to novel pharmacotherapeutic strategies. *Expert Opin Pharmacother*. 9:1845-1857.

Yasuhara, T.; Shingo, T.; Kobayashi, K.; Takeuchi, A.; Yano, A.; Muraoka, K.; Matsui, T.; Miyoshi, Y.; Hamada, H. & Date. I. (2004). Neuroprotective effects of vascular endothelial growth factor (VEGF) upon dopaminergic neurons in a rat model of Parkinson's disease. *Eur J Neurosci*. 19:1494-1504.

Yasuhara, T.; Shingo, T.; Muraoka, K.; wen Ji, Y.; Kameda, M.; Takeuchi, A.; Yano, A.; Nishio, S.; Matsui, T.; Miyoshi, Y.; Hamada, H. & Date. I. (2005). The differences between high and low-dose administration of VEGF to dopaminergic neurons of in vitro and in vivo Parkinson's disease model. *Brain Res*. 1038:1-10.

Zhang, F.; Tang, Z.; Hou, X.; Lennartsson, J.; Li, Y.; Koch, A.W.; Scotney, P.; Lee, C.; Arjunan, P.; Dong, L.; Kumar, A.; Rissanen, T.T.; Wang, B.; Nagai, N.; Fons, P.; Fariss, R.; Zhang, Y.; Wawrousek, E.; Tansey, G.; Raber, J.; Fong, G.H.; Ding, H.; Greenberg, D.A.; Becker, K.G.; Herbert, J.M.; Nash, A.; Yla-Herttuala, S.; Cao, Y.; Watts, R.J. & Li, X. (2009). VEGF-B is dispensable for blood vessel growth but critical for their survival, and VEGF-B targeting inhibits pathological angiogenesis. *Proc Natl Acad Sci U S A*. 106:6152-6157.

# Part 2

# Prevention, Protection and Monitoring of Neurodegeneration

# 4

# Extract of *Achillea fragrantissima* Downregulates ROS Production and Protects Astrocytes from Oxidative-Stress-Induced Cell Death

Anat Elmann[1], Alona Telerman[1], Sharon Mordechay[1],
Hilla Erlank[1], Miriam Rindner[1], Rivka Ofir[2] and Elie Beit-Yannai[3]
*[1]Department of Food Science, Volcani Center,*
*Agricultural Research Organization, Bet Dagan,*
*[2]Dead Sea & Arava Science Center and Department of Microbiology & Immunology*
*Ben-Gurion University of the Negev, Beer-Sheva,*
*[3]Department of Clinical Pharmacology, Faculty of Health Sciences,*
*Ben-Gurion University of the Negev, Beer-Sheva,*
*Israel*

## 1. Introduction

Oxidative damage plays a pivotal role in the initiation and progress of many human diseases and also in the development of acute and chronic pathological conditions in brain tissue (Halliwell, 2006; Hyslop et al., 1995; Ischiropoulos & Beckman, 2003; Minghetti, 2005). Compared with other tissues, the brain is particularly vulnerable to oxidative damage due to its high rate of oxygen utilization and high contents of oxidizable polyunsaturated fatty acids (Floyd, 1999; Sastry, 1985). In addition, certain regions of the brain are highly enriched in iron, a metal that is catalytically involved in the production of damaging reactive oxygen species (ROS) (Hallgren & Sourander, 1958). Although ROS are critical intracellular signaling messengers (Schrecka & Baeuerlea, 1991), excess of free radicals may lead to peroxidative impairment of membrane lipids and, consequently, to disruption of neuronal functions, and apoptosis. Among the ROS that are responsible for oxidative stress, $H_2O_2$ is thought to be the major precursor of highly reactive free radicals, and is regarded as a key factor in both neuronal (Vaudry et al., 2002) and astroglial cell death (Ferrero-Gutierrez et al., 2008). $H_2O_2$ is normally produced in reactions predominantly catalyzed by superoxide dismutase (SOD) and monoaminoxidases (MAO) A and B in the brain (Almeida et al., 2006; Duarte et al., 2007). As with both $Ca^{2+}$ and NO, $H_2O_2$ appears to play contradictory roles, in that it is potentially toxic at high concentrations, even though it is a central signaling compound at low concentrations (Miura et al., 2002). Brain cells have the capacity to produce peroxides, particularly $H_2O_2$, in large amounts (Dringen et al., 2005). Excess of $H_2O_2$ accumulates during brain injuries and neurodegenerative diseases, and can cross cell membranes to elicit its biological effects intracellularly (Bienert et al., 2006). Although $H_2O_2$ is generally poorly reactive, it forms highly toxic hydroxyl radicals, which may damage all the major classes of biological macromolecules in the cell, through iron- or copper ion-mediated oxidation of lipids, proteins, and nucleic acids. This capability can partly account for $H_2O_2$-mediated neuronal and glial cell death. $H_2O_2$ also induces differential protein activation, which indicates varied biological effects of this molecule. In the mammalian central nervous system (CNS), the transition metal zinc is an endogenous molecule that is localized exclusively to the synaptic vesicles of glutamatergic neurons and that has a special role in modulating synaptic transmission. Chelatable zinc is released into the synaptic cleft with the neurotransmitter during neuronal execution (Assaf & Chung, 1984), and under normal circumstances the robust release of zinc is transient and is efficiently cleared from the synaptic cleft to ensure the performance of successive stimuli. However, in pathological conditions, zinc dyshomeostasis, with consequently elevated levels of extracellular zinc has been recognized as an important factor in the resulting neuropathology (Choi & Koh, 1998; Cote et al., 2005; Li et al., 2009). In neurotransmission, the amount of zinc in the synaptic cleft is in the 10- to 30-µM range, but in pathological conditions that involve sustained neuronal depolarization, e.g., ischemia, stroke, or traumatic brain injury, the levels of extracellular zinc can increase to 100- to 400-µM, at which it can contribute to the resulting neuropathology (Frederickson et al., 2005; Li et al., 2001). *In vivo* and *in vitro* studies showed that, at concentrations that can be reached in the mammalian CNS during excitotoxic episodes, injuries or diseases, zinc is toxic to both neurons and astrocytes (Bishop et al., 2007; Hwang et al., 2008; Kim et al., 1999a; Kim et al., 1999b; Koh et al., 1996; Ryu et al., 2002; Sheline et al., 2000; Stork & Li, 2009). Zinc induces oxidative stress and ROS production, which contribute to both glial cell death (Ryu et al., 2002) and neuronal cell death (Kim et al. 1999a; Kim et al. 1999b). Zinc decreased the GSH content of primary cultures of astrocytes (Kim et al., 2003; Ryu et al., 2002), increased their GSSG content (Kim et al., 2003) and inhibited glutathione reductase activity in these cells (Bishop et al., 2007); furthermore, it slowed the clearance of exogenous $H_2O_2$ by astrocytes, and promoted intracellular production of ROS (Bishop et al., 2007). Thus, ROS generation, glutathione depletion and mitochondrial dysfunction may be key factors in $ZnCl_2$–induced glial toxicity (Ryu et al., 2002). Astrocytes are the most abundant glial cell type in the brain. They play important roles in maintenance of homeostasis, in provision of metabolic substrates for neurons, and also in coupling cerebral blood flow to neuronal activity. They are prominent in protecting neurons against oxidative stress and cell death, and in providing trophic supports such as the glial cell-line-derived neurotrophic factor (GDNF) (Sandhu et al., 2009). There is evidence that dysfunctional astrocytes can enhance neuronal degeneration by diminishing secretion of trophic factors (Takuma et al., 2004). The study of astrocytes is particularly important, in light of the co- existence of apoptotic death of neurons and astrocytes in damaged brains affected by ischemia and neurodegenerative diseases. Despite their high antioxidative activities, astrocytes exhibit a high degree of vulnerability, and are not resistant to the effects of ROS. They respond to substantial or sustained oxidative stress with increased intracellular $Ca^{2+}$, loss of mitochondrial potential, and decreased oxidative phosphorylation (Robb et al., 1999). Since astrocytes determine the brain's vulnerability to oxidative injury, and form a tight functional unit with neurons, once astrocyte energy metabolism and antioxidant capacity are impaired, astrocytic death may critically impair neuronal survival (Feeney et al., 2008; Lu et al., 2008). Thus, protection of astrocytes from oxidative insult appears essential to brain function maintenance. Many herb and plant extracts are used as folk medicines for various kinds of diseases and organ dysfunctions. *Achillea fragrantissima (Af;* Asteraceae) is a desert plant that for many years has been used as a hypoglycemic medicinal plant in traditional medicine in the Arabian region (Yaniv et al.,

1987), and for the treatment of gastrointestinal disturbances (Segal et al., 1987). The ingredient responsible for the anti-spasmolytic activity was found to be a flavone aglycone named cirsiliol (5,3',4'-trihydroxy-6,7-dimethoxyflavone) that was shown to antagonize the spasmodic effects, inhibit $Ca^{2+}$ influx and stimulate $Ca^{2+}$ release from intracellular stores (Mustafa et al., 1992). In addition, the hydro-alcoholic extract of *Af* was shown to have a remarkable antiviral activity against poliomyelitis-1 virus (Soltan & Zaki, 2009). However, the effects of *Af* in the context of brain injuries and neurodegenerative diseases, have not been studied to date. In a recent study we have found that the ethanolic extract of *Achillea fragrantissima* inhibited lipopolysaccharide (LPS) –induced nitric oxide (NO) production by activated primary microglial cells. This extract also inhibited LPS - elicited expression of the pro-inflammatory cytokines interleukin1β (IL-1β) and tumor necrosis factor-α (TNFα), as well as expression of the proinflammatory enzymes, cyclooxygenase-2 (COX-2) and nitric oxide synthase (iNOS) by these cells (in preparation). Since oxidative stress has become accepted as a suitable target for early therapeutic intervention in brain injuries and neurodegenerative diseases, the present study addressed the astroprotective and antioxidant activities of this plant extract.

## 2. Materials and methods

### 2.1 Reagents
Dulbecco's modified Eagle's medium (DMEM), Leibovitz-15 medium, glutamine, antibiotics (10,000 IU/ml penicillin and 10,000 µg/ml streptomycin), soybean trypsin inhibitor, fetal bovine serum (FBS) and Dulbecco's phosphate buffered saline (PBS) (without calcium and magnesium) were purchased from Biological Industries (Beit Haemek, Israel); dimethyl sulfoxide (DMSO) was obtained from Applichem (Darmstadt, Germany); Hydrogen peroxide was obtained from MP Biomedicals (Ohio, USA); 2,2'-Azobis(amidinopropane) (ABAP) was obtained from Wako chemicals (Richmond, VA), and other chemicals including $ZnCl_2$ and 2'7'-dichlorofluorescein diacetate (DCF) were purchased from Sigma Chemical Co. (St Louis, MO, USA).

### 2.2 Preparation of *Af* Extracts
The plant was collected in the Arava Valley and authenticated. The voucher specimens have been kept in as part of the Arava Rift Valley Plant Collection; VPC (Dead Sea & Arava Science Center, Central Arava Branch, Israel, http://www.deadseaarava-rd.co.il/) under the accession code AVPC0040. Freshly collected plants were dried at 40 °C for three days and extracted in ethanol (96%). The liquid phase was then evaporated off, and the dry material was dissolved in DMSO to a concentration of 100 mg/ml to produce the *Af* extract.

### 2.3 High performance liquid chromatography (HPLC) conditions
The ethanolic extract of *Af* was subjected to HPLC chromatography. Separation was made using reverse phase column (Betasil C-18, 5 µm, 250 × 0.46 mm; Thermo-Hypersil, UK) by gradient elution with water-acetic acid (97 : 3 V/V) and methanol as described previously (Chen et al., 2010), and detection at 360 nm (Blue line) and 280 nm (Red line) (Fig. 1).

### 2.4 Liquid chromatography–mass spectrometry (LC–MS) conditions
The ethanolic extract of *Af* was subjected to MS/MS (Fig. 2). The mass spectra were performed on a liquid chromatography–mass spectrometry (LC–MS) Agilent 1100LC series

(Wald- bronn, Germany) and Bruker Esquire 3000plus MS (Bremen, Germany) instrument, operated in the electrospray ionization (ESI) in a positive ion mode. A reverse phase column (BetasilC-18,5 mm, 250 mm x 0.46 mm, Thermo-Hypersil,UK) was used. The MS conditions

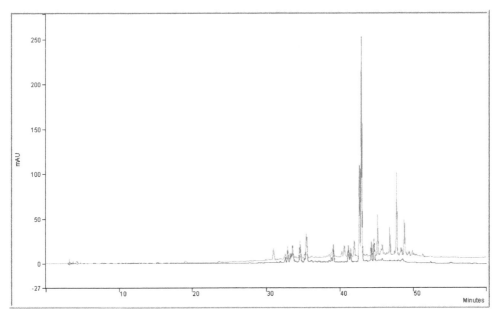

Fig. 1. HPLC analysis of the ethanolic extract of *Af*

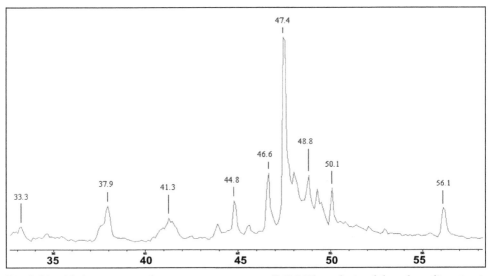

Fig. 2. Liquid chromatography–mass spectrometry (LC–MS) analysis of the ethanolic extract of *Af*

Extract of Achillea fragrantissima Downregulates ROS Production and Protects Astrocytes from
Oxidative-Stress-Induced Cell Death

93

were optimized as follows: API electron spray interface, positive mode polarity, a drying gas flow of 10L/min, an nebulizer gas pressure of 60psi,a drying gas temperature of 300°C, a fragmentor voltage of 0.4V and capillary voltage of 4.5kV.

Four main peaks were identified by ESI-MS: Compound 1, ($C_{27}H_{34}O_{14}Na$), r.t. 50.1, m/z 605 [M+Na+146+146], m/z 582 [M+H+146+146]+, ; suggested as epicatechin-rhamnoside. Compound 2, ($C_{28}H_{33}O_{13}$), r.t. 48.8- m/z 577 [M+H+146+146]+; suggested as Acacetin rhamnoside. Compound 3, ($C_{22}H_{22}O_{10}Na$ ), r.t. 47.4- m/z 469 [M+Na+162]+, , m/z 447 [M+H+162]+,; suggested as Acacetin-glucoside, m/z 285 [M+H]+ aglycon. Compound 4, ($C_{24}H_{25}O_{12}$), r.t. 46.6- m/z 465 [M+H+162]+, suggested as Quercetin-glucoside, m/z 303 [M+H]+ aglycon.

### 2.5 Preparation of primary glial cell cultures

Cultures of primary rat glial cells were prepared from cerebral cortices of 1- to 2-day-old neonatal Wistar rats. Briefly, meninges and blood vessels were carefully removed from cerebral cortices kept in Leibovitz-15 medium; brain tissues were dissociated by trypsinization with 0.5% trypsin (10 min, 37 °C, 5% $CO_2$); and cells were washed first with DMEM containing soybean trypsin inhibitor (100 μg/ml) and 10% FBS and then with DMEM containing 10% FBS. Cells were seeded in tissue culture flasks pre-coated with poly-D-lysine (20 μg/ml in 0.1 M borate buffer pH 8.4) and incubated at 37 °C in humidified air with 5% $CO_2$. The medium was changed on the second day and every second day thereafter. At the time of primary cell confluence (day 10), microglial and progenitor cells were discarded by shaking (180 RPM, 37 °C) the flasks on a horizontal shaking platform. Astrocytes were then replated on 24-well poly-D-lysine-coated plastic plates, at a density of $1 \times 10^5$/well, in DMEM (without phenol red) containing 2% FBS, 2 mM glutamine, 100 U/ml penicillin, and 100 μg/ml streptomycin.

The research was conducted in accordance with the internationally accepted principles for laboratory animal use and care, as found in the US guidelines, and was approved by the Institutional Animal Care and Use Committee of The Volcani Center, Agricultural Research Organization.

### 2.6 Treatment of astrocytes

Twenty four hours after plating, the original medium in which the cells were grown was aspirated off, and fresh medium was added to the cells. Dilutions of plant extracts first in DMSO and then in the growth medium were made freshly from stock solution just prior to each experiment and were used immediately. The final concentration of DMSO in the medium was 0.2%. Dilutions of $H_2O_2$ in the growth medium were made freshly from a 30% stock solution immediately prior to each experiment and were used immediately.

### 2.7 Determination of cell viability

Cell viability was determined using a commercial colorimetric assay (Roche Applied Science, Germany) according to the manufacturer's instructions. This assay is based on the measurement of lactate dehydrogenase (LDH) activity released from the cytosol of damaged cells into the incubation medium.

### 2.8 Evaluation of intracellular ROS production

Intracellular ROS production was detected using the non-fluorescent cell permeating compound, 2'7'-dichlorofluorescein diacetate (DCF-DA). DCF-DA is hydrolyzed by intracellular esterases and then oxidized by ROS to a fluorescent compound 2'-7'-DCF. Astrocytes were plated onto 24 wells plates (300,000 cells/well) and treated with DCF-DA (20 µM) for 30 min at 37⁰C. Following incubation with DCF, cultures were rinsed twice with PBS and then re-suspended (1) For measurement of $H_2O_2$-induced ROS: in DMEM containing 10% FBS, 8 mM HEPES, 2 mM glutamine, 100 U/ml penicillin, and 100 µg/ml streptomycin (2) For measurement of $ZnCl_2$ - induced ROS: in a defined buffer containing 116 mM NaCl, 1.8 mM $CaCl_2$, 0.8 mM $MgSO_4$, 5.4 mM KCl, 1 mM $NaH_2PO_4$, 14.7 mM $NaHCO_3$, and 10 mM HEPES, pH, 7.4. The fluorescence was measured in a plate reader with excitation at 485 nm and emission at 520 nm.

### 2.9 Cellular antioxidant activity of *Af* extract
Peroxyl radicals are generated by thermolysis of 2,2'-Azobis(amidinopropane) (ABAP) at physiological temperature. ABAP decomposes at approximately $1.36 \times 10^{-6} s^{-1}$ at 37°C, producing at most $1 \times 10^{12}$ radicals/ml/s (Bowry & Stocker, 1993; Niki et al., 1986; Thomas et al., 1997). Astrocytes were plated onto 24 wells plates (300,000 cells/well) and were incubated for 1 hr with *Af* extract. Then astrocytes were preloaded with DCF-DA for 30 min, washed, and ABAP (0.6 mM final concentration) was then added. The fluorescence, which indicates ROS levels, was measured in a plate reader with excitation at 485 nm and emission at 520 nm.

### 2.10 Differential pulse voltammetry analysis
Ethanolic extracts were obtained by dissolving 1 g of dry plant powder in 10 ml of ethanol overnight at room temperature. Before performing the differential pulse voltammetry (DPV) analysis, tetrabutylammonium perchlorate was added to the ethanolic extract to final concentration of 1% and the total reducing capacity of the *Af* extracts was analyzed, as described before (Butera et al., 2002). Briefly, the plant extract was placed in a cyclic voltammeter cell equipped with a working electrode (3.2 mm in diameters, glassy carbon), a reference electrode (Ag/AgCl), and an auxiliary electrode (platinum wire). The DPV potential was conducted at a scan rate of 40 mV/s, pulse amplitude 50 mV, sample width 17 ms, pulse width 50 ms, pulse period 200 ms. An electrochemical working station (CH Instruments Inc., 610B, Austin, TX, USA) was used. The output of the DPV experiments was a potential-current curve (Kohen et al., 1999).

### 2.11 Data analysis
Statistical analyses were performed with one-way ANOVA followed by Tukey-Kramer multiple comparison tests using Graph Pad InStat 3 for windows (GraphPad Software, San Diego, CA, USA).

## 3. Results

### 3.1 Protection by the *Af* extract of astrocytes from $H_2O_2$ -induced cell death
$H_2O_2$ exposure is used as a model of ischemia reperfusion. The concentration of $H_2O_2$ used in our experiments (175-200 microM) resembles the concentration reported by Hyslop *et al* to be the concentration of $H_2O_2$ that appears in the rat striatum under ischemic conditions (Hyslop et al., 1995). In order to characterize the astroprotective potential of the *Af* extract against $H_2O_2$ -induced oxidative stress, we have assessed changes in intracellular ROS production and in cell viability, using a model in which oxidative stress was induced by the

addition of this compound to cultured primary astrocytes. Exposure of normal primary astrocytes with $H_2O_2$ resulted in a time and concentration dependent astrocytic cell death 20 h later (data not shown). To find out whether the *Af* extract has a protective effect and to determine the optimal concentration of the extract needed for such an effect, astrocytes were pre-incubated with different concentrations of *Af* extract. $H_2O_2$ was then added, and cytotoxicity was determined after 20 h. Our results showed that the *Af* extract exerted a protective action against $H_2O_2$ -induced cell death in a dose-dependent manner (Fig. 3). No significant changes were observed in the viability of cells treated with similar concentrations of the *Af* extract in the absence of $H_2O_2$ (Fig. 3).

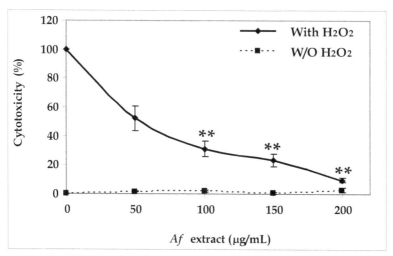

Fig. 3. Protection from $H_2O_2$-induced astrocytic cell death by different concentrations of the extract of *Af*

Astrocytes were treated with different concentrations of *Af* extract. $H_2O_2$ (200 µM) was added 2 h after the addition of *Af* extract. Cell death was determined 20 h later. Each point represents the means ± SEM of five experiments ($n = 20$). **$p < 0.001$ compared to cells treated with $H_2O_2$ alone.

### 3.2 *Af* extract inhibits $H_2O_2$- and $ZnCl_2$-induced ROS generation

In order to gain more insight into the mechanisms by which the *Af* extract might exert its protective effects, and to determine whether this extract could inhibit ROS production induced by $H_2O_2$ and $ZnCl_2$, we assessed the intracellular generation of ROS by these toxic molecules, and tested whether treatment of astrocytes with the *Af* extract affected intracellular ROS levels. For the study of preventive effects against intracellular ROS formation the cells were preloaded with the ROS indicator DCF-DA, and were pretreated with various concentrations of *Af* extract before the application of $H_2O_2$ or $ZnCl_2$ stress, and ROS formation was determined by reading fluorescence every hour for 4 h. As can be seen in Fig. 4A, $H_2O_2$ induced ROS production in astrocytes, with the maximum levels produced after 1 h. Pretreatment of astrocytes with the *Af* extract inhibited the $H_2O_2$-induced elevation of the levels of intracellular ROS in a dose-dependent manner (Fig. 4B). We also found that treatment with $ZnCl_2$ increased ROS generation in astrocytes, and that, similarly to the effect of the *Af* extract on $H_2O_2$-induced ROS, this extract greatly attenuated $ZnCl_2$-induced ROS generation (Fig. 5).

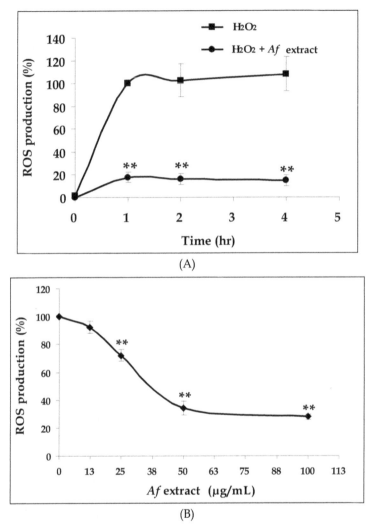

(A)

(B)

Fig. 4. The *Af* extract attenuates $H_2O_2$-induced ROS production in astrocytes

Astrocytes were preloaded with the redox - sensitive DCF-DA for 30 min and washed with PBS. Preloaded astrocytes were then pre-incubated for 2 h with various concentrations of *Af* extract. $H_2O_2$ (175 µM) was added to the culture and the fluorescence intensity representing ROS production was measured. (A) Pre-incubation with 100 µg/ml *Af* extract and measurements at the indicated time points (B) Pre-incubation with various concentrations of *Af* extract and measurements after 1 h. Each point represents the mean ± SEM of two experiments ($n=7$). **$p<0.001$ when ROS production following treatment with $H_2O_2$+*Af* extract was compared to cells treated with $H_2O_2$ alone at each of the equivalent time points.

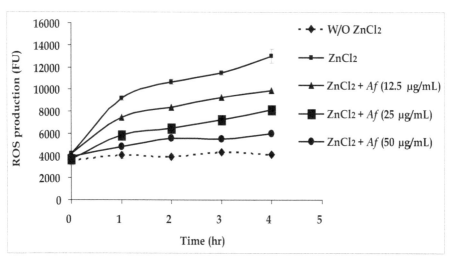

Fig. 5. Zinc induces ROS generation, and the *Af* extract attenuates ROS production following treatment of astrocytes with zinc

Astrocytes were preloaded with DCF-DA for 30 min and washed with PBS. They were then pre-incubated for 2 h with various concentrations of *Af* extract, after which, $ZnCl_2$ (50 μM) was added and the resulting fluorescence signal was measured at the indicated time points. Each point represents the mean ± SEM ($n$ = 7). $p<0.01$ when ROS production following treatment with $ZnCl_2+Af$ extract was compared to cells treated with $ZnCl_2$ alone at each of the equivalent time points

### 3.3 *Af* extract reduces 2,2'-azobis(amidinopropane) (ABAP)-mediated peroxyl radicals levels in astrocytes

In addition to $H_2O_2$, various other species, such as peroxynitrite (ONOO-), nitric oxide (NO·) and peroxyl radicals have been found to oxidize DCFH to DCF in cell culture (Wang & Joseph, 1999), therefore we have used the cellular antioxidant activity assay to measure the ability of compounds present in the *Af* extract to prevent formation of DCF by ABAP-generated peroxyl radicals (Wolfe & Liu, 2007). The kinetics of DCFH oxidation in astrocytes by peroxyl radicals generated from ABAP is shown in Fig. 6A, where it can be seen that ABAP generated radicals in a time-dependent manner, and that treatment of cells with *Af* extract moderated this induction. Fig. 6B shows that the increase in ROS–induced fluorescence was inhibited by *Af* extract in a dose-dependent manner. This indicates that compounds present in the *Af* extract entered the cells and acted as efficient intracellular hydroperoxyl radical scavengers.

### 3.4 Differential pulse voltammetry (DPV) analysis of *the* antioxidant capacity of *Af* extract

Extract antioxidant capacity was evaluated by differential pulse voltammetry approach (DPV). Voltammetric techniques of analysis are increasingly being used for the determination of many substances of pharmaceutical importance (Zapata-Urzua et al., 2010) as well as of fruit extracts (Butera et al., 2002). These techniques are based on the measurement of current that results from oxidation or reduction at an electrode surface following an applied potential

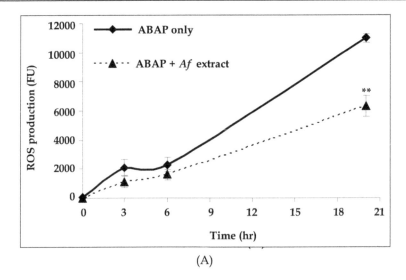

(A)

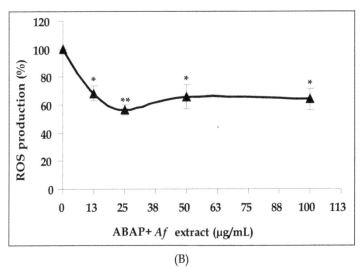

(B)

Fig. 6. Peroxyl radical - induced oxidation of DCFH to DCF in primary astrocytes, and the inhibition of oxidation by *Af* extract

Astrocytes were incubated for 1 h with *Af* extract. They were then preloaded with DCF-DA for 30 min and washed with PBS, after which, 0.6 mM ABAP was added and ROS levels were measured at the indicated time points. Each point represents mean ± SEM of two experiments ($n = 7$). **A**. *Af* extract at 25 µg/ml. **B**. ROS production was measured 20 h after the addition of ABAP *$p<0.01$, **$p<0.001$ compared to cells treated with ABAP only at the equivalent time points.

difference. The DPV technique has excellent resolving power, and is able to differentiate between peaks due to different electroactive species in the same solution which are no more that 50 mV apart (Smyth & Woolfson, 1987). In the present study we have used the DPV approach to analyze the total reducing capacity of the ethanolic *Af* extract. On the potential-current curve generated by DPV, the values of the potential are a characteristic of the antioxidant material and the values of the current are proportional to the amounts of the corresponding antioxidant. Analysis of the *Af* extract by DPV revealed two anodic waves that are caused by two major reducing groups of low-molecular-weight antioxidants, representing the total antioxidants in the extract (Fig. 7). The anodic wave potentials and their corresponding anodic currents, representing the amount of each antioxidant, are presented at Table 1.

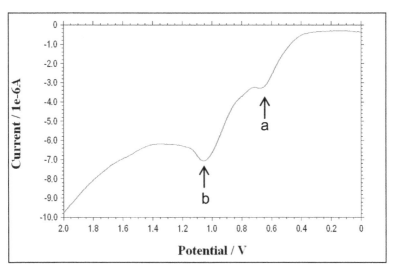

Fig. 7. Representative differential pulse voltammogram of the *Af* extract

Differential pulse voltammetry (DPV) was conducted from E = 0.0 V to final E = 2.0 V at a scan rate of 40 mV/s, pulse amplitude 50 mV, sample width 17 ms, pulse width 50 ms, pulse period 200 ms. Extracts were prepared in duplicate, and each sample was traced three times. a - first anodic wave; b - second anodic wave.

|  | Anodic wave a | Anodic wave b |
|---|---|---|
| **Potential (V ± SD)** | 0.625±0.003 | 1.039±0.024 |
| **Current (μA ± SD )** | 3.233±0.251 | 7.027±0.063 |

Table 1. Anodic potentials and currents of the ethanolic extracts of *Af*

## 4. Discussion

The main findings of the present study were that an ethanolic extract of the desert plant *Af* could protect primary cultures of rat brain astrocytes from $H_2O_2$ -induced cell death, and reduced the levels of intracellular ROS produced after treatment with $H_2O_2$, $ZnCl_2$ or ABAP. This protective effect of *Af* and the reduction in ROS levels might be mediated by its antioxidant activities (as was demonstrated by the DPV experiments) or by modulation of signals and processes induced by $H_2O_2$ and $ZnCl_2$. For example, it has been found, that $H_2O_2$ induced the phosphorylation of ERK1/2, AKT/protein kinase B and ATF-2 in C6 glioma cells (Altiok et al., 2006). It also has been demonstrated that cell death caused by zinc was accompanied by membrane translocation of protein kinase C-alpha (PKC-$\alpha$), phosphorylation of extracellular signal-regulated kinase (ERK), and activation of group IV calcium-dependent cytosolic phospholipase $A_2$ (cPLA$_2$) (Chang et al., 2010; Liao et al., 2011). It was also reported that $Zn^{2+}$ bound to and inhibited glutathione reductase and peroxidase, the major enzymes responsible for glutathione (GSH) metabolism and cellular antioxidative defense mechanisms (Mize & Langdon, 1962; Splittgerber & Tappel, 1979).

Hydrogen peroxide also decreased astrocyte membrane fluidity, induced cytoskeletal reorganization, decreased the activities of the antioxidant enzymes catalase and superoxide dismutase (SOD) (Naval et al., 2007), and increased formation of cytonemes and cell-to-cell tunneling nanotube (TNT)-like connections (Zhu et al., 2005). Thus, the *Af* extract might interfere with any or all of the described processes, and enhance the resistance of astrocytes to $ZnCl_2$ and $H_2O_2$ toxicity, and to oxidative stress. Moreover, defense of glial cells against oxidative damage would be essential for maintaining brain functions.

There are two opportunities for compounds present in *Af* extract to elicit their antioxidant effects in our model: they can act at the cell membrane and break peroxyl radical chain reactions at the cell surface; or they can be taken up by the cell and react intracellularly with ROS. Therefore, the efficiency of cellular uptake and/or membrane binding, combined with the radical-scavenging activity dictates the efficacy of the tested compounds. In order to discriminate between these possibilities, astrocytes were pre-incubated with ABAP, which generates ROS intracellularly. According to our results, which show that *Af* extract inhibited intracellular ROS levels, in addition to other possible activities, compounds present in *Af* extract could enter the cells and react with ROS intracellularly.

Because many low-molecular-weight antioxidants might contribute to the cellular antioxidant defense properties, we analyzed the total antioxidant content of the *Af* extract by the DPV method, which enabled us to demonstrate the presence of two reducing equivalents in the *Af* extract. The advantages of DPV over other voltammetric techniques include excellent sensitivity with a very wide useful linear concentration range for organic species ($10^{-6}$ to $10^{-3}$ M), short analysis times, simultaneous determination of several analytes, and ease of generating a variety of potential waveforms and measuring small currents.

Our LC-MS analysis identified quercetin-glucoside as one of the major peaks in the *Af* extract. Quercetin glycosides are widely consumed flavonoids that are found in many fruits and vegetables, e.g., onion, and, like other flavonoids, offer a wide range of potential health benefits, including prevention of atherosclerosis and cardiovascular diseases (Peluso, 2006; Terao et al., 2008). In recent years, intestinal absorption and metabolism of quercetin glucosides have been extensively investigated with regard to their bioavailability (Spencer et al., 2004; Walle, 2004). Quercetin glucosides are well absorbed by the small intestine because the presence of a glucose moiety significantly enhances absorption (Arts et al. 2004; Boyer et al., 2005; Hollman & Arts, 2000). In the process of intestinal absorption quercetin-glucosides are subjected to hydrolysis and subsequent conversion into conjugated glucuronides and/or sulfates (Murota & Terao, 2003). A variety of metabolites circulating in the blood-stream were identified (Day et al., 2001; Mullen et al., 2002), and some of them were found to possess a substantial antioxidant activity (da Silva et al., 1998; Manach et al., 1998). It was suggested that metabolites of quercetin glucosides accumulate in the aorta - a target site for its anti-atherosclerotic effect, and attenuate lipid peroxidation that occur in the aorta, along with the attenuation of hyperlipidemia (Kamada et al., 2005; Terao, 1999; Terao et al., 2008).

Two other compounds in the *Af* extract were also identified by LC-MS: acacetin 7-o-rhamnoside, which was also identified in the aerial parts of several plants (El-Wakil, 2007; Sharaf et al., 1997), and acacetin 7-o-glucoside, which was also found in the anti-inflammatory extract of Mcfadyena unguis-cati L. (Aboutabl et al., 2008). All four compounds identified by LC-MS analysis as major peaks in *Af* extract, namely epicatechin-rhamnoside, Acacetin rhamnoside, Acacetin-glucoside, and Quercetin-glucoside, are stable compounds, that under our experimental conditions (ethanol extraction, resolubilization in DMSO, and tissue culture experiments at 37°C and neutral pH) would not react chemically with each other. Chemical interactions between these compounds might occur under high temperatures and extreme pH values.

Several studies have revealed that some herbal medications and antioxidants show promise in prevention of neurodegenerative diseases (Iriti et al., 2010). Substances that can restrict and/or protect brain cells from oxidative stress show promise as potential tools in the therapy of various brain injuries and neurodegenerative diseases. Desert plants survive various stress conditions, including oxidative stress., therefore it is reasonable to suppose that various endogenous molecules present in these plants might also assist animal cells to cope with stresses that develop during pathological conditions.

## 5. Conclusions

In light of their antioxidant and astroprotective properties, we suggest that *Af* extracts might serve as a new source of beneficial phytochemicals, and should be further evaluated for nutraceutical development as polyvalent cocktails for prevention or treatment of various brain injuries and neurodegenerative diseases, in which oxidative stress and astrocytic cell death form part of the pathophysiology.

## 6. Acknowledgments

This work was supported by the Chief Scientist of the Ministry of Science, Israel, and by The Israel Science Foundation (grant No. 600/08).

## 7. References

Aboutabl, E.A., Hashem F.A., Sleem A.A., & Maamoon A.A. (2008). Flavonoids, anti-inflammatory activity and cytotoxicity of *Macfadyena Unguis-Cati* L. *The African Journal of Traditional, Complementary and Alternative medicines (AJTCAM)*, Vol.5, No. 1, pp.18-26, ISSN 0189-6016

Almeida, A.M., Bertoncini C.R., Borecky J., Souza-Pinto N.C., & Vercesi A.E. (2006). Mitochondrial DNA damage associated with lipid peroxidation of the mitochondrial membrane induced by Fe2+-citrate. *Anais da Academia Brasileira de Ciências*, Vol.78, No. 3, pp.505-514, ISSN 0001-3765

Altiok, N., Ersoz M., Karpuz V., & Koyuturk M. (2006). *Ginkgo biloba* extract regulates differentially the cell death induced by hydrogen peroxide and simvastatin. *NeuroToxicology*, Vol.27, No. 2, pp.158-163, ISSN 0161-813X

Arts, I.C., Sesink A.L., Faassen-Peters M., & Hollman P.C. (2004). The type of sugar moiety is a major determinant of the small intestinal uptake and subsequent biliary excretion of dietary quercetin glycosides. *British Journal of Nutrition,* Vol.91, No.6, pp.841-847, ISSN 0007-1145

Assaf, S.Y., & Chung S.H. (1984). Release of endogenous Zn2+ from brain tissue during activity. *Nature (London),* Vol.308, No. 5961, pp.734-736, ISSN 0028-0836

Bienert, G.P., Schjoerring J.K., & Jahn T.P. (2006). Membrane transport of hydrogen peroxide. *Biochimica et biophysica acta,* Vol.1758, No. 8, pp.994-1003, ISSN 0005-2736

Bishop, G.M., Dringen R., & Robinson S.R. (2007). Zinc stimulates the production of toxic reactive oxygen species (ROS) and inhibits glutathione reductase in astrocytes. *Free radical biology & medicine,* Vol.42, No. 8, pp.1222-1230, ISSN 0891-5849

Bowry, V.W., & Stocker R. (1993). Tochoferol-mediated oxidation. The prooxidant effect of vitamin E on the radical-initiated oxidation of human low density lipoproteins. *Journal of the American Chemical Society,* Vol.115, No. 14, pp.6029-6044, ISSN 0002-7863

Boyer, J., Brown D., & Liu R.H. (2005). In vitro digestion and lactase treatment influence uptake of quercetin and quercetin glucoside by the Caco-2 cell monolayer. *Nutrition Journal,* Vol.4, No. 1, pp.1, ISSN 1475-2891

Butera, D., Tesoriere L., Di Gaudio F., Bongiorno A., Allegra M., Pintaudi A.M., Kohen R., & Livrea M.A. (2002). Antioxidant activities of sicilian prickly pear (Opuntia ficus indica) fruit extracts and reducing properties of its betalains: betanin and indicaxanthin. *Journal of agricultural and food chemistry,* Vol.50, No. 23, pp.6895-6901, ISSN 0021-8561

Chang, C.Y., Ou Y.C., Kao T.K., Pan H.C., Lin S.Y., Liao S.L., Wang W.Y., Lu H.C., & Chen C.J. (2010). Glucose exacerbates zinc-induced astrocyte death. *Toxicology letters,* Vol.199, No. 1, pp.102-109, ISSN 0378-4274

Chen, H., Zuo Y., & Deng Y. (2010). Separation and determination of flavonoids and other phenolic compounds in cranberry juice by high-performance liquid chromatography. *Journal of Chromatography A,* Vol.913, No. 1-2, pp.387-395, ISSN 0021-9673

Choi, D.W., & Koh J.Y. (1998). Zinc and brain injury. *Annual review of neuroscience,* Vol.21, pp.347-375, ISSN 0147-006X

Cote, A., Chiasson M., Peralta M.R., 3rd, Lafortune K., Pellegrini L., & Toth K. (2005). Cell type-specific action of seizure-induced intracellular zinc accumulation in the rat hippocampus. *The Journal of physiology,* Vol.566, No. 3, pp.821-837, ISSN 0022-3751

da Silva, E.L., Piskula M.K., Yamamoto N., Moon J.H., & Terao J. (1998). Quercetin metabolites inhibit copper ion-induced lipid peroxidation in rat plasma. *FEBS letters,* Vol.430, No. 3, pp.405-408, ISSN 0014-5793

Day, A.J., Mellon F., Barron D., Sarrazin G., Morgan M.R., & Williamson G. (2001). Human metabolism of dietary flavonoids: identification of plasma metabolites of quercetin. *Free radical research,* Vol.35, No. 6, pp.941-952, ISSN 1071-5762

Dringen, R., Pawlowski P.G., & Hirrlinger J. (2005). Peroxide detoxification by brain cells. *Journal of neuroscience research,* Vol.79, No. 1-2, pp.157-165, ISSN 0360-4012

Duarte, T.L., Almeida G.M., & Jones G.D. (2007). Investigation of the role of extracellular H2O2 and transition metal ions in the genotoxic action of ascorbic acid in cell culture models. *Toxicology letters,* Vol.170, No. 1, pp.57-65, ISSN 0378-4274

El-Wakil, E.A. (2007). Phytochemical and molluscicidal investigations of Fagonia arabica. *Zeitschrift für Naturforschung C. A journal of biosciences,* Vol.62, No. 9-10, pp.661-667, ISSN 0939-5075

Feeney, C.J., Frantseva M.V., Carlen P.L., Pennefather P.S., Shulyakova N., Shniffer C., & Mills L.R. (2008). Vulnerability of glial cells to hydrogen peroxide in cultured hippocampal slices. *Brain research,* Vol.1198, pp.1-15, ISSN 0006-8993

Ferrero-Gutierrez, A., Perez-Gomez A., Novelli A., & Fernandez-Sanchez M.T. (2008). Inhibition of protein phosphatases impairs the ability of astrocytes to detoxify hydrogen peroxide. *Free radical biology & medicine,* Vol.44, No. 10, pp.1806-1816, ISSN 0891-5849

Floyd, R. (1999). Antioxidants, oxidative stress, and degenerative neurological disorders. *Experimental Biology and Medicine,* Vol.222, No. 3, pp.236-245, Print ISSN 1535-3702 Online ISSN 1535-3699

Frederickson, C.J., Koh J.Y., & Bush A.I. (2005). The neurobiology of zinc in health and disease. *Nature reviews. Neuroscience,* Vol.6, pp.449-462, ISSN 1471-003X (Print)1471-0048 (Electronic)

Hallgren, B., & Sourander P. (1958). The effect of age on the non-hem iron in the human brain. *Journal of neurochemistry,* Vol.3, pp.41-51, ISSN 1471-4159

Halliwell, B. (2006). Oxidative stress and neurodegeneration: where are we now? *Journal of neurochemistry,* Vol.97, No. 6, pp.1634-1658, ISSN 0022-3042

Hollman, P.C., & Arts L.C. (2000). Review: Flavonols, flavones and flavanols - nature, occurrence and dietary burden. *Journal of the Science of Food and Agriculture,* Vol.80, No. 7, pp.1081-1093, ISSN 0022-5142

Hwang, J.J., Lee S.J., Kim T.Y., Cho J.H., & Koh J.Y. (2008). Zinc and 4-hydroxy-2-nonenal mediate lysosomal membrane permeabilization induced by H2O2 in cultured hippocampal neurons. *Journal of Neuroscience,* Vol.28, No. 12, pp.3114-3122, ISSN 0270-6474

Hyslop, P.A., Zhang Z., Pearson D.V., & Phebus L.A. (1995). Measurement of striatal $H_2O_2$ by microdialysis following global forebrain ischemia and reperfusion in the rat: correlation with the cytotoxic potential of $H_2O_2$ in vitro. *Brain Resarch,* Vol.671, No. 2, pp.181-186, ISSN 0006-8993

Iriti, M., Vitalini S., Fico G., & Faoro F. (2010). Neuroprotective herbs and foods from different traditional medicines and diets. *Molecules (Basel, Switzerland),* Vol.15, No. 5, pp.3517-3555, ISSN 1420-3049

Ischiropoulos, H., & Beckman J.S. (2003). Oxidative stress and nitration in neurodegeneration: Cause, effect, or association? *Journal Of Clinical Investigation,* Vol.111, No. 2, pp.163-169, ISSN 0021-9738

Kamada, C., da Silva E.L., Ohnishi-Kameyama M., Moon J.H., & Terao J. (2005). Attenuation of lipid peroxidation and hyperlipidemia by quercetin glucoside in the aorta of high cholesterol-fed rabbit. *Free radical research,* Vol.39, No. 2, pp.185-194, ISSN 1071-5762

Kim, E.Y., Koh J.Y., Kim Y.H., Sohn S., Joe E., & Gwag B.J. (1999a). Zn2+ entry produces oxidative neuronal necrosis in cortical cell cultures. *The European journal of neuroscience,* Vol.11, No. 1, pp.327-334, ISSN 0953-816X

Kim, G.W., Gasche Y., Grzeschik S., Copin J.C., Maier C.M., & Chan P.H. (2003). Neurodegeneration in striatum induced by the mitochondrial toxin 3-nitropropionic acid: Role of matrix metalloproteinase-9 in early blood-brain barrier disruption? *Journal of Neuroscience*, Vol.23, No. 25, pp.8733-8742, ISSN 0270-6474

Kim, Y.H., Kim E.Y., Gwag B.J., Sohn S., & Koh J.Y. (1999b). Zinc-induced cortical neuronal death with features of apoptosis and necrosis: mediation by free radicals. *Neuroscience*, Vol.89, No. 1, pp.175-182, ISSN 0306-4522

Koh, J.Y., Suh S.W., Gwag B.J., He Y.Y., Hsu C.Y., & Choi D.W. (1996). The role of zinc in selective neuronal death after transient global cerebral ischemia. *Science (New York, N.Y.)*, Vol.272, No. 5264, pp.1013-1016, ISSN 0036-8075

Kohen, R., Beit-Yannai E., Berry E.M., & Tirosh O. (1999). Overall low molecular weight antioxidant activity of biological fluids and tissues by cyclic voltammetry. *Methods in enzymology*, Vol.300, Oxidants and Antioxidants Part B, pp.285–296, ISSN 0076-6879

Li, H., Swiercz R., & Englander E.W. (2009). Elevated metals compromise repair of oxidative DNA damage via the base excision repair pathway: implications of pathologic iron overload in the brain on integrity of neuronal DNA. *Journal of neurochemistry*, Vol.110, No. 6, pp.1774-1783, ISSN 0022-3042

Li, Y., Hough C.J., Suh S.W., Sarvey J.M., & Frederickson C.J. (2001). Rapid translocation of Zn(2+) from presynaptic terminals into postsynaptic hippocampal neurons after physiological stimulation. *Journal of neurophysiology*, Vol.86, No. 5, pp.2597-2604, ISSN 0022-3077

Liao, S.L., Ou Y.C., Lin S.Y., Kao T.K., Pan H.C., Chang C.Y., Lai C.Y., Lu H.C., Wang W.Y., & Chen C.J. (2011). Signaling cascades mediate astrocyte death induced by zinc. *Toxicology letters*, Vol.204, No. 2-3, pp.108-117, ISSN 0387-4274

Lu, M., Hu L.F., Hu G., & Bian J.S. (2008). Hydrogen sulfide protects astrocytes against $H_2O_2$-induced neural injury via enhancing glutamate uptake. *Free radical biology & medicine*, Vol.45, No. 12, pp.1705-1713, ISSN 0891-5849

Manach, C., Morand C., Crespy V., Demigne C., Texier O., Regerat F., & Remesy C. (1998). Quercetin is recovered in human plasma as conjugated derivatives which retain antioxidant properties. *FEBS letters*, Vol.426, No. 3, pp.331-336, ISSN 0014-5793

Minghetti, L. (2005). Role of inflammation in neurodegenerative diseases. *Current Opinion In Neurology*, Vol.18, No. 3, pp.315-321, ISSN 1350-7540

Miura, I., Miyamoto K., Nakamura K., & Watanabe Y. (2002). Hydrogen peroxide induced chemokine production in the glia-rich cultured cerebellar granule cells under acidosis. *Life sciences*, Vol.70, No. 7, pp.821-831, ISSN 0024-3205

Mize, C.E., & Langdon R.G. (1962). Hepatic glutathione reductase. I. Purification and general kinetic properties. *The Journal of biological chemistry*, Vol.237, No. 5, pp.1589-1595, ISSN (printed): 0021-9258 (electronic): 1083-351X.

Mullen, W., Graf B.A., Caldwell S.T., Hartley R.C., Duthie G.G., Edwards C.A., Lean M.E., & Crozier A. (2002). Determination of flavonol metabolites in plasma and tissues of rats by HPLC-radiocounting and tandem mass spectrometry following oral ingestion of [2-(14)C]quercetin-4'-glucoside. *Journal of Agriculture and Food Chemistry*, Vol.50, No. 23, pp.6902-6909, ISSN 0021-8561

Extract of Achillea fragrantissima Downregulates ROS Production and Protects Astrocytes from
Oxidative-Stress-Induced Cell Death

105

Murota, K., & Terao J. (2003). Antioxidative flavonoid quercetin: implication of its intestinal absorption and metabolism. *Archives of biochemistry and biophysics*, Vol.417, No. 1, pp.12-17, ISSN 0003-9861

Mustafa, E.H., Abu Zarga M., & Abdalla S. (1992). Effects of cirsiliol, a flavone isolated from Achillea fragrantissima, on rat isolated ileum. *General pharmacology*, Vol.23, No. 3, pp.555-560, ISSN 0306-3623

Naval, M.V., Gómez-Serranillos M.P., Carreteroa M.E., & Villara A.M. (2007). Neuroprotective effect of a ginseng (Panax ginseng) root extract on astrocytes primary culture. *Journal of ethnopharmacology*, Vol.112, No. 2, pp.262-270, ISSN 0378-8741

Niki, E., Saito M., Yoshikawa Y., Yamamoto Y., & Kamiya Y. (1986). Oxidation of lipids XII. Inhibition of oxidation of soybean phosphatidylcholine and methyl linoleate in aqueous dispersions by uric acid. *Bulletin of the Chemical Society of Japan*, Vol.59, pp.471-477, online ISSN: 1348-0634 print ISSN: 0009-2673

Peluso, M.R. (2006). Flavonoids attenuate cardiovascular disease, inhibit phosphodiesterase, and modulate lipid homeostasis in adipose tissue and liver. *Experimental biology and medicine (Maywood, N.J.)*, Vol.231, No. 8, pp.1287-1299, ISSN 1535-3702

Robb, S.J., Robb-Gaspers L.D., Scaduto R.C., Thomas A.P., & Connor J.R. (1999). Influence of calcium and iron on cell death and mitochondrial function in oxidatively stressed astrocytes. *Journal of neuroscience research*, Vol.55, No. 6, pp.674-686, ISSN 0360-4012

Ryu, R., Shin Y., Choi J.W., Min W., Ryu H., Choi C.R., & Ko H. (2002). Depletion of intracellular glutathione mediates zinc-induced cell death in rat primary astrocytes. *Experimental brain research*, Vol.143, No. 2, pp.257-263, ISSN 0014-4819

Sandhu, J.K., Gardaneh M., Iwasiow R., Lanthier P., Gangaraju S., Ribecco-Lutkiewicz M., Tremblay R., Kiuchi K., & Sikorska M. (2009). Astrocyte-secreted GDNF and glutathione antioxidant system protect neurons against 6OHDA cytotoxicity. *Neurobiology of disease*, Vol.33, No. 3, pp.405-414, ISSN 0969-9961

Sastry, P. (1985). Lipids of nervous tissue: composition and metabolism. *Progress in lipid resarch*, Vol.24, No. 2, pp.69-176, ISSN 0163-7827

Schrecka, R., & Baeuerlea P.A. (1991). A role for oxygen radicals as second messengers. *Trends in Cell Biology*, Vol.1, No. 2-3, pp.39-42, ISSN 0962-8924

Segal, R.A., Duddeck D.H., & Kajtar M. (1987). The sesquiterpene lactones from *A. fragrantissima*. *Tetrahedron*, Vol.43, No. 18, pp.4125-4132, ISSN 0040-4020

Sharaf, M., el-Ansari M.A., Matlin S.A., & Saleh N.A. (1997). Four flavonoid glycosides from Peganum harmala. *Phytochemistry (Oxford)*, Vol.44, No. 3, pp.533-536, ISSN 0031-9422

Sheline, C.T., Behrens M.M., & Choi D.W. (2000). Zinc-induced cortical neuronal death: contribution of energy failure attributable to loss of NAD(+) and inhibition of glycolysis. *Journal of Neuroscience*, Vol.20, No. 9, pp.3139-3146, ISSN 0270-6474

Smyth, W.F., & Woolfson A.D. (1987). Drug assays--the role of modern voltammetric techniques. *Journal of clinical pharmacy and therapeutics*, Vol.12, No. 2, pp.117-134, ISSN 0269-4727

Soltan, M.M., & Zaki A.K. (2009). Antiviral screening of forty-two Egyptian medicinal plants. *Journal of ethnopharmacology*, Vol.126, No. 1, pp.102-107, ISSN 0378-8741

Spencer, J.P., Abd-el-Mohsen M.M., & Rice-Evans C. (2004). Cellular uptake and metabolism of flavonoids and their metabolites: implications for their bioactivity. *Archives of biochemistry and biophysics*, Vol.423, No. 1, pp.148-161, ISSN 0003-9861

Splittgerber, A.G., & Tappel A.L. (1979). Inhibition of glutathione peroxidase by cadmium and other metal ions. *Archives of Biochemistry and Biophysics*, Vol.197, No. 2, pp.534-542, ISSN: 0003-9861

Stork, C.J., & Li Y.V. (2009). Rising zinc: a significant cause of ischemic neuronal death in the CA1 region of rat hippocampus. *Journal of cerebral blood flow and metabolism*, Vol.29, No. 8, pp.1399-1408, ISSN 0271-678X

Takuma, K., Baba A., & Matsuda T. (2004). Astrocyte apoptosis: implications for neuroprotection. *Progress in Neurobiology*, Vol.72, No.2, pp.111-127, ISSN 0301-0082

Terao, J. (1999). Dietary flavonoids as antioxidants in vivo: conjugated metabolites of (-)-epicatechin and quercetin participate in antioxidative defense in blood plasma. *The Journal of Medical Investigation*, Vol.46, No. 3-4, pp.159-168, ISSN 1343-1420

Terao, J., Kawai Y., & Murota K. (2008). Vegetable flavonoids and cardiovascular disease. *Asia Pacific journal of clinical nutrition*, Vol.17 Suppl 1, pp.291-293, ISSN 0964-7058

Thomas, M.J., Chen Q., Franklin C., & Rudel L.L. (1997). A comparison of the kinetics of low-density lipoprotein oxidation initiated by copper or by azobis (2-amidinopropane). *Free radical biology & medicine*, Vol.23, No. 6, pp.927-935, ISSN 0891-5849

Vaudry, D., Pamantung T.F., Basille M., Rousselle C., Fournier A., Vaudry H., Beauvillain J.C., & Gonzalez B.J. (2002). PACAP protects cerebellar granule neurons against oxidative stress-induced apoptosis. *European Journal of Neuroscience*, Vol.15, No. 9, pp.1451-1460, ISSN 0953-816X

Walle, T. (2004). Absorption and metabolism of flavonoids. *Free Radical Biology and Medicine*, Vol.36, No. 7, pp.829-937, ISSN 0891-5849

Wang, H., & Joseph J.A. (1999). Quantifying cellular oxidative stress by dichlorofluorescein assay using microplate reader. *Free Radical Biology and Medicine*, Vol.27, No. 5-6, pp.612-616, ISSN 0891-5849

Wolfe, K.L., & Liu R.H. (2007). Cellular antioxidant activity (CAA) assay for assessing antioxidants, foods, and dietary supplements. *Journal of Agriculture and Food Chemistry*, Vol.55, No. 22, pp.8896-8907, ISSN 0021-8561

Yaniv, Z., Dafni A., Friedman J., & Palevitch D. (1987). Plants used for the treatment of diabetes in Israel. *Joural of Ethnopharmacology*, Vol.19, No. 2, pp.145-151, ISSN 0378-8741

Zapata-Urzua, C., Perez-Ortiz M., Bravo M., Olivieri A.C., & Alvarez-Lueje A. (2010). Simultaneous voltammetric determination of levodopa, carbidopa and benserazide in pharmaceuticals using multivariate calibration. *Talanta (Oxford)*, Vol.82, No. 3, pp.962-968, ISSN 0039-9140

Zhu, D., Tan K.S., Zhang X., Sun A.Y., Sun G.Y., & Lee J.C. (2005). Hydrogen peroxide alters membrane and cytoskeleton properties and increases intercellular connections in astrocytes. *Journal of cell science*, Vol.118, Pt 16, pp.3695-3703, ISSN 0021-9533

# 5

# Acid-Sensing Ion Channels in Neurodegenerative Diseases: Potential Therapeutic Target

Chu Xiang-Ping[1], Wang John Q.[1] and Xiong Zhi-Gang[2]
*[1]Department of Basic Medical Science,*
*University of Missouri-Kansas City, Kansas City, Missouri;*
*[2]Department of Neurobiology,*
*Morehouse School of Medicine, Atlanta, Georgia;*
*USA*

## 1. Introduction

Under pathological conditions such as tissue inflammation, ischemic stroke, traumatic brain injury, and epileptic seizure, accumulations of lactic acid due to enhanced anaerobic glucose metabolism and the release of proton from ATP hydrolysis result in significant reduction of tissue pH, a condition termed acidosis. Acidosis can activate a distinct family of ion channels: acid-sensing ion channels (ASICs) (Waldmann et al., 1997b), which are heavily expressed in the peripheral sensory and central neurons (Waldmann & Lazdunski, 1998; Krishtal, 2003; Wemmie et al., 2006; Lingueglia, 2007; Xiong et al., 2006, 2007, 2008; Sluka et al., 2009). ASICs belong to the amiloride-sensitive degenerin/epithelial Na$^+$ channel (DEG/ENaC) superfamily (Kellenberger & Schild, 2002). Four genes (*ACCN1 - 4*) encoding at least six ASIC subunits have been cloned. Each subunit has two transmembrane domains with a large extracellular loop and short intracellular N- and C-termini (Waldmann et al., 1997b). Functional ASICs are trimeric complexes of these subunits (Jasti et al., 2007; Gonzales et al., 2009) and most of these subunits can form homomeric and/or heteromeric channels (Benson et al., 2002; Baron et al., 2002, 2008; Wemmie et al., 2002, 2003; Askwith et al., 2004; Chu et al., 2004, 2006; Xiong et al., 2004; Zha et al., 2006; Sherwood et al., 2011). ASICs are enriched in brain neurons (Alvarez de la Rosa et al., 2003; Wemmie et al., 2003; Xiong et al., 2004; Sherwood et al., 2011), where at least three (ASIC1a, ASIC2a and ASIC2b) of the seven subunits can be found. ASIC1a is the dominant subunit in brain and homomeric ASIC1a and heteromeric ASIC1a/2b channels are permeable to both Na$^+$ and Ca$^{2+}$ ions (Waldmann et al., 1997b; Yermolaieva et al., 2004; Zha et al., 2006; Sherwood et al., 2011). ASICs are inhibited by the diuretic amiloride, a non-specific ASIC blocker (Waldmann et al., 1997b). The tarantula toxin psalmotoxin 1 (PcTX1) blocks the homomeric ASIC1a (Escoubas et al., 2000) and heteromeric ASIC1a/2b (Sherwood et al., 2011) channels. The roles of ASICs in a variety of neurologic conditions are still under active investigation. ASIC1a channels localize at synapse and contribute to synaptic plasticity, learning/memory, and fear conditioning (Wemmie et al., 2002, 2003, 2004). Activation of Ca$^{2+}$-permeable homomeric ASIC1a and heteromeric ASIC1a/2b channels is involved in acidosis-mediated ischemic brain injury (Xiong et al., 2004; Pignataro et al., 2007; Sherwood et al., 2011). Moreover, ASIC1a channels play critical roles in neurodegenerative diseases such as multiple sclerosis (Friese et al., 2007; Vergo et al., 2011), Parkinson's (Arias et al., 2008) and Huntington's (Wong et al., 2008) disease and in seizures (Chang et al., 2007; Ziemann et al., 2008) and depression (Coryell et al., 2009). Thus, controlling their activation might ameliorate acidosis-mediated CNS disorders (Xiong et al., 2008). This chapter provides an overview of recent advance in electrophysiological properties as well as pharmacological profiles of ASICs, and their roles in neurodegenerative disorders.

## 2. Electrophysiological and pharmacological properties of ASICs

### 2.1 Electrophysiological properties of ASICs

The electrophysiological properties and pharmacological profiles of ASICs have been extensively explored in heterologous expression systems (Chu et al., 2004; Hesselager et al., 2004) and in neurons from different brain regions, such as cortex (Varming, 1998; Xiong et al., 2004; Chu et al., 2004, 2006), hippocampus (Baron et al., 2002; Askwith et al., 2004), striatum (Jiang et al., 2009), cerebellum (Allen & Attwell, 2002), retinal ganglion (Lilley et al., 2004), and spinal cord (Wu et al., 2004; Baron et al., 2008). Fig. 1 shows typical ASIC current mediated by homomeric ASIC1a, 1b, 2a, or 3 channels expressed in CHO cells.

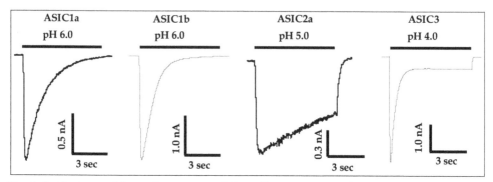

Fig. 1. Acid-triggered inward currents in CHO cells expressing indicated ASIC subunits

Homomeric ASIC1a channels have a pH for half-maximal activation (pH$_{50}$) between 6.2 and 6.8 (Babini et al., 2002; Benson et al., 2002; Chu et al., 2002; Jiang et al., 2009). Although the precise configuration of ASICs in native neurons is not clear, homomeric ASIC1a and heteromeric ASIC1a/2 channels are the major components in brain neurons (Wemmie et al., 2002; Askwith et al., 2004; Xiong et al., 2004; Jiang et al., 2009; Sherwood et al., 2011). For example, our recent studies have shown that rapid drops in extracellular pH from 7.4 to lower levels (e.g., 6.5, 6.0, 5.0 and 4.0) induced transient inward currents in cultured medium spiny neurons (MSNs) of the mouse striatum (Fig. 2A) (Jiang et al., 2009). The dose-response curve for activation of ASICs revealed a pH$_{50}$ value of 6.25 (Fig. 2B). This pH$_{50}$ value of ASICs in MSNs is comparable to that of homomeric ASIC1a channels (Walmann et al., 1997). The ASIC currents in MSNs had a linear I-V relationship with a reversal potential close to +60 mV (Fig. 2C, D), indicating that ASICs in MSNs are Na$^+$-selective.

In contrast to homomeric ASIC1a channels, the following properties distinguish rodent ASIC1b from ASIC1a: (1), although the amino acid sequence of approximately 2/3 of the

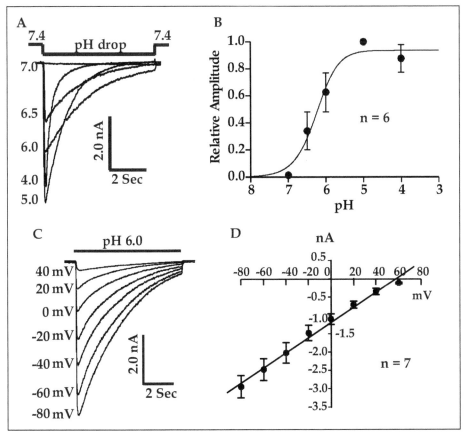

Fig. 2. Electrophysiological properties of ASICs in cultured mouse MSNs. (A) pH-dependent activation of ASIC currentsin in MSNs. (B) Dose-response curve for activation of the currents by pH drops. The $pH_{50}$ value is 6.25 and the Hill coeficient is 0.94. (C) The I-V relationship of acid-activated currents with different holding levels by decreasing the pH from 7.4 to 6.0 in MSNs. (D) The I-V curve. The extrapolated reversal potential is close to 60 mV, which is close to the sodium equilibrium potential

ASIC1a and ASIC1b proteins are identical, there are significant differences in the sequence for the first one third (about 172 amino acids) of the protein beginning at the N terminal; this sequence includes the intracellular N-terminus, the first transmembrane domain, and the proximal part of the ectodomain (Chen et al., 1998; Bassler et al., 2001); (2), the expression of ASIC1b in the nervous system is limited to peripheral sensory neurons, while ASIC1a is also expressed in the CNS; (3), rodent ASIC1b is impermeable to $Ca^{2+}$ while ASIC1a channels have significant $Ca^{2+}$ permeability; Interestingly, a recent study has shown that human ASIC1b channels are permeable to $Ca^{2+}$ (Hoagland et al., 2010); (4), the threshold for activation of ASIC1b current is lower than ASIC1a (~6.5 for ASIC1b and ~7.0 for ASIC1a) and it has lower $pH_{50}$ (5.9); (5), ASIC1b is potentiated by PcTx1(Chen et al., 2006), which is a specific inhibitor of ASIC1a.

Homomeric ASIC2a channels are relatively insensitive to proton, with a $pH_{50}$ of 4.4 (Price et al., 1996; Waldmann et al., 1996; Lingueglia et al., 1997). However, ASIC2a subunits can associate with ASIC1a to form heteromeric channels in brain (Askwith et al., 2004; Chu et al., 2004, 2006; Xiong et al., 2004; Jiang et al., 2009). Different from homomeric ASIC2a subunits, homomeric ASIC2b subunits do not form functional channels by themselves, but can associate with other ASIC subunits to form heteromultimeric channels (Lingueglia et al., 1997; Hesselager et al., 2004; Sherwood et al., 2011). For example, ASIC2b can be associated with ASIC1a to form functional channels and contribute to acidosis-induced neuronal injury (Sherwood et al., 2011).

ASIC3, like ASIC1b (Chen et al., 1998), is expressed primarily in peripheral sensory neurons (Waldmann et al., 1997a; Babinski et al., 1999; Wu et al., 2004; Lingueglia, 2007; Lin et al., 2008). In contrast to other subunits of ASICs, homomeric ASIC3 channels can respond to a large drop of extracellular pH with a transient inactivating current followed by a sustained component (Waldmann et al., 1997a; Sanilas et al., 2009) (Fig. 1). The transient currents are highly sensitive to protons, with a $pH_{50}$ of around 6.5 (Waldmann et al., 1997a; Hesselager et al., 2004). Electrophysiological studies have shown that ASIC3 subunits function as homomeric or heteromeric channels in sensory neurons (Sutherland et al., 2001; Benson et al., 2002; Deval et al., 2004, 2008; Lin et al., 2008; Hattori et al., 2009). They can sense extracellular acidification occurring in physiological and/or pathological processes, such as cutaneous touch, pain perception, inflammation and ischemia (Benson et al., 1999; Immke & McCleskey, 2001; Price et al., 2001; Sutherland et al., 2001; Mamet et al., 2003; Molliver et al., 2005; Sluka et al., 2007; Ikeuchi et al., 2009). For example, ASIC3 channels expressed in cardiac sensory neurons can respond to myocardial ischemia (Benson et al., 1999; Sutherland et al., 2001; Yagi et al., 2006). Further, cutaneous sensory neurons from rats display large ASIC3-like currents when stimulated by moderate acidosis (Deval et al., 2008). Consequently, it is generally accepted that ASIC3 is a sensor of moderate acidosis during ischemia and inflammatory pain in sensory neurons (Lingueglia, 2007).

ASIC4 subunits are expressed in pituitary gland. Similar to ASIC2b, they do not seem to form functional homomeric channels (Aropian et al., 2000; Grunder et al., 2000).

## 2.2 Pharmacological profiles of ASICs
### 2.2.1 Amiloride
Amiloride, the potassium-sparing diuretic agent, is a commonly used nonspecific blocker for ASICs. It inhibits the ASIC current and acid-induced increase in intracellular $Ca^{2+}$ ($[Ca^{2+}]_i$) with an $IC_{50}$ of 10–60 μM (Waldmann et al., 1997b; de Weille et al., 1998; Chen et al., 1998; Benson et al., 1999; Chu et al., 2002; Wu et al., 2004; Xiong et al., 2004; Yermolaieva et al., 2004; Jiang et al., 2009). For example, our recent study has shown that amiloride dose-dependently inhibited the ASIC currents in MSNs with an $IC_{50}$ of 13.6 μM (Fig. 3) (Jiang et al., 2009). Unlike the currents mediated by other homomeric ASICs, however, the sustained current mediated by homomeric ASIC3 channels is insensitive to amiloride (Waldmann et al., 1997b; Benson et al., 1999; Yagi et al., 2006). Based on the studies of ENaC, it is believed that amiloride inhibits ASICs by a direct blockade of the channel (Schild et al., 1997; Adams et al., 1999). The pre-TM II region of the channel is critical for the effect of amiloride. Mutation of Gly-430 in this region, for example, dramatically changed the sensitivity of ASIC2a current to amiloride (Champigny et al., 1998). Consistent with its inhibition on the ASIC current, amiloride has been shown to suppress acid-induced pain in peripheral

sensory system (Ugawa et al., 2002; Sluka et al., 2003; Jones et al., 2004; Dube et al., 2005), and acidosis-mediated injury of CNS neurons (Xiong et al., 2004; Yermolaieva et al., 2004). However, because of its nonspecificity for other ion channels (e.g., ENaC and T-type $Ca^{2+}$ channels) and ion exchange systems (e.g., $Na^+/H^+$ and $Na^+/Ca^{2+}$ exchanger), it is less likely that amiloride will be used as a future neuroprotective agent in human subjects. It is worth mentioning that the normal activity of $Na^+/Ca^{2+}$ exchanger, for example, is critical for maintaining the cellular $Ca^{2+}$ homeostasis and the survival of neurons against delayed calcium deregulation caused by glutamate receptor activation (Bano et al., 2005). Inhibition of $Na^+/Ca^{2+}$ exchange by amiloride may therefore compromise normal neuronal $Ca^{2+}$ handling, thus potentiating the glutamate toxicity (Bano et al., 2005).

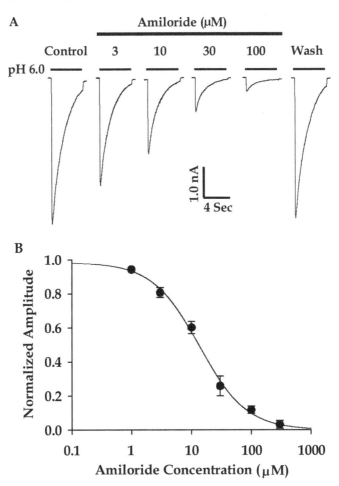

Fig. 3. Dose-dependent blockade of ASIC currents in cultured MSNs by amiloride, a non-specific ASIC blocker. (A) Amiloride dose-dependently inhibits the ASIC currents activated by pH 6.0. (B) Dose-inhibition curve of the acid-induced currents by amiloride. The $IC_{50}$ of amiloride is 13.6 µM

## 2.2.2 A-317567

A-317567, a small molecule structurally unrelated to amiloride, is another nonselective ASIC blocker (Dube et al., 2005). It inhibits the ASIC1a, ASIC2a, and ASIC3-like currents with an $IC_{50}$ of 2–30 µM. Unlike amiloride, which has no effect on the slow component of the ASIC3 current, A-317567 blocks both the fast and the sustained ASIC3 currents. Also different from amiloride, A-317567 does not show diuresis or natriuresis activity (Dube et al., 2005), suggesting that it is more specific for ASICs than amiloride. Its inhibition of sustained ASIC3 current suggests that it might be potent in reducing acidosis-mediated chronic pain. Indeed, A-317567 has been shown to be effective in suppressing the pain in a rat model of thermal hyperalgesia at a dose tenfold lower than amiloride (Dube et al., 2005).

## 2.2.3 PcTX1

Being a peptide toxin isolated from venom of the South American tarantula *Psalmopoeus cambridgei*, PcTX1 is a potent and specific inhibitor for homomeric ASIC1a channels (Escoubas et al., 2000). This toxin contains 40 amino acids cross-linked by three disulfide bridges. In heterologous expression systems, PcTX1 specifically inhibits the acid-activated current mediated by homomeric ASIC1a subunits with an $IC_{50}$ of 1 nM (Escoubas et al., 2000). At concentrations that effectively inhibit the ASIC1a current, it has no effect on the currents mediated by other configurations of ASICs (Escoubas et al., 2000), or known voltage-gated $Na^+$, $K^+$, $Ca^{2+}$ channels as well as several ligand-gated ion channels (Xiong et al., 2004). Unlike amiloride, which directly blocks the ASICs, PcTX1 acts as a gating modifier. It shifts the channel from its resting state toward the inactivated state by increasing its apparent affinity for protons (Chen et al., 2005). Recently, PcTX1 has also been shown to suppress heteromeric ASIC1a/2b channels (Sherwood et al., 2011).

## 2.2.4 APETx2

Being a peptide toxin isolated from sea anemone *Anthopleura elegantissima*, APETx2 is a potent and selective inhibitor for homomeric ASIC3 and ASIC3 containing channels (Diochot et al., 2004). The toxin contains 42 amino acids, also cross-linked by three disulfide bridges. It reduces transient peak acid-evoked currents mediated by homomeric ASIC3 channels (Diochot et al., 2004). In contrast to the peak ASIC3 current, the sustained component of the ASIC3 current is insensitive to APETx2. In addition to homomeric ASIC3 channels ($IC_{50}$ = 63 nM for rat and 175 nM for human), APETx2 inhibits heteromeric ASIC3/1a ($IC_{50}$ = 2 µM), ASIC3/1b ($IC_{50}$ = 900 nM), and ASIC3/2b ($IC_{50}$ = 117 nM). Homomeric ASIC1a, ASIC1b, ASIC2a, and heteromeric ASIC3/2a channels, on the other hand, are not sensitive to APETx2 (Diochot et al., 2004).

## 2.2.5 Nonsteroid anti-inflammatory drugs (NSAIDs)

NSAIDs are the most commonly used anti-inflammatory and analgesic agents. They inhibit the synthesis of prostaglandins (PGs), a main tissue inflammatory substance. A recent study demonstrated that NSAIDs also inhibit the activity of ASICs at their therapeutic doses for analgesic effects (Voilley et al., 2001). Ibuprofen and flurbiprofen, for example, inhibit ASIC1a containing channels with an $IC_{50}$ of 350 µM. Aspirin and salicylate inhibit ASIC3 containing channels with an $IC_{50}$ of 260 µM, whereas diclofenac inhibits the same channels with an $IC_{50}$ of 92 µM. In addition to a direct inhibition of the ASIC activity, NSAIDs also prevent inflammation-induced increase of ASIC expression in sensory neurons (Voilley et al., 2001).

## 2.2.6 Aminoglycosides (AGs)

AGs (streptomycin, neomycin and gentamicin) are a group of antibiotics that have been shown to block $Ca^{2+}$ channels (Zhou and Zhao, 2002), excitatory amino acid receptors (Pérez et al., 1991), and transient-receptor-potential V1 channels (Raisinghani and Premkumar, 2005). Recently, Garza et al determined the effect of AGs on proton-gated ionic currents in DRG neurons of the rat, and in human embryonic kidney (HEK)-293 cells (Garza et al., 2010). In DRG neurons, streptomycin and neomycin produced a significant, reversible reduction in the amplitude of proton-gated currents in a concentration-dependent manner. In addition, they slowed desensitization rates of ASIC currents. Gentamicin also showed a significant reversible action on the ASIC currents. In HEK-293 cells, streptomycin produced a significant reduction in the amplitude of the proton-gated current, whereas neomycin and gentamicin had no significant effect. These results indicate that ASICs are molecular targets for AGs, which may explain, in part, their effects on excitable cells. Moreover, AGs might potentially represent a novel class of molecules with high affinity, specificity, and selectivity for different ASIC subunits.

## 2.2.7 Diarylamidines

Diarylamidines have been widely used for the treatment of protozoan diseases such as trypanosomiasis and leishmaniasis since 1930s (Baraldi et al., 2004; Mishra et al., 2007). Recently, Chen and colleges found that four members of the diarylamidines, 4', 6-diamidino-2-phenylindole, diminazene, hydroxystilbamidine and pentamidine strongly inhibit ASIC currents in hippocampal neurons with $IC_{50}$ of 2.8, 0.3, 1.5 and 38 μM, respectively. The inhibitory concentration is much lower than amiloride. Sub-maximal concentrations of diminazene also potently accelerate desensitization of ASIC currents in hippocampal neurons. Diminazene blocks ASIC1a, -1b, -2a, and -3 currents expressed in CHO cells with a rank order of potency 1b > 3 > 2a > or = 1a. This study indicates that diarylamidines represent a novel class of non-amiloride ASIC blockers and suggests that diarylamidines as small molecules may be developed as therapeutic agents in the treatment of ASIC-involved diseases (Chen et al., 2010).

## 3. Activation of ASICs induces membrane depolarization and increases intracellular $Ca^{2+}$ in brain neurons

Since all ASICs are $Na^+$-selective channels which have a reversal potential near $Na^+$ equilibrium potential (+60 mV), activation of ASICs at normal resting potentials produces exclusively inward currents which result in membrane depolarization and the excitation of neurons (Baron et al., 2002; Wu et al., 2004; Jiang et al., 2009). For example, our recent study has shown that a minor drop in extracellular pH from 7.4 to 6.8 induces significant membrane depolarization, which accompanies trains of action potentials (Fig. 4) (Jiang et al., 2009). This acid-induced membrane depolarization is significantly attenuated by either amiloride or PcTX1 (Fig. 4). Tetrodotoxin, a voltage-gated $Na^+$ channel blocker, has little effect on the membrane depolarization but completely diminished the action potentials triggered by a drop in pH from 7.4 to 6.8. For homomeric ASIC1a channels, acid activation induces $Ca^{2+}$ entry directly through these channels (Walmann et al., 1997b; Chu et al., 2002; Xiong et al., 2004; Yermolaieva et al., 2004). In addition, the ASIC-mediated membrane depolarization may facilitate the activation of voltage-gated $Ca^{2+}$ channels and NMDA receptor-gated channels (Wemmie et al., 2002; Zha et al., 2006), further promoting neuronal excitation and $[Ca^{2+}]_i$ accumulation. The $Ca^{2+}$-permeability of ASICs in CNS neurons has been characterized using fluorescent $Ca^{2+}$ imaging and ion-substitution protocols (Xiong et al., 2004; Yermolaieva et al., 2004). In mouse cortical, striatal and hippocampal neurons, activation of ASICs by decreasing in extracellular pH induces increases in $[Ca^{2+}]_i$. This acid-induced increase in $[Ca^{2+}]_i$ could be recorded in the presence of a cocktail blocking other voltage-gated and ligand-gated $Ca^{2+}$ channels (Xiong et al., 2004; Jiang et al., 2009), indicating $Ca^{2+}$ entry directly through ASICs. The acid-induced increase in $[Ca^{2+}]_i$ is eliminated by specific and non-specific ASIC1a blockade, or by ASIC1 gene knockout (Xiong et al., 2004; Yermolaieva et al., 2004; Jiang et al., 2009). Consistent with the finding of fluorescent imaging, acid-activated inward current is activated when extracellular solution contains $Ca^{2+}$ as the only conducting cation (Xiong et al., 2004). Thus, homomeric ASIC1a channels constitute an additional and important $Ca^{2+}$ entry pathway for neurons.

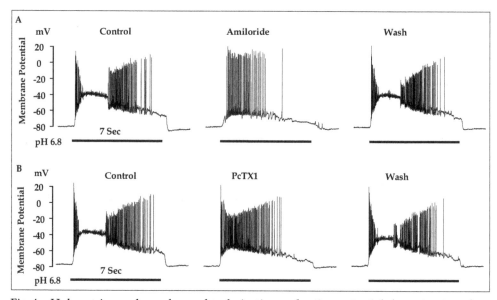

Fig. 4. pH drop triggered membrane depolarization and action potentials by activation of ASICs in cultured MSNs. Membrane depolarization by a drop in pH from 7.4 to 6.8 subsequently triggered trains of action potentials. The membrane depolarization was inhibited by amiloride (A) and PcTX1 (B)

## 4. Physiological implications of ASICs in the CNS

### 4.1 ASIC1a channels in synaptic plasticity, learning and memory

A change in pH at the synaptic cleft following synaptic release may render ASICs the opportunity to regulate synaptic transmission. The findings that ASICs are present at synaptic sites and can interact with postsynaptic density protein 95 as well as C kinase 1-interacting proteins (Hruska-Hageman et al., 2002; Wemmie et al., 2002; Zha et al., 2006, 2009) support this notion. Indeed, studies by Wemmie and coworkers have demonstrated that ASIC1a activation is involved in synaptic plasticity, learning and memory (Wemmie et al., 2002). They demonstrated that high frequency stimulation produces long-lasting potentiation of excitatory postsynaptic potentials (EPSP) in hippocampal slices from wild-type mice. However, the potentiation of EPSP decays rapidly to the baseline in slices from ASIC1a null mice. Further studies showed that the NMDA receptor antagonist D-2-Amino-5-phosphonovalerate inhibits EPSP summation in slices from wild-type but not ASIC1a-knockout mice, suggesting that the loss of ASIC1a impaired NMDA-receptor function. ASIC1a disruption does not impair presynaptic vesicle release, as evidenced by normal single evoked EPSPs and paired-pulse facilitation. Interestingly, a later study by Cho and Askwith demonstrated that the presynaptic release probability is increased in cultured hippocampal neurons from the ASIC1 knockout mice (Cho & Askwith, 2008). Although localizations of ASICs at neuronal cell body and postsynaptic sites have been clearly demonstrated (Wemmie et al., 2002; Zha et al., 2006), it remains to be determined whether ASICs are also expressed at presynaptic sites.

## 4.2 ASIC1a channels in fear-related behavior

ASIC1a is enriched in key structures of fear circuit (e.g. amygdala) (Wemmie et al., 2003). Thus, ASIC1a may influence fear responses. Indeed, Wemmie and colleagues demonstrated that ASIC1-null mice display significant deficits in cue and context fear conditioning (Wemmie et al., 2003). The loss of ASIC1a also reduces unconditioned fear in the open field test, during acoustic startle, and in response to predator odor (Coryell et al., 2007). Overexpressing ASIC1a, on the other hand, increases fear conditioning (Wemmie et al., 2004), but not unconditioned fear responses (Coryell et al., 2008).

Further studies by Wemmie's group suggest that activation of ASIC1a in brain chemosensors contributes to $CO_2$ induced fear-related behavior (Ziemann et al., 2009). It has long been known that breathing $CO_2$ triggers panic attacks in patients with panic disorder, and that these patients show an increased sensitivity to $CO_2$ inhalation (Papp et al., 1993). In addition, patients with increasing hypercarbia due to respiratory failure become extremely anxious. How can $CO_2$ inhalation contribute to fear behavior and related panic disorders? Wemmie and colleagues have provided evidence that ASIC1a channels are involved (Ziemann et al., 2009). They showed that inhaled $CO_2$ triggers a drop in brain pH and induces fear behavior in mice. Eliminating or inhibiting ASIC1a significantly limits this activity. Overexpressing ASIC1a in the amygdala rescues the $CO_2$-induced fear deficit in ASIC1a null mice. Buffering brain pH, on the other hand, attenuates fear behavior, whereas lowering pH in the amygdale reproduces the effect of $CO_2$. These studies provide a novel molecular mechanism underlying $CO_2$-induced intense fear and related anxiety/panic disorders and define the amygdala as an important chemosensor that detects hypercarbia/acidosis and initiates behavioral responses (Ziemann et al., 2009).

## 4.3 ASICs and retinal integrity

pH variations in the retina are involved in the fine-tuning of visual perception. Expression of ASICs in the retina suggests that they might play a role (Lilley et al., 2004). One study by Ettaiche suggested that ASIC2 is important for retinal function and likely protects against light-induced retinal degeneration. They showed that both photoreceptors and neurons of the mouse retina express ASIC2a and ASIC2b. Inactivation of the ASIC2 gene in mice leads to an increased rod electroretinogram of a- and b-waves, indicating an enhanced gain of visual transduction. ASIC2 knockout mice also show more sensitivity to light-induced retinal degeneration. Thus, ASIC2 is likely a negative modulator of rod phototransduction, and that functional ASIC2 channels are beneficial for the maintenance of retinal integrity (Ettaiche et al., 2004). However, since homomeric ASIC2a channels have an extremely low-sensitivity to protons (i.e. $pH_{50}$ of 4.4), it is not clear whether active channel activity is required for this role.

Further studies by Ettaiche and colleagues also suggested an involvement of ASIC1a in retinal physiology (Ettaiche et al., 2006). In situ hybridization and immunohistochemistry detected the expression of ASIC1a in the outer and inner nuclear layers (cone photoreceptors, horizontal cells, some amacrine and bipolar cells) and in the ganglion cell layer. ASIC1a knockdown by antisense oligonucleotides and ASIC1a blockade by relatively specific inhibitor PcTX1 decreased the photopic a- and b-waves and oscillatory potentials. This finding suggests that ASIC1a is involved in normal retinal activity. Interestingly, a recent study by Render and colleagues did not detect any remarkable morphological changes in cone photoreceptors in ASIC1a-/- mice, at least at 5 or 22-27 weeks of age (Render et al., 2010). Thus, the exact role of this subunit in retinal integrity and/or function remains to be determined.

In addition to ASIC1a and ASIC2, a potential role of ASIC3 in retinal function and survival has been reported (Ettaiche et al., 2009). Ettaiche and colleagues demonstrated the presence of ASIC3 in the rod inner segment of photoreceptors, in horizontal and some amacrine cells. ASIC3 is also detected in retinal ganglion cells (RGCs) but contributes little to ASIC currents recorded in cultured RGCs. At 2 - 3 months, knockout mice experienced a moderate enhancement of scotopic electroretinogram a-wave amplitude and a concomitant increase of b-wave amplitude without alteration of retinal structure. Older (8-month-old) mice had large reductions in scotopic a- and b-waves, respectively, and reductions in oscillatory potential amplitudes associated with complete disorganization of the retina and degenerating rod inner segments. At 8 and 12 months of age, GFAP and TUNEL staining revealed an up-regulation of GFAP expression in Müller cells and the presence of apoptotic cells in the inner and outer retina (Ettaiche et al., 2009). Thus, ASIC3 also appears to be required for the maintenance of retina integrity.

## 5. ASICs in neurodegenerative diseases

### 5.1 ASIC1 channels and multiple sclerosis

Multiple sclerosis is a neuroinflammatory disease associated with axonal degeneration. Although inflammation and demyelination are the primary features of CNS lesions, axonal degeneration correlates best with clinical deficits in individuals with this disease. It has been suggested that the inflammatory insult leads to axonal degeneration by causing neuronal mitochondrial dysfunction, energy failure and alteration of ion exchange mechanisms (Waxman, 2006). Since excessive accumulation of $Na^+$ and $Ca^{2+}$ ions is associated with axonal degeneration (Stys & LoPachin, 1998), Friese et al determined whether ASIC1a activation, which is known to cause accumulation of $Na^+$ and $Ca^{2+}$ ions, contributes to such process in inflammatory lesions of the CNS (Friese et al., 2007). They showed that in an experimental model of autoimmune encephalomyelitis (EAE), ASIC1 null mice exhibit a significantly reduced clinical deficit and axonal degeneration as compared to wild-type mice. Further, pH measurements in the spinal cord of EAE mice display tissue acidosis sufficient to open ASIC1. The ASIC1 gene disruption also shows protective effect in nerve explants in vitro. ASIC blockade by amiloride is equally neuroprotective in nerve explants and in EAE. Thus, ASIC1a may be a potential target for axon degeneration associated with multiple sclerosis.

More recently, Vergo et al., from the same group studied acute and chronic EAE and multiple sclerosis spinal cord and optic nerve tissues to examine the distribution of ASIC1 and its relationship with neuronal and glial damage (Vergo et al., 2011). They found that ASIC1 was upregulated in axons and oligodendrocytes within lesions from mice with acute EAE and from patients with active multiple sclerosis. The expression of ASIC1 was associated with axonal damage as indicated by co-localization with the axonal injury marker beta amyloid precursor protein. Moreover, blocking ASIC1 with amiloride protected both myelin and neurons from damage in the acute model, and when given either at disease onset or, more clinically relevant, at first relapse, ameliorated disability in mice with chronic-relapsing EAE. Together these findings suggest that blockade of ASIC1 has the potential to provide both neuro- and myelo-protective benefits in multiple sclerosis (Vergo et al., 2011).

### 5.2 ASICs and Parkinson's disease (PD)

PD is characterized by motor impairments and a loss of dopaminergic neurons in the substantia nigra (SNc) (Dauer & Przedborski, 2003). However, the mechanism of neuronal injury is not entirely clear. Previous studies have shown that the vulnerable neurons in this region also express ASIC1a (Wemmie et al., 2003; Pidoplichko & Dani, 2006). Given that PD, like ischemia, is associated with cerebral lactic acidosis, Arias et al tested the effect of ASIC blockade in a mouse model of PD induced by 1-methyl-4-phenyl-1,2,3,6-tetrahydropyridine (MPTP) treatment (Arias et al., 2008). As expected, amiloride was found to protect SNc neurons from MPTP-induced degeneration, and to preserve dopaminergic cell bodies in the SNc. Administration of PcTX venom resulted in a modest effect, attenuating the deficits in striatal DAT binding and dopamine. These findings suggest a potential role for ASICs in the pathogenesis of Parkinson's disease.

### 5.3 ASICs and Huntington's disease (HD)

HD is a fatal neurodegenerative disorder. Energy metabolism deficit and acidosis have been observed in both *in vitro* and *in vivo* models of HD as well as in the brains of HD patients (Wong et al., 2008). To examine the potential involvement of ASICs in the pathology of HD, Wong et al tested effect of amiloride derivative benzamil both *in vitro* and *in vivo* (Wong et al., 2008). They showed that benzamil markedly reduced the huntingtin-polyglutamine (htt-polyQ) aggregation in an inducible cellular system. In addition, the effect of benzamil was recapitulated in the R6/2 animal model of HD. Further experimentation showed that benzamil alleviated the inhibition of ubiquitin-proteasome system (UPS) activity, resulting in enhanced degradation of soluble htt-polyQ specifically in its pathological range. Blocking the expression of ASIC1a with siRNA also enhanced UPS activity, resulting in decreased htt-polyQ aggregation in the striatum of R6/2 mice. Thus, targeting ASIC1a might be an alternative approach to combat HD and other polyQ-related disorders.

### 5.4 ASIC1a and Alzheimer's disease (AD)

Based on ASIC1a channels in synaptic plasticity and learning/memory, a recent preliminary study has suggested that a reduced function of ASIC1a channels may contribute to the learning and memory deficit associated with AD (Maysami et al., 2009). In this study, Maysami et al showed that acid-activated currents in mouse cortical neurons and in CHO cells expressing ASIC1a are inhibited by nanomolar concentrations of amyloid beta peptide, a critical player for the pathology of AD. In addition to a reduction of current amplitude, amyloid beta peptide also slows down the activation of the channels. Thus, restoring the activity of ASIC1a channels could be a new intervention for AD.

## 5.5 ASICs in depression-related behavior

Depression disorders are a highly prevalent condition among adults in general population but the molecular pathways underlying depression are poorly understood. Recent studies by Coryell and colleagues have linked ASIC function to depression-related behavior (Coryell et al., 2009). They demonstrated that genetically disrupting ASIC1a in mice produced antidepressant-like effects in the forced swim test, the tail suspension test, and following unpredictable mild stress. Pharmacologically inhibiting ASIC1a also had antidepressant-like effects. The effects of ASIC1a disruption in the forced swim test were independent and additive to those of several commonly used antidepressants. Restoring ASIC1a to the amygdale of ASIC1a null mice reversed the forced swim test effects. The mechanism underlying the involvement of ASIC1a in depression-related behavior is not clear. It is likely that brain-derived neurotrophic factor (BDNF) is involved since both ASIC1a disruption and inhibition interfere with the ability of stress to reduce BDNF in the hippocampus. Thus, antagonists of ASIC1a channels may have potential for combating human depression.

## 5.6 ASICs and anxiety disorders

Anxiety disorders are debilitating neuropsychiatric disorders. Current treatments for anxiety disorders include pharmacological agents such as benzodiazepines and selective serotonin reuptake inhibitors. These agents, while effective in many patients, can induce a variety of side effects. Thus, it is necessary to develop a new generation of effective and better-tolerated anxiolytic agents. In this regard, Dwyer et al have shown that ASIC1a inhibitors have an effect in preclinical rodent models of autonomic and behavioral parameters of anxiety (Dwyer et al., 2009). In the stress-induced hyperthermia model, acute administration of ASIC inhibitors PcTX1, A-317567, and amiloride prevented stress-induced elevations in core body temperature. In the four-plate test, acute treatment with PcTX1 and A-317567 produced dose-dependent increases in the number of punished crossings. Further experiment showed that infusion of A-317567 into the amygdala significantly elevated the extracellular levels of GABA, but not glutamate, in this brain region. These findings suggest that ASIC inhibition has anxiolytic-like effects in some behavioral models and that GABAergic mechanisms are involved in the effects.

A recent study also suggests an involvement of ASIC3 in anxiety-like behavior (Wu et al., 2010). Although it is widely accepted that ASIC3 is predominately distributed in the peripheral nervous system, its expression has been found in rat hypothalamus (Meng et al., 2009). Study by Wu and colleagues also reported the expression of ASIC3 in the sensory mesencephalic trigeminal nucleus of mouse brain (Wu et al., 2010). However, whether ASIC3 plays any functional role in the brain was unclear. Wu et al showed that, in anxiety behavior tasks, ASIC3 null mice spent more time in the open arms of an elevated plus maze than did their wild-type littermates. ASIC3 null mice also displayed less aggressiveness toward intruders but more stereotypic repetitive behaviors during resident-intruder testing than did wild-type littermates. Therefore, loss of ASIC3 produces behavioral changes in anxiety and aggression in mice, which suggests that ASIC3-dependent sensory activities might be related to the central process of emotion modulation (Wu et al., 2010).

Although the studies from ASIC1a and ASIC3 knockout mice indicated that ASICs contribute to neuropsychiatric disorders such as depression and anxiety, whether these neurological conditions are associated with significant change in local or global pH in the CNS remains to be determined.

### 5.7 ASICs in acidosis-mediated ischemic neuronal injury

During neurological conditions such as brain ischemia, increased anaerobic glycolysis due to reduced oxygen supply leads to lactic acid accumulation (Rehncrona, 1985). Accumulation of lactic acid, alone with increased $H^+$ release from ATP hydrolysis, causes a decrease in pH, resulting in brain acidosis. During brain ischemia, for example, extracellular pH falls to 6.5 or lowers (Rehncrona, 1985; Nedergaard et al., 1991).

Acidosis has long been known to play an important role in ischemic brain injury (Tombaugh & Sapolsky, 1993; Siesjo, et al., 1996), and a direct correlation of brain acidosis with infarct size has been described (Siesjo, 1988). However, the exact mechanism underlying acidosis-mediated neuronal injury remained uncertain. Severe acidosis may cause non-selective denaturation of proteins and nucleic acids (Kalimo et al., 1981); trigger cell swelling through stimulation of $Na^+/H^+$ and $Cl^-/HCO_3^-$ exchangers, which leads to cellular edema and osmolysis (Kimelberg et al., 1990); hinder postischemic metabolic recovery by inhibiting mitochondrial energy metabolism and impairing postischemic blood flow via vascular edema (Hillered et al., 1985). The stimulation of pathologic free radical formation by acidosis has also been described (Rehncrona et al., 1989). At the neurotransmitter level, profound acidosis inhibits astrocytic glutamate uptake, which may contribute to excitatory neuronal injury (Swanson et al., 1995). Marked acidosis, with tissue pH<5.5, may influence neuronal vulnerability indirectly by damaging glial cells (Giffard et al., 1990).

The widespread expression of ASIC1a in the brain, its activation by pH drops to the level commonly seen during ischemia, and its demonstrated role in intracellular $Ca^{2+}$ accumulation suggested a potential involvement of these channels in the pathology of brain injury. Indeed, a number of recent studies have demonstrated an important role for ASIC1a activation in acidosis-mediated neuronal injury (Xiong et al., 2004; Yermolaieva et al., 2004; Gao et al., 2005; Pignataro nt al., 2007; Sherwood et al., 2009, 2011; Gu et al., 2010; Jetti et al., 2010; Li et al., 2010; Mari et al., 2010). In cultured mouse and human cortical neurons, for example, activation of ASICs by acid incubation induced glutamate receptor-independent neuronal injury inhibited by specific ASIC1a blockade, and/or by ASIC1 gene knockout (Xiong et al., 2004; Li et al., 2010). In rodent models of brain ischemia, intracerebroventricular injection of ASIC1a blocker/inhibitor reduced the infarct volume from transient or permanent focal ischemia by up to 60%(Xiong et al., 2004; Pignataro et al., 2007). Similarly, ASIC1 gene knockout produced significant neuroprotection in mice (Xiong et al., 2004). The protection by ASIC1a blockade had a time window of efficacy of up to 5 hours, and the protection persists for at least 7 days (Pignataro nt al., 2007).

More recently, Sherwood et al., found that ASIC2b subunit can form functional channels with ASIC1a in cultured hippocampal neurons, and that the heteromeric ASIC1a/2b channels are calcium-permeable (Sherwood et al., 2011). Further, activation of heteromeric ASIC1a/2b channels contributes to acidosis-induced neuronal death. These data indicate that ASIC2, like ASIC1a, plays a role in acidosis-induced neuronal death and implicate the ASIC1a/2b subtype as a novel pharmacological target to prevent neuronal injury after stroke (Sherwood et al., 2011).

Since activation of NMDA receptors and subsequent $Ca^{2+}$ toxicity have been known to play an important role in ischemic brain injury, the outcome of co-application of both antagonists has also been investigated. Compared to ASIC1a or NMDA blockade alone, co-application of NMDA and ASIC antagonists produced additional neuroprotection, and the presence of ASIC1a blockade prolonged the time window of effectiveness of NMDA blockade (Pignataro nt al., 2007). Thus, ASIC1a represents a novel pharmacological target for ischemic brain injury.

In contrast to ASIC1a, a study by Johnson and colleagues suggests that an increased ASIC2a expression could provide protection against ischemic injury (Johnson et al., 2001). They showed an increased ASIC2a expression in neurons that survived global ischemia. This may be explained by the possibility that increased ASIC2a expression favors the formation of heteromeric ASIC1a/ASIC2a channels with reduced acid-sensitivity and no $Ca^{2+}$ permeability.

## 5.8 ASIC activation and epileptic seizure activity

A significant drop of brain pH during intense neuronal excitation or seizure activity (Urbanics et al., 1978; Somjen et al., 1984; Simon et al., 1985, 1987; Chesler & Chan, 1988; Chesler & Kaila, 1992) suggests that ASIC activation might occur and activated ASICs then play a role in the generation/maintenance of epileptic seizures. However, the exact role of ASIC activation in seizure generation, propagation, and termination seems controversial.

Babinski and colleagues first reported a change of ASIC1a and ASIC2b expression in the hippocampal area following pilocarpine-induced epilepticus (Biagini et al., 2001), suggesting that the channels containing ASIC1a and ASIC2b subunits might play a role in the pathology of epilepsy.

Later on, a number of studies showed that amiloride, a commonly used non-selective ASIC blocker, has an anticonvulsant property *in vivo* in pilocarpine and pentylenetetrazole models of seizures (Ali et al., 2004, 2006; N'Gouemo, 2008), suggesting that ASIC activation might be proconvulsant. However, since amiloride also inhibits a number of other channels and ion exchange systems, these findings do not define ASICs as a specific target for amiloride to achieve its anti-epileptic action.

Using a number of *in vitro* epilepsy models, a preliminary study by Chang et al provided additional evidence that ASIC1a activation might be proconvulsant (Chang et al., 2007). In a cell culture model of epilepsy, brief withdrawal of the NMDA antagonist kynurenic acid induces a dramatic increase in the firing of action potentials, in addition to a sustained membrane depolarization. ASIC blockade by amiloride and the selective ASIC1a blocker PcTX1 significantly inhibited the increase of neuronal firing and the sustained membrane depolarization. In hippocampal slices, high frequency electrical stimulation or removal of extracellular $Mg^{2+}$ triggers spontaneous seizure-like bursting. Bath perfusion of amiloride and PcTX1 decreased the amplitude and the frequency of these seizure-like bursting activities. Similarly, slices prepared from the brains of ASIC1a knockout mice demonstrated a reduced sensitivity to low extracellular $Mg^{2+}$-induced or stimulation-evoked seizure activities (Chang et al., 2007).

In contrast, studies by Ziemann and colleagues, performed largely *in vivo*, have suggested that activation of ASIC1a channels is involved in the termination of epileptic seizure activity (Ziemann et al., 2008). An interesting finding by Ziemann and colleagues was that the level of ASIC1a expression is higher in GABAergic interneurons than in excitatory neurons (Ziemann et al., 2008). Therefore, acidosis generated during seizures might produce more

ASIC activation in inhibitory interneurons and facilitate GABAergic transmission, resulting in seizure termination.

The inconsistent data on the role of ASICs in epileptic seizures may result from the use of different epilepsy models. The different ages of animals used may also contribute to the inconsistency since expression and function of ASICs in CNS neurons undergo dramatic developmental changes (Li et al., 2010). In addition, the finding that hippocampal interneurons are highly diverse with dramatically different expression level of ASICs (Weng et al., 2010) adds additional complexity to this subject.

## 6. Conclusion

ASICs represent new biological components in peripheral sensory and CNS neurons. Increasing evidence indicates the involvement of these channels in both physiological and pathological processes of CNS (Grunder & Chen, 2010). Therefore, targeting these channels may provide novel and effective therapeutic interventions for a number of CNS diseases. In addition to establishing ASIC-specific small molecule antagonists that can easily pass through the blood brain barrier, alternative strategies may consider targeting endogenous modulators that are known to influence the expression and/or activity of these channels.

## 7. References

Adams, C.M.; Snyder, P.M. & Welsh, M.J. (1999). Paradoxical Stimulation of a DEG/ENaC Channel by Amiloride. *Journal of Biological Chemistry*, Vol. 274, No. 22, pp.15500-15504, ISSN 0021-9258

Akopian, A.N.; Chen, C.C.; Ding, Y. Cesare, P. & Wood, J.N. (2000). A New Member of the Acid-Sensing Ion Channel Family. *Neuroreport,* Vol.11, No.10, pp. 2217 – 2222, ISSN 0959-4956

Ali, A.; Ahmad, F.J.; Pillai, K.K. & Vohora, D. (2004). Evidence of the Antiepileptic Potential of Amiloride With Neuropharmacological Benefits in Rodent Models of Epilepsy and Behavior. *Epilepsy & Behavior,* Vol. 5, No. 3, pp. 322-328, ISSN 1525-5050

Ali, A.; Pillai, K.P.; Ahmad, F.J.; Dua, Y. & Vohora, D. (2006). Anticonvulsant Effect of Amiloride in Pentetrazole-Induced Status Epilepticus in Mice. *Pharmacological Reports,* Vol. 58, No.2, pp. 242-245, ISSN 1734-1140

Allen, N.J. & Attwell, D. (2002). Modulation of ASIC Channels in Rat Crebellar Purkinje Nurons by Ichemia-Rlated Sgnals. *Journal of Phsiology,* Vol. 543, No. 2, pp. 521 – 529, ISSN 0022-3751

Alvarez de la Rosa, D.; Canessa, C.M.; Fyfe, G.K. & Zhang, P. (2000). Structure and Regulation of Amiloride Sensitive Sodium Channels. *Annual Review of Physiology,* Vol. 62, No.1, pp.573-594, ISSN 0066-4278

Arias, R.L.; Sung, M.L.; Vasylyev, D.; Zhang, M.Y.; Albinson, K.; Kubek, K.; Kagan, N.; Beyer, C.; Lin, Q.; Dwyer, J.M.; Zaleska, M.M.; Bowlby, M.R.; Dunlop, J. & Monaghan, M. (2008). Amiloride is Neuroprotective in an MPTP Model of Parkinson's Disease. *Neurobiology of Disease,* Vol. 31, No. 3, pp. 334-341, ISSN 0969-9961

Askwith, C.C.; Wemmie, J.A.; Price, M.P.; Rokhlina, T. & Welsh, M.J. (2004). Acid-Sensing Ion Channel 2 (ASIC2) Modulates ASIC1 H+-Activated Currents in Hippocampal

Neurons. *Journal of Biological Chemistry*, Vol. 279, No. 18, pp.18296-18305, ISSN 0021-9258

Babini, E.; Paukert, M.; Geisler, H.S. & Grunder, S. (2002). Alternative Splicing and Interaction with Di- and Polyvalent Cations Control the Dynamic Range of Acid-Sensing Ion Channel 1 (ASIC1). *Journal of Biological Chemistry*, Vol. 277, No. 44, pp.41597-41603, ISSN 0021-9258

Bano, D.; Young, K.W.; Guerin, C.J.; Lefeuvre, R.; Rothwell, N.J.; Naldini, L.; Rizzuto, R.; Carafoli, E. & Nicotera, P. (2005). Cleavage of the Plasma Membrane $Na^+/Ca^{2+}$ Exchanger in Excitotoxicity. *Cell*, Vol. 120,No.2, pp. 275-285, ISSN 0092-8674

Baraldi, P.G.; Bovero, A.; Fruttarolo, F.; Preti, D.; Tabrizi, M.A.; Pavani, M.G. & Romagnoli, R. (2004). DNA Minor Groove Binders as Potential Antitumor and Antimicrobial Agents. *Medicinal Research Reviews*, Vol. 24, No. 4, pp. 475-528, ISSN 0198-6325

Baron, A.; Voilley, N.; Lazdunski, M. & Lingueglia, E. (2008). Acid Sensing Ion Channels in Dorsal Spinal Cord Neurons. *Journal of Neuroscience*, Vol.28, No.6, pp.1498-1508, ISSN 0270-6474

Baron, A.; Waldmann, R. & Lazdunski, M. (2002). ASIC-Like, Proton-Activated Currents in Rat Hippocampal Neurons. *Journal of Physiology*, Vol. 539, No.2, pp.485-494, ISSN 0022-3751

Bässler, E.L.; Ngo-Anh, T.J.; Geisler, H.S.; Ruppersberg, J.P. & Gründer, S. (2001). Molecular and Functional Characterization of Acid-Sensing Ion Channel (ASIC) 1b. *Journal of Biological Chemistry*, Vol. 276, No. 36, pp. 33782-33787, ISSN 0021-9258

Benson, C.J.; Eckert, S.P. & McCleskey, E.W. (1999). Acid-Evoked Currents in Cardiac Sensory Neurons: A Possible Mediator of Myocardial Ischemic Sensation. *Circulation Research*, Vol. 84, No. 8, pp. 921-928, ISSN 0009-7330

Benson, C.J.; Xie, J.; Wemmie, J.A.; Price, M.P.; Henss, J.M.; Welsh, M.J. & Snyder, P.M. (2002). Heteromultimers of DEG/ENaC Subunits Form $H^+$-Gated Channels in Mouse Sensory Neurons. *Proceedings of National Academy of Science U.S.A.*, Vol. 99, No. 4, pp. 2338-2343, ISSN 0027-8424

Benveniste, M. & Dingledine, R. (2005). Limiting Stroke-Induced Damage by Targeting an Acid Channel. *New England Journal of Medicine*, Vol. 352, No. 1, pp. 85-86, ISSN 0028-4793

Biagini, G.; Babinski, K.; Avoli, M.; Marcinkiewicz, M. & Seguela, P. (2001). Regional and Subunit Specific Down-Regulation of Acid-Sensing Ion Channels in the Pilocarpine Model of Epilepsy. *Neurobiology of Disease*, Vol. 8, No. 1, pp.45-58, ISSN 0969-9961

Champigny, G.; Voilley, N.; Waldmann, R. & Lazdunski, M. (1998). Mutations Causing Neurodegeneration in Caenorhabditis Elegans Drastically Alter the PH Sensitivity and Inactivation of the Mammalian $H^+$-Gated $Na^+$ Channel MDEG1. *Journal of Biological Chemistry*, Vol. 273, No. 25, pp. 15418-15422, ISSN 0021-9258

Chang, S.Y.; Li, M.H.; Li, T.F.; Chu, X.P.; Lan, J.Q.; Thomson, S.; Jessick, V.; Meller, R.; Simon, R.P. & Xiong, Z.G. (2007). Involvement of Acid-Sensing Ion Channels in the Generation of Epileptic Seizure Activity [abstract]. 37th *Society for Neuroscience Annual Meeting*, 257.5. ISBN 0-916110-04-4, San Diego, California, USA, November 3-7, 2007

Chen, C.C.; England, S.; Akopian, A.N. & Wood, J.N. (1998). A Sensory Neuron Specific, Proton-Gated Ion Channel. *Proceedings of National Academy of Science U.S.A.*, Vol. 95, No. 17, pp.10240 – 10245, ISSN 0027-8424

Chen, X.; Kalbacher, H. & Gründer, S. (2006). Interaction of Acid-Sensing Ion Channel (ASIC) 1 with the Tarantula Toxin Psalmotoxin 1 is State Dependent. *Journal of General Physiology*, Vol.127, No.3, pp.267-76, ISSN 0022-1295

Chen, X.; Kalbacher, H. & Gründer, S. (2005). The Tarantula Toxin Psalmotoxin 1 Inhibits Acid-Sensing Ion Channel (ASIC) 1a by Increasing its Apparent $H^+$ Affinity. *Journal of General Physiology*, Vol.126, No.1, pp. 71-79, ISSN 0022-1295

Chen, X.; Qiu, L.; Li, M.; Dürrnagel, S.; Orser, B.A.; Xiong, Z.G. & MacDonald, J. F. (2010). Diarylamidines: High Potency Inhibitors of Acid-Sensing Ion Channels. *Neuropharmacology*, Vol. 58, No. 7, pp.1045-1053, ISSN 0028-3908

Chesler, M. & Chan, C.Y. (1988). Stimulus-Induced Extracellular PH Transients in the In Vitro Turtle Cerebellum. *Neuroscience*, Vol. 27, No. 3, pp. 941-948, ISSN 0306-4522

Chesler, M. & Kaila, K. (1992). Modulation of PH by Neuronal Activity. *Trends in Neuroscience*, Vol, 15, No. 10, pp. 396-402, ISSN 0166-2236

Cho, J.H. & Askwith, C.C. (2008). Presynaptic Release Probability Is Increased in Hippocampal Neurons From ASIC1 Knockout Mice. *Journal of Neurophysiology*, Vol. 99, No. 2, pp.426-441, ISSN 0022-3077

Chu, X.P.; Close, N.; Saugstad, J.A. & Xiong, Z.G. (2006). ASIC1a-Specific Modulation of Acid-Sensing Ion Channels in Mouse Cortical Neurons by Redox Reagents. *Journal of Neuroscience*, Vol. 26, No. 20, pp. 5329 – 5339, ISSN 0270-6474

Chu, X.P.; Miesch, J.; Johnson, M.; Root, L.; Zhu, X.M.; Chen, D.; Simon, R.P. & Xiong, Z.G. (2002). Proton-Gated Channels in PC12 Cells. *Journal of Neurophysiology*, Vol. 87, No. 5, pp.2555-2561, ISSN 0022-3077

Chu, X.P.; Wemmie, J.A.; Wang, W.Z.; Zhu, X.M.; Saugstad, J.A.; Price, M.P.; Simon, R.P. & Xiong, Z.G. (2004). Subunit-Dependent High-Affinity Zinc Inhibition of Acid-Sensing Ion Channels. *Journal of Neuroscience*, Vol.24, No. 40, pp. 8678 – 8689, ISSN 0270-6474

Coryell, M.W.; Wunsch, A.M.; Haenfler, J.M.; Allen, J.E.; McBride, J.L.; Davidson, B.L. & Wemmie, J.A. (2008). Restoring Acid-Sensing Ion Channel-1a in the Amygdala of Knock-out Mice Rescues Fear Memory but not Unconditioned Fear Responses. *Journal of Neuroscience*, Vol. 28, No. 51, pp. 13738-13741, ISSN 0270-6474

Coryell, M.W.; Wunsch, A.M.; Haenfler, J.M.; Allen, J.E.; Schnizler, M.; Ziemann, A.E.; Cook, M.N.; Dunning, J.P.; Price, M.P.; Rainier, J.D.; Liu, Z.; Light, A.R.; Langbehn, D.R. & Wemmie, J.A. (2009). Acid-Sensing Ion Channel-1a in the Amygdala, a Novel Therapeutic Target in Depression-Related Behavior. *Journal of Neuroscience*, Vol. 29, No. 17, pp. 5381-5388, ISSN 0270-6474

Coryell, M.W.; Ziemann, A.E.; Westmoreland, P.J.; Haenfler, J.M.; Kurjakovic, Z.; Zha, X.M.; Price, M.; Schnizler, M.K. & Wemmie, J.A. (2007). Targeting ASIC1a Reduces Innate Fear and Alters Neuronal Activity in the Fear Circuit. *Biological Psychiatry.* Vol.62, No. 10, pp.1140-1148, ISSN 0006-3223

Dauer, W. & Przedborski, S. (2003). Parkinson's Disease: Mechanisms and Models. *Neuron*, Vol. 39, No. 6, pp. 889-909, ISSN 0896-6273

Deval, E.; Noël, J.; Lay, N.; Alloui, A.; Diochot, S.; Friend, V.; Jodar, M.; Lazdunski, M. & Lingueglia, E. (2008). ASIC3, A Sensor of Acidic and Primary Inflammatory Pain. *EMBO Journal*, Vol. 27, No. 22, pp. 3047– 3055, ISSN 0261-4189

Diochot, S.; Baron, A.; Rash, L.D.; Deval, E.; Escoubas, P.; Scarzello, S.; Salinas, M. & Lazdunski, M. (2004). A New Sea Anemone Peptide, APETx2, Inhibits ASIC3, A Major Acid-Sensitive Channel in Sensory Neurons. *EMBO Journal*, Vol. 23, No.7, pp.1516-1525, ISSN 0261-4189

Deval, E.; Salinas, M.; Baron, A.; Lingueglia, E. & Lazdunski, M. (2004). ASIC2b-Dependent Regulation of ASIC3, An Essential Acid-Sensing Ion Channel Subunit in Sensory Neurons via the Partner Protein PICK-1. *Journal of Biological Chemistry*, Vol. 279, No. 19, pp. 19531-19539, ISSN 0021-9258

de Weille, J.R.; Bassilana, F.; Lazdunski, M. & Waldmann, R. (1998). Identification, Functional Expression and Chromosomal Localisation of a Sustained Human Proton-Gated Cation Channel. *FEBS Letters*, Vol.433, No.3, pp.257-60, ISSN 0014-5793

Dubé, G.R.; Lehto, S.G.; Breese, N.M.; Baker, S.J.; Wang, X.; Matulenko, M.A.; Honoré, P.; Stewart, A.O.; Moreland, R.B. & Brioni, J.D. (2005). Electrophysiological and In Vivo Characterization of A-317567, a Novel Blocker of Acid Sensing Ion Channels. *Pain*, Vol. 117, No. 1-2, pp. 88-96. ISSN 0885-3294

Dwyer, J.M.; Rizzo, S.J.; Neal, S.J.; Lin, Q.; Jow, F.; Arias, R.L.; Rosenzweig-Lipson, S.; Dunlop, J. & Beyer, C.E. (2009). Acid Sensing Ion Channel (ASIC) Inhibitors Exhibit Anxiolytic-Like Activity in Preclinical Pharmacological Models. *Psychopharmacology (Berl)*, Vol.203, No. 1, pp. 41-52, ISSN 1432-2072

Escoubas, P.; de Weille, J.R.; Lecoq, A.; Diochot, S.; Waldmann, R.; Champigny, G.; Moinier, D.; Ménez, A. & Lazdunski, M. (2000). Isolation of a Tarantula Toxin Specific for a Class of Proton-Gated Na+ Channels. *Journal of Biological Chemistry*, Vol. 275, No. 33, pp. 25116-25121, ISSN 0021-9258

Ettaiche, M.; Deval, E.; Cougnon, M.; Lazdunski, M. & Voilley, N. (2006). Silencing Acid-Sensing Ion Channel 1a Alters Cone-Mediated Retinal Function. *Journal of Neuroscience*, Vol. 26, No. 21, pp.5800-5809, ISSN 0270-6474

Ettaiche, M.; Deval, E.; Pagnotta, S.; Lazdunski, M. & Lingueglia, E. (2009). Acid-Sensing Ion Channel 3 in Retinal Function and Survival. *Investigative Ophthalmology & Visual Science*, Vol. 50, No.5, pp. 2417-2426, ISSN 0146-0404

Ettaiche, M.; Guy, N.; Hofman, P.; Lazdunski, M. & Waldmann, R. (2004). Acid-Sensing Ion Channel 2 is Important For Retinal Function and Protects Against Light-Induced Retinal Degeneration. *Journal of Neuroscience*, Vol. 24, No. 5, pp. 1005-1012, ISSN 0270-6474

Friese, M.A.; Craner, M.J.; Etzensperger, R.; Vergo, S.; Wemmie, J.A.; Welsh, M.J.; Vincent, A. & Fugger, L. (2007). Acid-Sensing Ion Channel-1 Contributes to Axonal Degeneration in Autoimmune Inflammation of the Central Nervous System. *Nature Medicine*, Vol.13, No. 12, pp.1483-1489, ISSN 1078-8956

Gao, J.; Duan, B.; Wang, D.G.; Deng, X.H.; Zhang, G.Y.; Xu, L. & Xu, T.L. (2005). Coupling Between NMDA Receptor and Acid-Sensing Ion Channel Contributes to Ischemic Neuronal Death. *Neuron*, Vol. 48, No.4, pp.635-646, ISSN 0896-6273

Garza, A.; López-Ramírez, O.; Vega, R. & Soto, E. (2010). The Aminoglycosides Modulate the Acid-Sensing Ionic Channel Currents in Dorsal Root Ganglion Neurons from the Rat. *Journal of Pharmacology & Experimental Therapeutics*, Vol. 332, No. 2, pp. 489-499. ISSN 0022-3565

Giffard, R.G.; Monyer, H. & Choi, D.W. (1990). Selective Vulnerability of Cultured Cortical Glia to Injury by Extracellular Acidosis. *Brain Research*, 1990; Vol. 530, No.1, pp. 138-141, ISSN 0006-8993

Gonzales, E.B.; Kawate, T. & Gouaux, E. (2009). Pore Architecture and Ion Sites in Acid-Sensing Ion Channels and P2X Receptors. *Nature*, Vol. 460, No. 7255, pp.599-604, ISSN 0028-0836

Grunder, S. & Chen, X. (2010). Structure, Function, and Pharmacology of Acid-Sensing Ion Channels (ASICs): Focus on ASIC1a. *International Journal of Physiology, Pathophysiology and Pharmacology*, Vol. 2, No.2 , pp. 73-94, ISSN 1944-8171

Grunder, S.; Geissler, H.S.; Bassler, E.L. & Ruppersberg, J.P. (2000). A New Member of Acid-Sensing Ion Channels from Pituitary Gland. *Neuroreport*, Vol.11, No.8, pp. 1607 – 1611, ISSN 0959-4956

Gu, L.; Liu, X.; Yang, Y.; Luo, D. & Zheng, X. (2010). ASICs Aggravate Acidosis-Induced Injuries During Ischemic Reperfusion. *Neuroscience Letters*, Vol. 479, No. 1, pp. 63-68, ISSN 0304-3940

Hattori, T.; Chen, J.; Harding, A.M.; Price, M.P.; Lu, Y.; Abboud, F.M. & Benson, C.J. (2009). ASIC2a and ASIC3 Heteromultimerize to Form PH-Sensitive Channels in Mouse Cardiac Dorsal Root Ganglia Neurons. *Circulation Research*, Vol. 105, No.3, pp. 279-286, ISSN 0009-7330

Hesselager, M.; Timmermann, D.B. & Ahring, P.K. (2004). PH Dependency and Desensitization Kinetics of Heterologously Expressed Combinations of Acid-Sensing Ion Channel Subunits. *Journal of Biological Chemistry*, Vol. 279, No. 12, pp. 11006-11015, ISSN 0021-9258

Hillered, L.; Smith, M.L. & Siesjo, B.K. (1985). Lactic Acidosis and Recovery of Mitochondrial Function Following Forebrain Ischemia in the Rat. *Journal of Cerebral Blood Flow & Metabolism*, Vol. 5, No. 2, pp.259-266, ISSN 0271-678X

Hoagland, E.N.; Sherwood, T.W.; Lee, K.G.; Walker, C.J. & Askwith, C.C. (2010). Identification of a Calcium Permeable Human Acid-Sensing Ion Channel 1 Transcript Variant. *Journal of Biological Chemistry*, Vol. 285, No. 53, pp. 41852-41862, ISSN 0021-9258

Huang, Y. & McNamara, J.O. (2004). Ischemic Stroke: "Acidotoxicity" is a Perpetrator. *Cell*, Vol. 118, No.6, pp.665-666, ISSN 0092-8674

Hruska-Hageman, A.M.; Wemmie, J.A.; Price, M.P. & Welsh, M.J. (2002). Interaction of the Synaptic Protein PICK1 (Protein Interacting with C Kinase 1) with the Non-Voltage Gated Sodium Channels BNC1 (Brain $Na^+$ Channel 1) and ASIC (Acid-Sensing Ion Channel). *Biochemical Journal*, Vol. 361, No. 3, pp. 443-450, ISSN 0264-6021

Ikeuchi, M.; Kolker, S.J. & Sluka, K.A. (2009). Acid-Sensing Ion Channel 3 Expression in Mouse Knee Joint Afferents and Effects of Carrageenan-Induced Arthritis. *Journal of Pain*, Vol.10, No. 3, pp. 336 – 342, ISSN 1256-5900

Immke, D.C. & McCleskey, E.W. (2001). Lactate Enhances the Acid-Sensing Na+ Channel on Ischemia-Sensing Neurons. *Nature Neuroscience*, Vol.4, No. 9, pp. 869-870, ISSN 1097- 6256

Jasti, J.; Furukawa, H.; Gonzales, E.B. & Gouaux, E. (2007). Structure of Acid-Sensing Ion Channel 1 at 1.9 A Resolution and Low pH. *Nature*, Vol. 449, No. 7160, pp.316-323, ISSN 0028-0836

Jetti, S.K.; Swain, S.M.; Majumder, S.; Chatterjee, S.; Poornima, V. & Bera, A.K. (2010). Evaluation of the Role of Nitric Oxide in Acid Sensing Ion Channel Mediated Cell Death. *Nitric Oxide*, Vol. 22, No. 3, pp. 213-219, ISSN 1089-8603

Jiang, Q.; Li, M.H.; Papasian, C.J.; Branigan, D.; Xiong, Z.G.; Wang, J.Q. & Chu, X.P. (2009). Characterization of Acid-Sensing Ion Channels in Medium Spiny Neurons of Mouse Striatum. *Neuroscience*, Vol.162, No.1, pp. 55 – 66, ISSN 0306-4522

Johnson, M.B.; Jin, K.; Minami, M.; Chen, D. & Simon, R.P. (2001). Global Ischemia Induces Expression of Acid-Sensing Ion Channel 2a in Rat Brain. *Journal of Cerebral Blood Flow & Metabolism*, Vol. 21, No. 6, pp.734-740, ISSN 0271-678X

Jones, N.G.; Slater, R.; Cadiou, H.; McNaughton, P. & McMahon, S.B. (2004). Acid-Induced Pain and its Modulation in Humans. *Journal of Neuroscience*, Vol.24, No. 48, pp. 10974 – 10979, ISSN 0270-6474

Kalimo, H.; Rehncrona, S.; Soderfeldt, B.; Olsson, Y. & Siesjo, B.K. (1981). Brain Lactic Acidosis and Ischemic Cell Damage: 2. Histopathology. *Journal of Cerebral Blood Flow & Metabolism*, Vol. 1, No. 3, pp.313-327, ISSN 0271-678X

Kellenberger, S. & Schild, L. (2002). Epithelial Sodium Channel/Degenerin Family of Ion Channels: a Variety of Functions for a Shared Structure. *Physiological Review*, Vol. 82, No. 3, pp. 735 – 767, ISSN 0031-9333

Kimelberg, H.K.; Barron, K.D.; Bourke, R.S.; Nelson, L.R. & Cragoe, E.J. (1990). Brain Anti-cytoxic Edema Agents. *Progress in Clinical and Biological Research* Vol. 361, No.1, pp. 363-385, ISSN 0361-7742

Krishtal, O. (2003). The ASICs: Signaling Molecules? Modulators? *Trends in Neuroscience*, Vol, 26, No. 9, pp. 477-483, ISSN 0166-2236

Li, M.; Inoue, K.; Branigan, D.; Kratzer, E.; Hansen, J.C.; Chen, J.W.; Simon, R.P. & Xiong, Z.G. (2010). Acid-Sensing Ion Channels in Acidosis-Induced Injury of Human Brain Neurons. *Journal of Cerebral Blood Flow & Metabolism*, Vol. 30, No. 6, pp.1247-1260, ISSN 0271-678X

Li, M.; Kratzer, E.; Inoue, K.; Simon, R.P. & Xiong, Z.G. (2010). Developmental Change in the Electrophysiological and Pharmacological Properties of Acid-Sensing Ion Channels in CNS Neurons. *Journal of Physiology*, Vol. 588, No.20, pp.3883-3900, ISSN 0022-3751

Lilley, S.; LeTissier, P. & Robbins, J. (2004). The Discovery and Characterization of a Proton-Gated Sodium Current in Rat Retinal Ganglion Cells. *Journal of Neuroscience*, Vol. 24, No. 5, pp. 1013 – 1022, ISSN 0270-6474

Lin, Y.W.; Min, M.Y.; Lin, C.C.; Chen, W.N.; Wu, W.L.; Yu, H.M. & Chen, C.C. (2008). Identification and Characterization of a Subset of Mouse Sensory Neurons That Express Acid-Sensing Ion Channel 3. *Neuroscience*, Vol.151, No.2, pp.544-557, ISSN 0306-4522

Lingueglia, E. (2007). Acid-Sensing Ion Channels in Sensory Perception. *Journal of Biological Chemistry*, Vol. 282, No. 24, pp. 17325–17329, ISSN 0021-9258

Lingueglia, E.; de Weille, J.R.; Bassilana, F.; Heurteaux, C.; Sakai, H.; Waldmann, R. & Lazdunski, M. (1997). A Modulatory Subunit of Acid Sensing Ion Channels in Brain and Dorsal Root Ganglion Cells. *Journal of Biological Chemistry*, Vol. 272, No. 47, pp. 29778–29783, ISSN 0021-9258

Lu, Y.; Ma, X.; Sabharwal, R.; Snitsarev, V.; Morgan, D.; Rahmouni, K.; Drummond, H.A.; Whiteis, C.A.; Costa, V.; Price, M.; Benson, C.; Welsh, M.J.; Chapleau, M.W. & Abboud, F.M. (2009). The Ion Channel ASIC2 is Required for Baroreceptor and Autonomic Control of the Circulation. *Neuron*, Vol. 64, No.6, pp. 885-897, ISSN 0896-6273

Mamet, J.; Lazdunski, M. & Voilley, N. (2003). How Nerve Growth Factor Drives Physiological and Inflammatory Expressions of Acid-Sensing Ion Channel 3 in Sensory Neurons. *Journal of Biological Chemistry*, Vol. 278, No. 49, pp. 48907 – 48913, ISSN 0021-9258

Mari, Y.; Katnik, C. & Cuevas, J. (2010). ASIC1a Channels are Activated by Endogenous Protons During Ischemia and Contribute to Synergistic Potentiation of Intracellular Ca(2+) Overload During Ischemia and Acidosis. *Cell Calcium*, Vol. 48, No. 1, pp. 70-82, ISSN 0143-4160

Maysami, S.; Branigan, D.; Simon, R.P. & Xiong, Z,G. (2009). Amyloid Beta Peptide Modulates the Activity of Acid-Sensing Ion Channels in Neurons [abstract]. 39th *Society for Neuroscience Annual Meeting*, 237.8. ISBN 0-916110-04-4, Chicago, Illinois, USA, October 17-21, 2009

Meng, Q.Y.; Wang, W.; Chen, X.N.; Xu, T.L. & Zhou, J.N. (2009). Distribution of Acid-Sensing Ion Channel 3 in the Rat Hypothalamus. *Neuroscience*, Vol. 159, No. 3, pp.1126-1134, ISSN 0306-4522

Mishra, J.; Saxena, A. & Singh, S. (2007). Chemotherapy of Leishmaniasis: Past, Present and Future. *Current Medicinal Chemistry*, Vol. 14, No. 10, pp. 1153-1169, ISSN 0929-8673

Molliver, D.C.; Immke, D.C.; Fierro, L.; Paré, M.; Rice, F.L. & McCleskey, E.W. (2005). ASIC3, An Acid-Sensing Ion Channel, is Expressed in Metaboreceptive Sensory Neurons. *Molecular Pain*, Vol.1, No. 1, pp. 35, ISSN 1744-8069

Nedergaard, M.; Kraig, R.P.; Tanabe, J. & Pulsinelli, W.A. (1991). Dynamics of Interstitial and Intracellular PH in Evolving Brain Infarct. *American Journal of Physiology*, Vol. 260, No. 3, pp. R581-R588, ISSN 0363-6119

N'Gouemo, P. (2008). Amiloride Delays the Onset of Pilocarpine-Induced Seizures in Rats. *Brain Research*, Vol. 1222, No. 1, pp. 230-232, ISSN 0006-8993

Papp, L.A.; Klein, D.F. & Gorman, J.M. (1993). Carbon Dioxide Hypersensitivity, Hyperventilation, and Panic Disorder. *American Journal of Psychiatry*, Vol. 150, No. 8, pp. 1149-1157, ISSN 0002-953X

Pidoplichko, V.I. & Dani, J.A. (2006). Acid-Sensitive Ionic Channels in Midbrain Dopamine Neurons are Sensitive to Ammonium, Which May Contribute to Hyperammonemia Damage. *Proceedings of National Academy of Science U.S.A.*, Vol. 103, No. 30, pp. 11376-11380, ISSN 0027-8424

Pignataro, G.; Simon, R.P. & Xiong, Z.G. (2007). Prolonged Activation of ASIC1a and the Time Window for Neuroprotection in Cerebral Ischaemia. *Brain*, Vol. 130, No.1, pp.151-158, ISSN 0006-8950

Pérez, M.E.; Soto, E. & Vega, R. (1991). Streptomycin Blocks the Postsynaptic Effects of Excitatory Amino Acids on the Vestibular System Primary Afferents. *Brain Research*, Vol. 563, No. 1-2, pp. 221-226, ISSN 0006-8993

Price, M.P.; Lewin, G.R.; McIlwrath, S.L.; Cheng, C.; Xie, J.; Heppenstall, P.A.; Stucky, C.L.; Mannsfeldt, A.G.; Brennan, T.J.; Drummond, H.A.; Qiao, J.; Benson, C.J.; Tarr, D.E.; Hrstka, R.F.; Yang, B.; Williamson, R.A. & Welsh, M.J. (2000). The Mammalian Sodium Channel BNC1 is Required for Normal Touch Sensation. *Nature*, Vol. 407, No. 6807, pp. 1007-1011, ISSN 0028-0836

Price, M.P.; McIlwrath, S.L.; Xie, J.; Cheng, C.; Qiao, J.; Tarr, D.E.; Sluka, K.A.; Brennan, T.J.; Lewin, G.R. & Welsh, M.J. (2001). The DRASIC Cation Channel Contributes to the Detection of Cutaneous Touch and Acid Stimuli in Mice. *Neuron*, Vol. 32, No. 6, pp. 1071-1083, ISSN 0896-6273

Price, M.P.; Snyder, P.M. & Welsh, M.J. (1996). Cloning and Expression of a Novel Human Brain Na+ Channel. *Journal of Biological Chemistry*, Vol. 271, No.14, pp.7879-7882, ISSN 0021-9258

Raisinghani, M. & Premkumar, L.S. (2005). Block of Native and Cloned Vanilloid Receptor 1 (TRPV1) by Aminoglycoside Antibiotics. *Pain*, Vol. 113, No. 1-2, pp. 123-33, ISSN 0885-3924

Rehncrona, S. (1985). Brain Acidosis. *Annals of Emergency Medicine*, Vol.14, No. 8, pp. 770-776, ISSN 0196-0644

Rehncrona, S.; Hauge, H.N. & Siesjo, B.K. (1989). Enhancement of Iron Catalyzed Free Radical Formation by Acidosis in Brain Homogenates: Differences in Effect by Lactic Acid and $CO_2$. *Journal of Cerebral Blood Flow & Metabolism*, Vol. 9, No. 1, pp. 65-70, ISSN 0271-678X

Render, J.A.; Howe, K.R.; Wunsch, A.M.; Guionaud, S.; Cox, P.J. & Wemmie, J.A. (2010). Histologic Examination of the Eye of Acid-Sensing Ion Channel 1a Knockout Mice. *International Journal of Physiology,Pathophysiology and Pharmacology*, Vol. 2, No.2 , pp. 69-72, ISSN 1944-8171

Salinas, M.; Lazdunski, M. & Lingueglia, E. (2009). Structural Elements for the Generation of Sustained Currents by the Acid Pain Sensor ASIC3. *Journal of Biological Chemistry*, Vol. 284, No., pp. 31851– 31859, ISSN 0021-9258

Schild, J.H. & Kunze, D.L. (1997). Experimental and Modeling Study of Na+ Current Heterogeneity in Rat Nodose Neurons and Its Impact on Neuronal Discharge. *Journal of Neurophysiology*, Vol. 78, No.6, pp.3198-209, ISSN 0022-3077

Sherwood, T.W. & Askwith, C.C. (2009). Dynorphin Opioid Peptides Enhance Acid-Sensing Ion Channel 1a Activity and Acidosis-Induced Neuronal Death. *Journal of Neuroscience*, Vol.29, No. 45, pp.14371-14380, ISSN 0270-6474

Sherwood, T.W.; Lee, K.G.; Gormley, M.G. & Askwith, C.C. (2011). Heteromeric Acid-Sensing Ion Channels (ASICs) Composed of ASIC2b and ASIC1a Display Novel Channel Properties and Contribute to Acidosis-Induced Neuronal Death. *Journal of Neuroscience*, Vol. 31, No. 26, pp. 9723-9734, ISSN 0270-6474

Siesjo, B.K. (1988). Acidosis and Ischemic Brain Damage. *Neurochemical Pathology* Vol. 9, No. pp.31-88, ISSN 0734-600X

Siesjo, B.K.; Katsura, K. & Kristian, T. (1996). Acidosis-Related Damage. *Advance in Neurology,* Vol. 71, No. 1, pp.209-233, ISSN 0091-3952

Simon, R.P.; Copeland, J.R.; Benowitz, N.L.; Jacob, P. III. & Bronstein, J. (1987). Brain Phenobarbital Uptake During Prolonged Status Epilepticus. *Journal of Cerebral Blood Flow & Metabolism,* Vol. 7, No. 6, pp. 783-788, ISSN 0271-678X

Simon, R.P.; Benowitz, N.; Hedlund, R. & Copeland, J. (1985). Influence of the Blood-Brain PH Gradient on Brain Phenobarbital Uptake During Status Epilepticus. *Journal of Pharmacology & Experimental Therapeutics,* Vol. 234, No. 3, pp. 830-835, ISSN 0022-3565

Sluka, K.A.; Price, M.P.; Breese, N.M.; Stucky, C.L.; Wemmie, J.A. & Welsh, M.J. (2003). Chronic Hyperalgesia Induced by Repeated Acid Injections in Muscle is Abolished by the Loss of ASIC3, but not ASIC1. *Pain,* Vol. 106, No.3, pp. 229-239, ISSN 0885-3924

Sluka, K.A.; Radhakrishnan, R.; Benson, C.J.; Eshcol, J.O.; Price, M.P.; Babinski, K.; Audette, K.M.; Yeomans, D.C. & Wilson, S.P. (2007). ASIC3 in Muscle Mediates Mechanical, but not Heat, Hyperalgesia Associated with Muscle Inflammation. *Pain,* Vol. 129, No. 1-2, pp. 102 – 112, ISSN 0885-3294

Sluka, K.A.; Winter, O.C. & Wemmie, J.A. (2009). Acid-Sensing Ion Channels: A New Target for Pain and CNS Diseases. *Current Opinion in Drug Discovery & Development,* Vol. 12, No.5, pp.693-704, ISSN 1367-6733

Somjen, G.G. (1984). Acidification of Interstitial Fluid in Hippocampal Formation Caused by Seizures and by Spreading Depression. *Brain Research,* Vol. 311, No. 1, pp. 186-188, ISSN 0006-8993

Stys, P.K. & LoPachin, R.M. (1998). Mechanisms of Calcium and Sodium Fluxes in Anoxic Myelinated Central Nervous System Axons. *Neuroscience,* Vol. 82, No. 1, pp. 21-32, ISSN

Sutherland, S.P.; Benson, C.J.; Adelman, J.P. & McCleskey, E.W. (2001). Acid-Sensing Ion Channel 3 Matches the Acid-Gated Current in Cardiac Ischemia-Sensing Neurons. *Proceedings of National Academy of Science U.S.A.,* Vol.98, No. 2, pp.711-766, ISSN 0027-8424

Swanson, R.A.; Farrell, K. & Simon, R.P. (1995). Acidosis Causes Failure of Astrocyte Glutamate Uptake During Hypoxia. *Journal of Cerebral Blood Flow & Metabolism,* Vol. 15, No. 3, pp. 417-424, ISSN 0271-678X

Tombaugh, G.C. & Sapolsky, R.M. (1993). Evolving Concepts About the Role of Acidosis in Ischemic Neuropathology. *Journal of Neurochemistry,* Vol. 61, No. 3, pp. 793-803, ISSN 0022-3042

Ugawa, S.; Ueda, T.; Ishida, Y.; Nishigaki, M.; Shibata, Y. & Shimada, S. (2002). Amiloride-Blockable Acid-Sensing Ion Channels are Leading Acid Sensors Expressed in Human Nociceptors. *Journal of Clinical Investigation,* Vol.110, No. 8, pp.1185-1190, ISSN 0021-9738

Ugawa, S.; Yamamoto, T.; Ueda, T.; Ishida, Y.; Inagaki, A.; Nishigaki, M. & Shimada, S. (2003). Amiloride-Insensitive Currents of the Acid-Sensing Ion Channel-2a

(ASIC2a)/ASIC2b Heteromeric Sour-Taste Receptor Channel. *Journal of Neuroscience*, Vol. 23, No. 9, pp. 3616-3622, ISSN 0270-6474

Urbanics, R.; Leniger-Follert, E. & Lubbers, D.W. (1978). Time Course of Changes of Extracellular $H^+$ and $K^+$ Activities During and After Direct Electrical Stimulation of the Brain Cortex. *Pflugers Archiv*, Vol. 378, No.1, pp. 47-53, ISSN 0365-267X

Varming, T. (1999). Proton-Gated Ion Channels in Cultured Mouse Cortical Neurons. *Neuropharmacology*, Vol. 38, No.12 , pp. 1875-1881, ISSN 0028-3908

Vergo, S.; Craner, M.J.; Etzensperger, R.; Attfield, K.; Friese, M.A.; Newcombe, J.; Esiri. M. & Fugger, L. (2011). Acid-Sensing Ion Channel 1 is Involved in Both Axonal Injury and Demyelination in Multiple Sclerosis and Its Animal Model. *Brain*, Vol.134, No. 2, pp. 571-584, ISSN 0006-8950

Voilley, N.; de Weille, J.; Mamet, J. & Lazdunski, M. (2001). Nonsteroid Anti-Inflammatory Drugs Inhibit Both the Activity and the Inflammation-Induced Expression of Acid-Sensing Ion Channels in Nociceptors. *Journal of Neuroscience*, Vol. 21, No. 20, pp. 8026-8033, ISSN 0270-6474

Waldmann, R.; Bassilana, F.; de Weille, J.; Champigny, G.; Heurteaux, C. & Lazdunski, M. (1997a). Molecular Cloning of a Non-Inactivating Proton-Gated Na+ Channel Specific for Sensory Neurons. *Journal of Biological Chemistry*, Vol. 272, No. 34, pp. 20975–20978, ISSN 0021-9258

Waldmann, R. & Lazdunski, M. (1998). H(+)-Gated Cation Channels: Neuronal Acid Sensors in the ENaC/DEG Family of Ion Channels. *Current Opinion in Neurobiology*, Vol. 8, No.3, pp. 418-424, ISSN 0959- 4388

Waldmann, R.; Champigny, G.; Bassilana, F.; Heurteaux, C. & Lazdunski, M. (1997b). A Proton-Gated Cation Channel Involved in Acid-Sensing. *Nature*, Vol. 386, No. 6621, pp.173-177, ISSN 0028-0836

Waldmann, R.; Champigny, G.; Voilley, N.; Lauritzen, I. & Lazdunski, M. (1996). The Mammalian Degenerin MDEG, An Amiloride-Sensitive Cation Channel Activated by Mutations Causing Neurodegeneration in Caenorhabditis Elegans. *Journal of Biological Chemistry*, Vol. 271, No. 18, pp. 10433–10436, ISSN 0021-9258

Waxman, S.G. (2006). Axonal Conduction and Injury in Multiple Sclerosis: the Role of Sodium Channels. *Nature Reviews Neuroscience*, Vol. 7, No.12, pp. 932-941, ISSN 1741-0048

Wemmie, J.A.; Askwith, C.C.; Lamani, E.; Cassell, M.D.; Freeman, J.H., Jr. & Welsh, M.J. (2003). Acid Sensing Ion Channel 1 is Localized in Brain Regions with High Synaptic Density and Contributes to Fear Conditioning. *Journal of Neuroscience*, Vol. 23, No. 13, pp.5496-5502, ISSN 0270-6474

Wemmie, J.A.; Chen. J.; Askwith, C.C.; Hruska-Hageman, A.M.; Price, M.P.; Nolan, B.C.; Yoder, P.G.; Lamani, E.; Hoshi, T.; Freeman, J.H. & Welsh, M.J. (2002). The Acid-Activated Ion Channel ASIC Contributes to Synaptic Plasticity, Learning, and Memory. *Neuron*, Vol. 34, No.3, pp.463-477, ISSN 0896-6273

Wemmie, J.A.; Coryell, M.W.; Askwith, C.C.; Lamani, E.; Leonard, A.S.; Sigmund, C.D. & Welsh, M.J. (2004). Overexpression of Acid-Sensing Ion Channel 1a in Transgenic Mice Increases Acquired Fear-Related Behavior. *Proceedings of National Academy of Science U.S.A.*, Vol. 101, No. 10, pp.3621-3626, ISSN 0027-8424

Wemmie, J.A.; Price, M.P. & Welsh, M.J. (2006). Acid-Sensing Ion Channels: Advances, Questions and Therapeutic Opportunities. *Trends in Neuroscience*, Vol. 29, No. 10, pp. 578-586, ISSN 0166-2236

Weng, J.Y.; Lin, Y.C. & Lien, C.C. (2010). Cell Type-Specific Expression of Acid-Sensing Ion Channels in Hippocampal Interneurons. *Journal of Neuroscience*, Vol. 30, No. 19, pp.6548-6558, ISSN 0270-6474

Wong, H.K.; Bauer, P.O.; Kurosawa, M.; Goswami, A.; Washizu, C.; Machida, Y.; Tosaki, A.; Yamada, M.; Knopfel, T.; Nakamura, T. & Nukina, N. (2008). Blocking Acid-Sensing Ion Channel 1 Alleviates Huntington's Disease Pathology via an Ubiquitin-Proteasome System Dependent Mechanism. *Human Molecular Genetics*, Vol.17, No. 20, pp. 3223-3235, ISSN 0964-6906

Wu, L.J.; Duan, B.; Mei, Y.D.; Gao, J.; Chen, J.G.; Zhuo, M.; Xu, L.; Wu, M. & Xu, T.L. (2004). Characterization of Acid-Sensing Ion Channels in Dorsal Horn Neurons of Rat Spinal Cord. *Journal of Biological Chemistry*, Vol. 279, No. 42, pp. 43716–43724, ISSN 0021-9258

Wu, W.L.; Lin, Y.W.; Min, M.Y. & Chen, C.C. (2010). Mice Lacking Asic3 Show Reduced Anxiety-Like Behavior on the Elevated Plus Maze and Reduced Aggression. *Genes, Brain and Behavior*, Vol. 9, No. 6, pp. 603-614, ISSN 1601-1848

Xiong, Z.G.; Chu, X.P. & Simon, R.P. (2007). Acid Sensing Ion Channels--Novel Therapeutic Targets for Ischemic Brain Injury. *Frontier in Bioscience*, Vol. 12, No. pp. 1376-1386, ISSN 1093-9946

Xiong, Z.G.; Zhu, X.M.; Chu, X.P.; Minami, M.; Hey, J., Wei, W.L.; MacDonald, J.F.; Wemmie, J.A.; Price, M.P.; Welsh, M.J. & Simon, R.P. (2004). Neuroprotection in Ischemia: Blocking Calcium Permeable Acid-Sensing Ion Channels, *Cell*, Vol. 118, No.6, pp. 687-698, ISSN 0092-8674

Xiong, Z.G.; Pignataro, G.; Li, M.; Chang, S.Y. & Simon, R.P. (2008). Acid-Sensing Ion Channels (ASICs) as Pharmacological Targets for Neurodegenerative Diseases. *Current Opinion in Pharmacology*, Vol.8, No. 1, pp.25-32, ISSN 1471- 4892

Xu, T.L. & Xiong, Z.G. (2007). Dynamic Regulation of Acid-Sensing Ion Channels by Extracellular and Intracellular Modulators. *Current Medicinal Chemistry*, Vol. 14, No.16, pp.1753-1763, ISSN 0929-8673

Yagi, J.; Wenk, H.N.; Naves, L.A. & McCleskey, E.W. (2006). Sustained Currents Through ASIC3 Ion Channels at the Modest pH Changes that Occur During Myocardial Ischemia. *Circulation Research*, Vol.99, No. 5, pp. 501 – 509, ISSN 0009-7330

Yermolaieva, O.; Leonard, A.S.; Schnizler, M.K.; Abboud, F.M. & Welsh, M.J. (2004). Extracellular Acidosis Increases Neuronal Cell Calcium by Activating Acid-Sensing Ion Channel 1a. *Proceedings of National Academy of Science U.S.A.*, Vol. 101, No. 17, pp.6752-6757, ISSN 0027-8424

Zha, X.M.; Costa, V.; Harding, A.M.; Reznikov, L.; Benson, C.J. & Welsh, M.J. (2009). ASIC2 Subunits Target Acid-Sensing Ion Channels to the Synapse via an Association with PSD-95. *Journal of Neuroscience*, Vol. 29, No. 26, pp. 8438 – 8446, ISSN 0270-6474

Zha, X.M.; Wemmie, J.A.; Green, S.H. & Welsh, M.J. (2006). Acid-Sensing Ion Channel 1A is a Postsynaptic Proton Receptor That Affects the Density of Dendritic Spines. *Proceedings of National Academy of Science U.S.A.*, Vol. 103, No. 44, pp. 16556-16561, ISSN 0027-8424

Zhou, Y. & Zhao, Z.Q. (2002). Effects of Neomycin on High-Threshold Ca(2+) Currents and Tetrodotoxin-Resistant Na(+) Currents in Rat Dorsal Root Ganglion Neuron. *European Journal of Pharmacology,* Vol. 450, No. 1, pp. 29-35, ISSN 0014-2999

Ziemann, A.E.; Allen, J.E.; Dahdaleh, N.S.; Drebot, I.I.; Coryell, M.W.; Wunsch, A.M.; Lynch, C.M.; Faraci, F.M.; Howard, M.A. III; Welsh, M.J. & Wemmie, J.A. (2009). The Amygdala is a Chemosensor that Detects Carbon Dioxide and Acidosis to Elicit Fear Behavior. *Cell,* Vol.139, No. 5, pp.1012-1021, ISSN 0092-8674

Ziemann, A.E.; Schnizler, M.K.; Albert, G.W.; Severson, M.A.; Howard, M.A. III.; Welsh, M.J. & Wemmie, J.A. (2008). Seizure Termination by Acidosis Depends on ASIC1a. *Nature Neuroscience,* Vol.11, No.7, pp. 816-822, ISSN 1097- 6256

# 6

# Immunization with Neural-Derived Peptides as a Potential Therapy in Neurodegenerative Diseases

Humberto Mestre and Antonio Ibarra
*Universidad Anahuac Mexico Norte*
*Mexico*

## 1. Introduction

There is a nosological dilemma when it comes to classifying what comprises a neurodegenerative disease (NDD). Degeneration – purely speaking – is to go from a higher to a lower level of functioning; it is deterioration from normalcy. Neurons are the functional elements of the nervous system. Then degeneration of the nervous system consists of a decrease or loss in the function of neurons. Not necessarily an atrophy, which consists of the death of a particular population of neurons. Clinically, NDD are comprised of progressive dementias, progressive ataxias, disorders in posture and movement, muscle weakness, and progressive blindness. The common characteristic in all of these pathologies is their chronicity. Each and every one of the aforementioned diseases consists of a chronic progression towards the loss of a particular function. However, this definition does not include a limit on temporality. Nosologically speaking neurodegeneration could include several other pathologies from an acute time frame. NDD can further be divided into an acute and chronic classification. Chronic diseases such as: amyotrophic lateral sclerosis (ALS), Alzheimer disease (AD) and Parkinson disease (PD) were the common conception of NDD. The latter was sustained until acute traumatic injuries to the central nervous system (CNS) were found to cause generalized inflammation and other phenomena that lead to degeneration. Examples of CNS injury that cause this secondary degeneration are: global or focal cerebral ischemia (stroke), spinal cord injury (SCI), and traumatic brain injury (TBI). The similarities in neurodegenerative processes between these and chronic NDD allows us to classify them within acute NDD. Neurodegeneration previously consisted of progressive atrophic disorders but has now expanded into the study of all pathophysiological processes that deteriorate the CNS. As a whole, NDD are the cause of many deaths around the world. In the US, stroke, traumatic injuries (such as: SCI and TBI), AD, and PD are within the top 15 causes of mortality, averaging 350,000 deaths per year (Xu et al., 2007). Although NDD have an elevated mortality their greatest impact is on morbidity, affecting 50 million Americans each year and generating a large amount of federal spending (Brown et al., 2005). Every year $144 billion USD are spent on AD alone, and that is excluding the spending required for the other 600 neurological disorders that have been described (Alzheimer's Association, 2010; Meek et al., 1998). The elevated prevalence and incidence require a large initiative to research the hallmarks of these diseases. Until now, our understanding of NDD is quite complex but there is still a lot to uncover. Research is normally directed towards the NDD with the most impact on society such as: ALS, AD and PD. Due to the increased availability of information on the previous diseases this chapter will only discuss these diseases within the chronic NDD section. In order to find treatment opportunities for each one of these diseases we must first understand the basic pathophysiology. ALS is a progressive degeneration of upper and lower motor neurons in the brain and spinal cord. This atrophy eliminates the brain's control over muscle movements and causes them to weaken and become paralyzed. Progressive muscular paralysis causes the inability to move, swallow, and eventually, breathe (Angelov et al., 2003). AD is a progressive disorder characterized by memory loss and severe cognitive decline. This degeneration is caused by excessive accumulations of extracellular amyloid beta peptide, which forms plaques in the hippocampus and cerebral cortex, leading to neuronal death (Frenkel et al., 2005; Butovsky et al., 2006). PD is a chronic progressive disease characterized by motor symptoms (tremor, rigidity and bradykinesia) and nonmotor symptoms (e.g. autonomic, mood and cognitive). These clinical hallmarks are attributed to the degeneration of nigrostraital dopaminergic neurons and other structures in the brainstem, cortex, and subcortex (Laurie et al., 2007). Multiple sclerosis (MS) is an inflammatory autoimmune CNS demyelinating disease that is thought to be perpetrated by myelin-reactive lymphocytes. Demyelination of the CNS causes the loss of function of the affected tract (Stuve et al., 2006). MS is considered an autoimmune disease and not a NDD because there is no direct neuronal death only demyelination. The nosology of NDD excludes MS from our study but it still shares very similar immune pathophysiology and most of the therapies mentioned are derived or designed for use in MS. The inflammatory component of acute injury to the CNS provided new insight into the autoimmune response propagated after a CNS insult. These findings gave immune cells a crucial role in the protection and regeneration of the injured CNS, as well as a role in chronic progressive NDD. Further insight into the immunological component of neurodegenerative diseases provides us with new mechanisms where we are able to intervene in order to resolve these disorders. One of these mechanisms is protective autoimmunity (PA). PA is a new concept where autoreactive mechanisms are being modulated in order to promote neuroprotection. Dr. Michal Schwartz from the Weizmann Institute of Science in Israel originally conceived this concept. Infiltration of immune cells after CNS injury was traditionally regarded as pathological. This view was based on the fact that immune cell-infiltration has been exclusively identified with inflammation, and that inflammation is generally harmful to the injured CNS. However, recent studies indicate that a well-controlled innate and adaptive immune response is essential for the repair of the injured tissue. These results brought about research into immunomodulatory therapies in several NDD. In acute NDD and MS, recent findings have suggested that the inflammatory response is strongly modulated by an autoimmune reaction directed against neural constituents, specifically against myelin basic protein (MBP), one of the most abundant and immunogenic proteins in the CNS (Butovsky et al., 2001; Ibarra et al., 2003; Popovich et al., 1996; Sospedra & Martin, 2005). Dr. Schwartz started to modulate the action of myelin-specific autoreactive lymphocytes by immunizing with MBP. This strategy improved tissue preservation, neuronal survival and motor recovery after acute SCI (Hauben et al., 2000a; Hauben et al., 2000b). PA also proved to be a T cell-dependent response that is genetically determined (Kipnis et al., 2001) and triggered as a physiological response to CNS trauma (Yoles et al., 2001). However, immunizing animals with self-antigens (i.e. MBP) induced an autoimmune disease known as experimental autoimmune encephalomyelitis (EAE, animal model of MS). Therefore, a different way of eliciting PA had to be obtained in order to prevent this complication. Studies suggested that immunizing with a weaker version of the self-antigen could solve the problem, these type of antigens became known as altered peptide ligands (APL). Vaccinating with APL would generate PA without degenerative autoimmunity. In the study of NDD, APL were derived from neural constituents and were therefore coined under the term neural-derived peptides (NDP). The success in the development of these immunomodulatory peptides has inspired a lot of research into their possible therapeutic applications in both chronic and acute NDD. These applications will be described in detail throughout this chapter.

## 2. Role of immune cells and their potential therapeutic effect

The CNS has long been considered to be an immunologically privileged location. The blood-brain barrier (BBB) was thought to maintain blood-borne cells of both the innate and adaptive immune system out of the CNS. This hypothesis assumed that microglia were the only innate immune cells of the CNS. During damage, microglia became activated and functioned as destructive inflammatory cells indistinguishable from infiltrating macrophages. Immune cells were thought to contribute to the increase in tissue damage during CNS disease (Bethea et al., 1998; Blight, 1992; Dusart et al., 1994; Popovich et al., 1997). The idea was supported by the following: i) CNS trauma activates T lymphocytes against neural constituents, and ii) the passive transfer of myelin autoreactive T cells caused EAE in previously healthy rats (Popovich et al., 1996). The notion was sustained in such a way that the complete inhibition of these responses was proposed as a potential therapeutic intervention, and remains to this day as the predominant clinical approach (Lopez-Vales et al., 2005; Popovich et al., 1999). However, it is now clear that these cells have a pivotal role in CNS repair (Hammarberg et al., 2000; Hashimoto et al., 2007; Hendrix & Nitsch, 2007; Moalem et al., 1999; Rapalino et al., 1998; Turrin & Rivest, 2006; Yin et al., 2003). In the healthy CNS the microglia is in a resting state where its morphology consists of a small cell soma and numerous branching processes, known as resting/ramified state. The ramifications are dynamic structures that enable the cell to sample and monitor its microenvironment (Nimmerjahn et al., 2005; Raivich, 2005). Resting microglia express CD45 (leukocyte common antigen), CD14, and CD11b/CD18 (Kreutzberg, 1996). Under duress, microglial expression patterns are modified from a monitoring role to one of protection and repair. Microglia begin to express key surface receptors such as: CD1, lymphocyte function-associated antigen 1 (LFA-1), intracellular adhesion molecule 1 (ICAM-1), and vascular cell adhesion molecule 1 (VCAM-1). Besides changing their surface receptor repertoire they begin to secrete: inflammatory cytokines such as TNFα and interleukins IL-1β and IL-6, chemokines like macrophage inflammatory protein (MIP-1α), monocyte chemoattractant protein (MCP-1), and interferon inducible protein 10 (IP-10). This change in microenvironment changes the resting/ramified state of the microglia into an amoeboid/phagocytic state. The activated state of microglia has beneficial functions during NDD such as: scavenging neurotoxins, removing cellular debris, and the secretion of trophic factors that promote neuronal survival (Frank-Cannon et al., 2009). During CNS injury, if microglia come in contact with products of the adaptive immune response such as interferon gamma (IFN-γ) and IL-4 it will acquire a phenotype that has antigen presenting cell (APC)-like qualities. This phenotype expresses major histocompatibility complex II (MHC-II) and B 7.2 receptors, giving it the ability to interact with elements of the adaptive immune response. As an APC, microglia can hold dialogue with T cells and are capable of releasing neurotrophic factors (BDNF, NT-3, NGF) and scavenging toxic neurotransmitters and reactive oxygen species (ROS) that endanger the tissue (Li et al., 2007; Schwartz et al., 2003). However, the chronic and uncontrolled activation of microglia increases the permeability of the BBB and elevates the amount of infiltrating blood-borne immune cells (Schmid et al., 2009). This promotes the activation of microglial cells into a destructive phenotype characterized by the production of high levels of nitric oxide (NO, a potent free radical), as well as TNFα, and cyclooxygenase 2 (COX2) (Franciosi et al., 2005; Lee et al., 2007; Shaked et al., 2004). In this phenotype microglia express low amounts of MHC-II and are thus incapable of communicating with the adaptive immune system, an important condition to promote neuroprotection (Schwartz et al., 2003; Shaked et al., 2004). In addition, T lymphocytes are recruited in small amounts and very late. The lack of T cell-mediated activation of microglia results in an uncoordinated release of additional pro-inflammatory cytokines, exacerbating the damage (Bethea et al., 1999; Lopez-Vales et al., 2006; Pan et al., 2003; Resnick et al., 1998; Schwartz et al., 2003; Vanegas & Schaible, 2001). The best way to elicit a T cell-mediated activation of microglial cells is through neural autoreactive T cells. This assures that T cells arrive to the CNS and activate microglia into their protective phenotype propagating the beneficial effects mentioned above (Figure 1). PA has proven to yield clinical improvements in the treatment of several NDD.

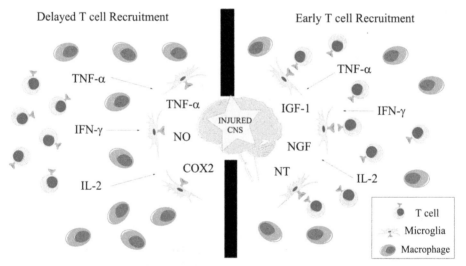

Fig. 1. T cell recruitment into the injured CNS

*Left panel:* An uncontrolled response where T cells are recruited very late allows the activation of microglia into a destructive phenotype. This is characterized by the release of nitric oxide (NO) and proinflammatory molecules like tumor necrosis factor alfa (TNF-α) and cyclooxygenase-2 (COX2). Under these circumstances, T cells intensify the inflammatory response and exacerbate neurodegeneration. *Right panel:* When the autoreactive response is elicited by immunizing with NDP there is an earlier and larger arrival of T cells. With this approach, microglial cells undergo a T cell-mediated activation into a protective phenotype. This regulated activation releases molecules that promote neuroprotection and neuroregeneration such as: neurotrophins (NT), nerve growth factor (NGF), and insulin-like growth factor 1 (IGF-1). The early arrival of T cells due to immunization with NDP regulates the response so that we can obtain the benefits and not the detriments of the immune response.

## 3. Modulation of the immune response using neural-derived peptides

Immunomodulation is an idea from the past that looks more promising than ever. It is a change in the body's normal physiological immune response to a specific antigen. This modulation changes the way the immune system would normally respond to an event and replaces it with an alternate desired response. The modification of immune responses is different from agents that suppress the immune response (such as corticosteroids). Immunomodulation has already become a reality. For example, IFN-γ is used in patients with chronic granulomatous disease (Farhoudi et al., 2003), IFN-β is used in patients with multiple sclerosis (Kumpfel et al., 2007), and IL-2 in patients with AIDS and metastatic melanoma (Davey et al., 1997; Terando et al., 2003). Aside from this, numerous vaccines use adjuvants to achieve the desired immune response (Partidos et al., 2004; Petrovsky & Aguilar, 2004). Modulation of the immune response as a therapeutic strategy is a promising alternative for several diseases. PA allows us to speculate that it is better to modulate the immune response rather than eliminating it. In chronic NDD, patients require a competent immune response to fend off pathogens and evade complications due to infections. The ablation of the immune response is usually done with steroids or immunosuppressants, which severely affect the patient's ability to initiate an adequate immune response. In the acute form of NDD the immune system is vital in the return to homeostasis. Immune cells extract cellular debris, reestablish blood flow, secrete neurotrophic factors and eliminate pathogens. All these beneficial effects are lost when the immune response is inhibited using immunosuppressant therapy. Accordingly, it seems only logical that the immune response is essential in NDD. In line with this, it is realistic to envision that the harmful effects exerted by immune cells could be reverted or changed to promote beneficial actions. In order to achieve this goal, it is crucial to avoid or at least diminish the activation of microglial cells by means of the classic pathway (destructive phenotype). For this purpose, an earlier and larger arrival of T cells to the site of injury should be promoted. The opportune and adequate arrival of these cells will favor the activation of microglia under the bases of a protective phenotype (Shaked et al., 2004). A simple way of making this possible is by immunizing with the same antigen that induces the autoreactive response: neural antigens. With this approach, an important number of microglial cells will acquire the protective phenotype and will then release molecules that instead of increasing damage will promote neuroprotection. Thus, we will obtain the benefits and not the detriments of this immune response. The present strategy proposes the modulation of the immunological response by boosting an autoreactive reaction. This could be a bit conflicting for general understanding since it is common to associate autoimmunity with disease. However, at present, it is very clear that autoimmunity is a physiological phenomenon perfectly compatible with homeostasis (Schwartz & Cohen, 2000). Furthermore, autoimmunity has been proposed as a useful and beneficial event (Hauben et al., 2005). Therefore, PA is a protective strategy where autoimmunity is the main player in providing beneficial effects during CNS injury.

## 4. Modulation of protective autoimmunity with no risk of autoimmune disease

As it was mentioned before, the possibility of inducing an autoimmune disease after vaccination with neural constituents is perhaps the main complication of this therapy. In order to solve this issue, immunizations are done with NDP. NDP are analogs of immunogenic epitopes with one (or a few) substitution(s) at specific amino acid positions of neural peptides (NP). The variation between the amino acid sequence is essential for contact with the T cell receptor (TCR) during antigen processing. This variation allows them to compete for TCR binding and to interfere with the necessary sequence of events required for T cell activation. The interference caused by NDP in TCR antigen recognition could affect T cell differentiation or induce a state of anergy (Nel & Slaughter, 2002). The specificity and avidity of the TCR with its ligand is determined by the primary sequence of the antigenic peptide. That particular sequence affects its binding to the complementary-determining regions of the TCR and the peptide-binding groove of the HLA molecule (Garboczi et al., 1996). A small variation in amino acid sequence can alter its ability to interact with either the MHC-II or TCR receptor molecule. This competition thereby converts an agonist peptide into a partial agonist or even an antagonist (Jameson & Bevan, 1995). Agonist peptides engage in high-affinity interactions with the TCR and induce a robust T cell response; whereas partial agonists or antagonists engage in lower affinity interactions that lead to altered or inhibitory responses (Jameson & Bevan, 1995; Kersh & Allen, 1996). Stimulation of naïve CD4+ T cells with an agonist peptide induces sufficient assembly of signaling complexes to allow activation of the IL-2 promoter and support a Th1 differentiation pathway. In contrast, the signals generated by APL activation are generally insufficient to induce IL-2 synthesis and therefore will not cause activation. That lack of IL-2 production might induce an anergic state or a skewing of the Th1/Th2 differentiation (Nel & Slaughter, 2002). Some APL are already being explored for neurological diseases (Figure 2). These peptides are derived from MBP-encephalitogenic epitopes. A group of them (G91, A96 and A91) have already been tested in animal models (Hauben et al., 2001). Importantly, immunized animals did not present clinical signs of EAE. A91 is a peptide derived from MBP (sequence 87-99), where the lysine residue at position 91 is replaced for alanine. This NDP cross-reacts with the original encephalitogenic epitope of MBP but it activates weak self-reactive T cells thus inducing autoimmunity without developing EAE. Immunizing with A91 inhibits EAE but neither causes anergy nor clonal deletion (Gaur et al., 1997). During antigenic presentation, A91 works as a partial agonist that instead of inducing a Th1 response promotes a Th2 differentiation pathway. This preference for the Th2 phenotype may be responsible for the elimination of the Th1-dependent response observed in EAE. Studies also indicate that post-injury injection of bone marrow-derived dendritic cells pulsed with A91, induce the same significant beneficial effects (Hauben et al., 2003). This indicates that the APC properties of the dendritic cell are enough to activate anti-A91 CD4+ T cells that are responsible for the elevated neuroprotection. To further support the use of immunomodulatory NDP, our laboratory examined the effects of combining immunizations with A91 and methylprednisolone (MP). The use of corticosteroids, such as MP, is the only therapeutic agent currently available for the treatment of a variety of NDD, primarily CNS trauma. In our study, a high dose of MP was administered together with an A91 immunization after SCI. As expected, MP eliminated the beneficial effects of A91. Nevertheless, when vaccination with A91 was delayed for 48 h after injury, there was no interference with its effect by the anti-inflammatory action of MP injected immediately after

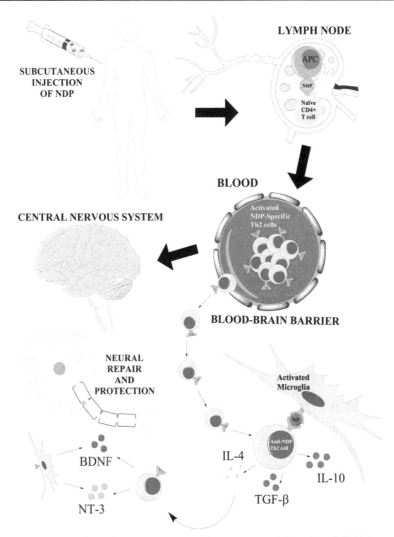

Fig. 2. Immunization with NDP causes repair and protection of the injured CNS Immunizing with NDP causes a peculiar adaptive immune response. The similarity of NDP with neural peptides (NP) causes T cell activation to deviate towards a Th2 phenotype. These NDP-reactive T cells are released into systemic blood flow where they can hone towards the site of injury. Once these autoreactive T cells infiltrate into the CNS, they come in contact with glial cells and activate microglia into a neuroprotective phenotype. Activated microglia function as antigen presenting cells (APC) and present NP to anti-NDP Th2 cells producing anti-inflammatory cytokines like interleukin- 4 and -10 (IL-4, IL-10) and transforming growth factor beta (TGF-β). This T cell-mediated anti-inflammatory effect further ameliorates the degenerative phenomena developed after CNS insult. These cells have also been shown to produce neurotrophic factors implicated in neuroregeneration like neurotrophin-3 (NT-3) and brain-derived neurotrophic factor (BDNF)

SCI (Ibarra et al., 2004). This finding suggests that vaccination with A91 is neuroprotective even if administered 48 h after injury, and that the effect of MP over the immune system is transient and does not interfere with later therapy even if that treatment is immune related. These results offer another interesting benefit of NDP-induced PA, and that is the clinical plausibility of these therapies. In the clinical setting, CNS trauma and pathology is diagnosed long after the moment of incidence. NDP-induced PA is functional even when administered 48 h after the development of NDD and works as an adjuvant in traditional clinical treatment protocols (MP administration post-CNS trauma). It appears that the beneficial effect of the vaccination with A91 will not necessarily be neutralized by concomitant treatment with MP. It is worth mentioning that one of the most prevailing adverse effects observed after NDP immunization is immediate-type hypersensitivity reactions. This undesirable effect is generally associated with the immune deviation toward Th2 phenotype. These observations should stimulate further research into which patients are most likely to benefit from this therapy. Taking into consideration all of the data, therapeutic vaccination with NDP appears to be a promising strategy that could be adapted for treatment in several NDD.

## 5. Effect of immunizing with neural-derived peptides

In the study of neuroprotection, the term autoreactivity is immediately associated with increased cell death, inhibition of neuroprotective mechanisms and a worse clinical outcome after CNS injury. However, our understanding of the immune system's role in the pathological CNS has changed drastically in the last couple of years. The old school of thought indicated that the immune response was responsible for the exacerbation of neurodestructive phenomenon, so the first line of defense was immunosuppression. The recent findings of PA suggested that the immune response was not only needed after an insult to the CNS but it also had a beneficial neuroprotective role in most NDD. This radical change in information forces us to reevaluate the existing treatment protocols for all NDD. If PA is present in a number of CNS diseases then the use of NDP immunizations is a reasonable treatment option. The use of NDP-induced PA results in the generation of a prevalent Th2 phenotype. These cell types have shown to have the most overwhelming neuroprotective effect in the CNS. The influential roles that these cells have on the outcome of disease have made them the goal of therapy development. The increase in Th2-inducing interventions has been studied in ALS, AD, PD, SCI, TBI, and stroke; it has even been proposed as a treatment for neurodevelopmental disorders such as Rett syndrome (Ben-Zeev et al., 2011). There are many different approaches to the induction of autoreactive Th2 lymphocytes some of these are: glatiramer acetate (GA, Coplymer-1, Cop-1, Copaxone), A91, poly-YE, p472 (Nogo-A-derived peptide). However, the only FDA-approved use of NDP-induced PA is GA under the brand name Copaxone for the treatment of MS. GA, also known as Cop-1, is the most studied of all APL-based therapies. Cop-1 is a synthetic polypeptide consisting of the amino acids tyrosine, glutamate, alanine and lysine that shows cross-reactivity with MBP (Schori et al., 2001; Kipnis & Schwartz, 2002). While the exact mechanism of Cop-1 is still not clearly elucidated, there is reason to believe that it induces Th2 differentiation, which later goes on to mediate neuroprotection (Aharoni et al., 2003; Aharoni et al., 2000). Although Th2 induction is the primary effect, immunization with Cop-1 also results in a Th1 cell deviation. This effect may seem paradoxical in nature but these pro-inflammatory Th1 cells are responsible for a sustained release of BDNF, NT-3, and NT-4

(Ziemssen, 2002, 2005). This Th1-mediated effect also induces astrocyte and neuronal production of these neurotrophic factors through a bystander effect (Aharoni et al., 2005). However, the effect of Cop-1 is not only mediated by its direct effect on CD4+ lymphocytes but also of its effect on APC, especially dendritic cells (DC). A recent study demonstrated that Cop-1 induced a Th2 response by modulating the APC function of DC. They demonstrated that DC exposed to Cop-1 during maturation had an impaired capacity of secreting IL-17p70 (the main Th1-polarizing cytokine). This effect resulted in the induction of a population with an increased frequency of effector Th2 cells that secreted IL-4 (Sanna et al., 2006; Vieira et al., 2003). Although the main components of NDP-induced PA are superficially understood, more research initiatives should be taken to better understand the therapeutic potential of these peptides. Most of the studies published use Cop-1 as the NDP, but the use of alternate peptide sequences such as A91 must be better understood. Nonetheless, there should be a constant effort to develop shorter, cheaper and more efficacious peptide sequences so that the true potential of NDP can be unlocked. Few studies have been conducted on the use of NDP in NDD.

## 5.1 Chronic neurodegenerative diseases
### 5.1.1 Amyotrophic lateral sclerosis
There have been many attempts to halt the progression of ALS by blocking different mediators of cytotoxicity (Ludolph et al., 2000). Because not all ALS patients have the defective SOD1 gene, motor neuron death is taken as the hallmark of disease because it is common to all cases of ALS. The animal model of ALS is acute peripheral nerve axotomy (Liu & Martin, 2001; Martin et al., 2000). The only drug currently used to slow down the progression of ALS is riluzole. Riluzole blocks the release of the excitatory neurotransmitter glutamate that can be toxic in elevated concentrations and is fundamental to ALS pathophysiology (Doble & Kennel, 2000; Meininger et al., 2000). In this study conducted by Angelov *et al.*, mice treated with Cop-1 (using a different regimen than MS) show more motor neuron survival in the acute and chronic phases of ALS (Angelov et al., 2003). In the study, mice were subjected to a unilateral facial nerve axotomy. They were then immunized with Cop-1 and assessed. The results showed that vaccination with Cop-1 protected against motor neuron death induced after facial nerve axotomy. Transection of the facial nerve in the adult mouse is known to cause an easily visible late degeneration of axotomized motor neurons (Sendtner et al., 1996). Eight weeks after axotomy, mice immunized with Cop-1 had significantly larger numbers of motor neurons compared to PBS-immunized controls. Studies also indicated that immunization with Cop-1 preserved the activity of axotomized motor neurons. The study concluded that there was an elevated preservation of facial nerve motor neurons but the next step was to confirm that these were still functional. Using biometrical analysis of the mice's whisking patterns they found that Cop-1-treated animals exhibited significantly better facial nerve functionality than controls. The previous results demonstrated that Cop-1-immunized ALS mice benefited from improved motor neuron survival and the preservation of their function after facial nerve axotomy. A mice strain that expresses human mutant SOD1 gene develops a motor disease that closely resembles human ALS. The loss of motor function eventually causes death because of the lack of muscular respiratory control. Angelov *et al.* concluded that treatment with Cop-1 immunizations resulted in an increased survival of the ALS mice. Immunizations with Cop-1 proved to be an adequate and efficacious therapy in an animal model of ALS. A small phase II study was held in human patients with ALS that finished with inconclusive results.

Most patients demonstrated adverse reactions at the site of immunization and elevated lymphocyte proliferation. Although the results showed promise, efforts must be taken to increase the sample size and scrutinize the possible mechanisms through which Cop-1 exerts its protective effects (Gordon et al., 2006). These small but conclusive examples of NDP-induced PA in ALS provide us with enough proof to understand the possible therapeutic advantages. The study of Cop-1 in ALS is still in its beginning and should therefore be a priority in the coming years for NDD researchers. The maximal benefits of PA in ALS have not yet been achieved.

### 5.1.2 Alzheimer disease

Previous studies proved that immunotherapy in AD via amyloid beta (Aβ) antibodies reduced the levels of Aβ plaques in transgenic mice. However, a human trial with Aβ antibodies caused severe adverse reactions in the form of meningoencephalitis (Nicoll et al., 2003; Orgogozo et al., 2003). A study done by Frenkel et al. postulated that meningoencephalitis was very similar to EAE. They decided to test if amyloid precursor protein-transgenic (APP-Tg) mice were more susceptible to develop EAE. They concluded that EAE lowered the levels of Aβ in APP-Tg mice using antibody-independent mechanisms. As a follow-up they decided to see if they could achieve the low Aβ levels without causing EAE. GA or Cop-1 was an FDA-approved treatment for relapsing-remitting MS and was known to cause an autoreactive response without developing EAE. They were able to reproduce the amyloid load achieved in EAE using immunization with GA (Frenkel et al., 2005). Butovsky et al performed a more directed study, towards the analysis of PA in AD. This work found that Aβ activated microglia supports neurogenesis when stimulated by IL-4. This means that a Th2 phenotype will result in the overexpression of IL-4 and increased neurogenesis after microglial activation with Aβ. Vaccination with autoreactive T cells besides aiding in neurogenesis helped in the elimination of the Aβ plaque in APP-Tg mice. The increase in neurogenesis and the removal of the Aβ plaques resulted in the counteraction of the cognitive decline normally seen in AD (Butovsky et al., 2006). The vaccination with NDP has proven to be of paramount importance in the treatment of yet another NDD. This data is also an indicator of the urgency with which these therapies should be developed, standardized, and translated into clinical trials where they can bear fruits to human disease.

### 5.1.3 Parkinson disease

Immunological studies in PD are controversial. The animal model is 1-methyl-4-phenyl-1,2,3,6-tetrahydropyridine (MPTP) intoxication (Benner et al., 2004; Laurie et al., 2006). This intoxication depletes dopaminergic neurons in the substantia nigra pars compacta (SNpc), simulating PD. The complication arises because MPTP toxicity also destroys the animal's immune system, causing significant changes in spleen size and diminished numbers of CD3+ T cells 7 days after intoxication (Benner et al., 2004). The alterations in normal immune response impede the researcher's ability to analyze the role of the immune system in PD. However, researchers bypass this complication by cell subset replacements. The use of NDP in PD has been briefly evaluated by several studies from the same laboratory. All studies use the MPTP toxicity model of PD and use adoptive transfer of T cells from Cop-1-immunized mice. In the first study of Benner et al. Cop-1-immunity was found to confer dopaminergic neuroprotection after MPTP intoxication. Animals that received the adoptive transfer of

Cop-1-reactive T cells exhibited a much smaller reduction in the number of SNpc dopaminergic neurons. For the functional analysis of dopaminergic circuits they quantified tyrosine hydroxylase (TH) density. The loss of TH density was significantly less in Cop-1-immunized mice than in controls. Unfortunately, even in Cop-1 immunized mice, the loss of TH density was up to 72%. However, the conclusion was that Cop-1-reactive T cell passive immunization protected neuronal dopamine metabolism as well as structural neuronal elements and its projections. Complementary analysis stated that transferred lymphocytes were readily observed both in ventral midbrains and striata of MPTP mice. The study was also interested in evaluating microglial activation due to the fact that these cells are considered to be pathological in this NDD. To assess microglial activation they analyzed the Mac-1 gene using real time RT-PCR. Results showed that Cop-1 splenocytes are capable of attenuating MPTP-induced microglial reactions and in turn limiting their neurodestructive processes. In accordance to previously demonstrated concepts, the beneficial effects of Cop-1 immunizations were T cell-dependent. Treatment with NDP also increased the expression of the neurotrophic factor GDNF. All results demonstrate the beneficial effects of immunizing with Cop-1 in PD (Benner et al., 2004). A similar study by Laurie et al. corroborated the results observed by Benner and co-workers. Although similar results were obtained, the latter was able to recollect new data. The study concluded that anti-Cop-1 CD4+ T cell transfer into MPTP intoxicated mice exerted its reparative effects in a dose dependent manner. Also this study attributed the neuroprotection to a particular subset of T lymphocytes, CD4+ T cells. This further implicated T helper cells as the main player in PA. In order to support that PA is T cell-dependent, authors' transplanted Cop-1 specific antibodies to MPTP intoxicated mice to see if this conferred neuroprotection, as expected the effects of Cop-1 are CD4+ T cell-dependent (Laurie et al., 2006). This study reiterates the outstanding potential that NDP-induced PA holds in the outcome of PD. Nonetheless, this topic deserves more investigation as to identify the effect of a normal functional immune system and not just the evaluation through substitution studies.

## 5.2 Acute neurodegenerative diseases
### 5.2.1 Cerebral ischemia
Immunization with NDP has also proved to be beneficial in cases of focal and global cerebral ischemia. There have been several studies of oral and nasal tolerization with neural constituents (Becker et al., 1997; Frenkel et al., 2003); however, only a few have resorted to NDP. There are primarily two studies that analyze the effects of this Th2-induced response after middle cerebral artery occlusion. The first by Ziv et al. used poly-YE, a high molecular weight (22 to 45 kDa) copolymer that was shown to exert modulatory effects on the immune system (Cady et al., 2000; Vidovic & Matzinger, 1988). This peptide demonstrated abilities to downregulate regulatory T cell functions and allows effector T cell activation. The study showed that a single immunization with poly-YE produced long-lasting clinical and behavioral benefits, along with neuroprotection and increased neurogenesis, starting from the subacute phase. They also found that poly-YE was beneficial even when administered 24 hours after occlusion. The effects of poly-YE immunization were long lasting as animals showed less residual impairment against controls even after 6 weeks. Histological analysis indicated that poly-YE attenuated cell loss in the hippocampus where PBS-treated rats showed large numbers of necrotic cells. The reduction in cell necrosis induced by poly-YE was so dramatic that the ipsilateral and contralateral sides were indistinguishable.

Immunization with poly-YE had a significant neuroprotective effect after stroke, but authors' also wanted to evaluate its neuroregenerative properties. They found that poly-YE promotes neurogenesis after stroke as they saw an overall increase in the number of newly formed neurons in the dentate gyri of treated animals. The results presented in this study showed that the administrations of poly-YE as late as 24 hours after the induction of ischemic stroke greatly improved subsequent recovery. It had a positive effect on the neurological outcome of stroke, delayed degeneration, and enhanced the repair of damaged structures. Also, the therapeutic window (24 hours) seemed to be significantly wider than most of the current candidate therapies for stroke, giving it much more clinically translational value (Ziv et al., 2007). A separate study in our laboratory examined the effect of Cop-1 immunizations on the outcome of ischemic stroke, using the middle cerebral artery occlusion model. Results suggested that Cop-1 significantly improved the neurological outcome of animals after stroke. Histolopathological assessment also demonstrated a decrease in infarct size and infarct volume in Cop-1-treated animals (Ibarra et al., 2007). The results of both studies do not necessarily elucidate the mechanisms through which NDP-induced PA exerts its protective effects in focal cerebral ischemia but they provide evidence of its neuroprotective, and even neuroregenerative, properties. These studies provide NDP-induced PA with another consequential benefit, and that is the wide therapeutic window. Immunizations with NDP in the treatment of stroke require exhaustive research before they reach clinical trial potential but these preliminary results are an enormous step closer.

### 5.2.2 Traumatic CNS injury

Traumatic CNS injury can be broken down into two compartments: TBI and SCI. A study by Kipnis et al. found that immunizing with Cop-1 after traumatic brain injury had a better outcome on neurological and histological evaluations after injury (Kipnis et al., 2003). TBI triggers self-destructive processes, like other injuries to the CNS. Kipnis et al. studied mice with closed head injury and determined that the immune system plays a key role in the spontaneous recovery. The trauma-induced deficit was reduced, both functionally and anatomically, by post-traumatic vaccination with Cop-1. Several studies have been published on the use of NDP in SCI. Hauben et al. used immunization with a variety of myelin-associated peptides, including those derived from Nogo-A, can be used to evoke a T cell-mediated response that promotes recovery. They show that neuronal degeneration after incomplete spinal cord contusion in rats was substantially reduced, and hence recovery was significantly promoted, by posttraumatic immunization with Nogo-A-derived, p472 (Hauben et al., 2001). Our laboratory has also demonstrated the beneficial effect of immunizing with NDP (A91) on motor recovery and neuronal survival after SCI (Martiñon et al., 2007). Furthermore, we have determined some of the mechanisms of action of NDP-induced PA. In a recent study we found that immunization with Cop-1 and A91 exerted its neuroprotective effect through the inhibition of lipid peroxidation (LP). Animals were immunized with A91 seven days before injury. With the aim of inducing the functional elimination of CNS-specific T cells, animals were tolerized against SC-protein extract and thereafter subjected to a SCI. The lipid-soluble fluorescent products were used as an index of LP and were assessed after injury. Immunization with NDP reduced LP after SCI. Functional elimination of CNS-specific T cells avoided the beneficial effect induced by PA (Ibarra et al., 2010). A consequential study hypothesized that LP was caused by an unregulated production of ROS seen after CNS injury. The main ROS produced during the secondary phase of damage after trauma is NO. When NO is produced in an unregulated fashion it can react with other free radicals such as superoxide anion and produce peroxynitrite a powerful neurotoxic substance. We determined that the decrease in lipid peroxidation was caused by an inhibition in the synthesis of NO after immunization with NDP after SCI (unpublished data). Our results supported our hypothesis and allowed us to corroborate the data with expression analysis. We used real time RT-PCR to also demonstrate a reduction in the expression of the enzyme implicated in post-injury synthesis of NO, the inducible form of nitric oxide synthase (iNOS) (unpublished data). By determining that A91 reactive T cells also secrete NT-3 and IL-4 after SCI, making them a Th2 phenotype, we further substantiate the PA hypothesis. Immunizing with NDP deviates the Th response down a Th2 pathway increasing the synthesis of molecules such as IL-4 and IL-10 and secretion of neurotrophic factors like NT-3. Finally, we have found that the severity of injury would determine the strength and the effect of the PA response (unpublished data). This new data adds more factors into the induction of an autoreactive response. Our study noticed that animals that sustained a non-complete injury to the spinal cord had an increased recovery when immunized with A91. These autoreactive T cells also secreted BDNF and had greater recognition for A91 in vitro. On the other hand, animals that sustained complete or severe SCI did not recover even after A91-immunization. Unexpectedly, these animals did not even possess a clonal response to A91, meaning they were not even able to recognize the antigen in vivo, even with an adjuvant. This indicates that animals that sustained a severe or complete injury to the spinal cord are severely immunosuppressed and may therefore not engage a true PA response (unpublished data). This data that has just surfaced indicates that the neuroimmunological components of CNS disease require much more research in order to elucidate this unknown mechanisms. Even further, we must continue to delve into this immunosuppression caused by severe injury. The study of the body's physiology under duress shows us some of the mechanisms it possesses that could help in regenerating the CNS during disease. Immunization with NDP has proven to be an excellent therapeutical intervention in SCI and several other NDD, providing it with reasonable necessity to continue research on the topic.

## 6. Improving the beneficial effect of protective autoimmunity

Even though the positive effect of immunizing with NDP has rendered significant results, it is possible to potentiate this effect. The improvement of this strategy would yield a better functional recovery and, thereby, a better quality of life for NDD-affected individuals. It is clear that several damaging mechanisms take place during the acute phase of injury. Unfortunately, NDP-induced PA develops after a few days of immunization. Before PA sets in, the neural tissue is unprotected; therefore, the best approach is a combination of neuroprotective strategies. A therapeutic intervention tailored to each specific time point of injury pathophysiology. This approach will ameliorate one or more of the destructive events and may improve the functional outcome even more than PA alone. Excessive production of ROS from the beginning of CNS injury causes lipid peroxidation LP (Hall, 1994). Peroxidation of membrane lipids affects the integrity of the cell membrane and is the most damaging mechanism. The unregulated synthesis of free radicals offers a potential intervention route for the treatment of NDD. An example of this is the use of glutathione monoethyl ester (GSHE). This cell-permeant derivative of glutathione (GSH) is an antioxidant that limits the effect of ROS on the bi-lipid membrane. GSH has shown neuroprotective properties after SCI (Guizar-Sahagun et al., 2005; Santoscoy et al., 2002). Aside from this effect, GSH supports the proliferation, growth, and differentiation of immune cells. Moreover, GSH is actually required for many specific T cell functions, including DNA replication and IL-2 synthesis (Kidd., 1997). The amount of GSH determines the magnitude of the immunological response (Droge et al., 1994) as well as its depletion inhibits normal function (Kidd, 1997). According to the data presented above, the addition of GSHE to NDP immunizations could significantly improve neuroprotection. The antioxidant properties of GSH will cover the overproduction of ROS from the beginning of injury while it could also assist in inducing a better PA response. A previous work carried out in our laboratory, examined the effect of this combination and demonstrated that the addition of GSHE to NDP immunizations induced earlier and better motor recovery after SCI compared to immunizations alone (Martinon et al., 2007). This effect was observed in animals subjected to either a contusive or a compressive SCI. The substantial improvement observed in treated animals allowed them to attain weight-supported plantar steps. This recovery is of great relevance when translating this treatment into a clinical setting. Motor improvement significantly correlated with increased axonal myelination as well as a marked survival of rubrospinal neurons. Besides finding adjuvant therapies for NDP-induced PA we wanted to see if multiple immunizations would increase the beneficial effect. We examined the effect of double immunizations and their effect on PA. Contrary to our expectations, double immunizations abolished the neuroprotective effect of single dose NDP-induced PA. The findings support the notion that the second immunization after SCI has a negative effect on PA. Rather than strengthening the protective effect, it eliminated it. This phenomenon was probably secondary to anergy since double immunization did not induce cell death (Martinon et al., 2007). According to the present data, the use of NDP and GSHE in SCI is a promising strategy. Further studies are necessary in order to establish the efficacy of this therapy and its potential applications into other NDD. Another attempt of synergistic therapeutic interventions is the use of GA with IFN-β-1a in MS (Lublin & Reingold, 2001). The development of adjuvant and synergistic therapies will aid in the optimization of NDP-induced PA allowing us to tackle the pathophysiology of several NDD.

## 7. Conclusion

The concept of PA revolutionized the way we saw the immune system in several different diseases. We figured out that it was more important to modulate the response than to eliminate it. With the logarithmic explosion in knowledge we must now hold these conclusions. The use of NDP and their effect on the immune response have proven to be helpful in several different pathologies, particularly in NDD. Using the information that we have recollected across the years, the mechanisms through which NDP-induced PA exerts its effects is everyday less obscure. Unfortunately, due to hypersensitivity reactions and heterogeneous responses among patients NDP have not been taken to their maximum potential. Unfortunately, PA is developed under the bases that the immune system is healthy and will function normally following an insult to the CNS. However, MS is an autoimmune disease, a case where the immune system is fatally skewed. This paradox forces us to adopt a revolutionary idea such as PA and apply it to NDD. The application of NDP-induced PA to the field of NDD can yield insurmountable results and therefore we urge the scientific community to aid in continuing to shed light on these once obscure mechanisms in order to make this therapeutic intervention efficacious and safe. The ultimate goal is to help the suffering and the complications of human disease.

## 8. References

Aharoni, R.; Eilam, R.; Domev, H.; Labunskay, G.; Sela, M. & Arnon, R. (2005). The immunomodulator glatiramer acetate augments the expression of neurotrophic factors in brains of experimental autoimmune encephalomyelitis mice. *Proceedings of the National Academy of Sciences of the United States of America*, Vol.102, No.52, (December 2005), pp. 19045-19050, ISSN 0027-8424

Aharoni, R.; Kayhan, B.; Eilam, R.; Sela, M. & Arnon, R. (2003). Glatiramer acetate-specific T cells in the brain express T helper 2/3 cytokines and brain-derived neurotrophic factor in situ. *Proceedings of the National Academy of Sciences of the United States of America*, Vol.100, No.24, (November 2003), pp. 14157-14162, ISSN 0027-8424

Aharoni, R.; Teitelbaum, D.; Leitner, O.; Meshorer, A.; Sela, M. & Arnon, R. (2000). Specific Th2 cells accumulate in the central nervous system of mice protected against experimental autoimmune encephalomyelitis by copolymer 1. *Proceedings of the National Academy of Sciences of the United States of America*, Vol.97, No.21, (October 2000), pp. 11472-11477, ISSN 0027-8424

Alzheimer's Association. (2010). Alzheimer's disease facts and figures. *Alzheimer's & dementia*, Vol.6, No.2, (March 2010), pp. 158-194. ISSN 1552-5279

Angelov, D.N.; Waibel, S.; Guntinas-Lichius, O.; Lenzen, M.; Neiss, W.F.; Tomov, T.L.; Yoles, E.; Kipnis, J.; Schori, H.; Reuter, A.; Ludolph, A. & Schwartz, M. (2003). Therapeutic vaccine for acute and chronic motor neuron diseases: implications for amyotrophic lateral sclerosis. *Proceedings of the National Academy of Sciences of the United States of America*, Vol.100, No.8, (April 2003), pp. 4790-4795, ISSN 0027-8424

Becker, K.J.; McCarron, R.M.; Ruetzler, C.; Laban, O.; Sternberg, E.; Flanders, K.C. & Hallenbeck, J.M. (1997). Immunologic tolerance to myelin basic protein decreases stroke size after transient focal cerebral ischemia. *Proceedings of the National Academy of Sciences of the United States of America*, Vol.94, No.20, (September 1997), pp. 10873-10878, ISSN 0027-8424

Ben-Zeev, B.; Aharoni, R.; Nissenkorn, A. & Arnon, R. (2011). Glatiramer acetate (GA, Copolymer-1) an hypothetical treatment option for Rett syndrome. *Medical Hypotheses*, Vol.76, No.2, (February 2011), pp. 190-193, ISSN 1532-2777

Benner, E.J.; Mosley, R.L.; Destache, C.J.; Lewis, T.B.; Jackson-Lewis, V.; Gorantla, S.; Nemachek, C.; Green, S.R.; Przedborski, S. & Gendelman, H.E. (2004). Therapeutic immunization protects dopaminergic neurons in a mouse model of Parkinson's disease. *Proceedings of the National Academy of Sciences of the United States of America*, Vol.101, No.25, (June 2004), pp. 9435-9440, ISSN 0027-8424

Bethea, J.R.; Castro, M.; Keane, R.W.; Lee, T.T.; Dietrich, W.D. & Yezierski, R.P. (1998). Traumatic spinal cord injury induces nuclear factor-kappaB activation. *The Journal of Neuroscience*, Vol.18, No.9, (May 1998), pp. 3251-3260, ISSN 0270-6474

Bethea, J.R.; Nagashima, H.; Acosta, M.C.; Briceno, C.; Gomez, F.; Marcillo, A.E.; Loor, K.; Green, J. & Dietrich, W.D. (1999). Systemically administered interleukin-10 reduces tumor necrosis factor-alpha production and significantly improves functional recovery following traumatic spinal cord injury in rats. *Journal of Neurotrauma*, Vol.16, No.10, (October 1999), pp. 851-863, ISSN 0897-7151

Blight, A.R. (1992). Macrophages and inflammatory damage in spinal cord injury. *Journal of Neurotrauma,* Vol.9, No.1, (March 1992), pp. 83-91, ISSN 0897-7151

Brown, R.C.; Lockwood, A.H. & Sonawane, B.R. (2005). Neurodegenerative diseases: an overview of environmental risk factors. *Environmental health perspectives,* Vol.113, No.9, (September 2005), pp. 1250-1256, ISSN 0091-6765

Butovsky, O.; Hauben, E. & Schwartz, M. (2001). Morphological aspects of spinal cord autoimmune neuroprotection: colocalization of T cells with B7--2 (CD86) and prevention of cyst formation. *The FASEB journal,* Vol.15, No.6, (April 2001), pp. 1065-1067, ISSN 0892-6638

Butovsky, O.; Koronyo-Hamaoui, M.; Kunis, G.; Ophir, E.; Landa, G.; Cohen, H. & Schwartz, M. (2006). Glatiramer acetate fights against Alzheimer's disease by inducing dendritic-like microglia expressing insulin-like growth factor 1. *Proceedings of the National Academy of Sciences of the United States of America,* Vol.103, No.31, (August 2006), pp. 11784-11789, ISSN 0027-8424

Cady, C.T.; Lahn, M.; Vollmer, M.; Tsuji, M.; Seo, S.J.; Reardon, C.L.; O'Brien, R.L. & Born, W.K. (2000). Response of murine gamma delta T cells to the synthetic polypeptide poly-Glu50Tyr50. *Journal of Immunology,* Vol.165, No.4, (August 2000), pp. 1790-1798, ISSN 0022-1767

Davey, R.T.,Jr.; Chaitt, D.G.; Piscitelli, S.C.; Wells, M.; Kovacs, J.A.; Walker, R.E.; Falloon, J.; Polis, M.A.; Metcalf, J.A.; Masur, H.; Fyfe, G. & Lane, H.C. (1997). Subcutaneous administration of interleukin-2 in human immunodeficiency virus type 1-infected persons. *The Journal of infectious diseases,* Vol.175, No.4, (April 1997), pp. 781-789, ISSN 0022-1899

Doble, A. & Kennel, P. (2000). Animal models of amyotrophic lateral sclerosis. *Amyotrophic lateral sclerosis and other motor neuron disorders,* Vol.1, No.5, (December 2001), pp. 301-312, ISSN 1466-0822

Droge, W.; Schulze-Osthoff, K.; Mihm, S.; Galter, D.; Schenk, H.; Eck, H.P.; Roth, S. & Gmunder, H. (1994). Functions of glutathione and glutathione disulfide in immunology and immunopathology. *The FASEB journal,* Vol.8, No.14, (November 1994), pp. 1131-1138, ISSN 0892-6638

Dusart, I.; Morel, M.P. & Sotelo, C. (1994). Parasagittal compartmentation of adult rat Purkinje cells expressing the low-affinity nerve growth factor receptor: changes of pattern expression after a traumatic lesion. *Neuroscience,* Vol.63, No.2, (November 1994), pp. 351-356, ISSN 0306-4522

Farhoudi, A.; Siadati, A.; Atarod, L.; Tabatabaei, P.; Mamishi, S.; Khotaii, G.; Armin, Sh. & Shirvani, F. (2003). Para Vertebral Abscess and Rib Osteomyelitis due to Aspergillous Fumigatus in a Patient with Chronic Granulomatous Disease. *Iranian journal of allergy, asthma, and immunology,* Vol.2, No.1, (March 2007), pp. 13-15, ISSN 1735-1502

Franciosi, S.; Choi, H.B.; Kim, S.U. & McLarnon, J.G. (2005). IL-8 enhancement of amyloid-beta (Abeta 1-42)-induced expression and production of pro-inflammatory cytokines and COX-2 in cultured human microglia. *Journal of neuroimmunology,* Vol.159, No.1-2, (February 2005), pp. 66-74, ISSN 0165-5728

Frank-Cannon, T.C.; Alto, L.T.; McAlpine, F.E. & Tansey, M.G. (2009). Does neuroinflammation fan the flame in neurodegenerative diseases? *Molecular neurodegeneration,* Vol.4, (n.d.), pp. 47, ISSN 1750-1326

Frenkel, D.; Huang, Z.; Maron, R.; Koldzic, D.N.; Hancock, W.W.; Moskowitz, M.A. & Weiner, H.L. (2003). Nasal vaccination with myelin oligodendrocyte glycoprotein reduces stroke size by inducing IL-10-producing CD4+ T cells. *Journal of immunology*, Vol.171, No.12, (December 2003), pp. 6549-6555, ISSN 0022-1767

Frenkel, D.; Maron, R.; Burt, D.S. & Weiner, H.L. (2005). Nasal vaccination with a proteosome-based adjuvant and glatiramer acetate clears beta-amyloid in a mouse model of Alzheimer disease. *The Journal of clinical investigation*, Vol.115, No.9, (September 2005), pp. 2423-2433, ISSN 0021-9738

Garboczi, D.N.; Ghosh, P.; Utz, U.; Fan, Q.R.; Biddison, W.E. & Wiley, D.C. (1996). Structure of the complex between human T-cell receptor, viral peptide and HLA-A2. *Nature*, Vol.384, No.6605, (November 1996), pp. 134-141, ISSN 0028-0836

Gaur, A.; Boehme, S.A.; Chalmers, D.; Crowe, P.D.; Pahuja, A.; Ling, N.; Brocke, S.; Steinman, L. & Conlon, P.J. (1997). Amelioration of relapsing experimental autoimmune encephalomyelitis with altered myelin basic protein peptides involves different cellular mechanisms. *Journal of neuroimmunology*, Vol.74, No.1-2, (April 1997), pp. 149-158, ISSN 0165-5728

Gordon, P.H.; Doorish, C.; Montes, J.; Mosley, R.L.; Diamond, B.; Macarthur, R.B.; Weimer, L.H.; Kaufmann, P.; Hays, A.P.; Rowland, L.P.; Gendelman, H.E.; Przedborski, S. & Mitsumoto, H. (2006). Randomized controlled phase II trial of glatiramer acetate in ALS. *Neurology*, Vol.66, No.7, (April 2006), pp. 1117-1119, ISSN 0028-3878

Guizar-Sahagun, G.; Ibarra, A.; Espitia, A.; Martinez, A.; Madrazo, I. & Franco-Bourland, R.E. (2005). Glutathione monoethyl ester improves functional recovery, enhances neuron survival, and stabilizes spinal cord blood flow after spinal cord injury in rats. *Neuroscience*, Vol.130, No.3, (n.d.), pp. 639-649, ISSN 0306-4522

Hall, E.D.; McCall, J.M. & Means, E.D. (1994). Therapeutic potential of the lazaroids (21-aminosteroids) in acute central nervous system trauma, ischemia and subarachnoid hemorrhage. *Advances in pharmacology*, Vol.28, (n.d.), pp. 221-268, ISSN 1054-3589

Hammarberg, H.; Lidman, O.; Lundberg, C.; Eltayeb, S.Y.; Gielen, A.W.; Muhallab, S.; Svenningsson, A.; Linda, H.; van Der Meide, P.H.; Cullheim, S.; Olsson, T. & Piehl, F. (2000). Neuroprotection by encephalomyelitis: rescue of mechanically injured neurons and neurotrophin production by CNS-infiltrating T and natural killer cells. *The Journal of Neuroscience*, Vol.20, No.14, (July 2000), pp. 5283-5291, ISSN 0270-6474

Hashimoto, M.; Sun, D.; Rittling, S.R.; Denhardt, D.T. & Young, W. (2007). Osteopontin-deficient mice exhibit less inflammation, greater tissue damage, and impaired locomotor recovery from spinal cord injury compared with wild-type controls. *The Journal of Neuroscience*, Vol.27, No.13, (March 2007), pp. 3603-3611, ISSN 0270-6474

Hauben, E.; Butovsky, O.; Nevo, U.; Yoles, E.; Moalem, G.; Agranov, E.; Mor, F.; Leibowitz-Amit, R.; Pevsner, E.; Akselrod, S.; Neeman, M.; Cohen, I.R. & Schwartz, M. (2000). Passive or active immunization with myelin basic protein promotes recovery from spinal cord contusion. *The Journal of Neuroscience*, Vol.20, No.17, (September 2000), pp. 6421-6430, ISSN 0270-6474

Hauben, E.; Gothilf, A.; Cohen, A.; Butovsky, O.; Nevo, U.; Smirnov, I.; Yoles, E.; Akselrod, S. & Schwartz, M. (2003). Vaccination with dendritic cells pulsed with peptides of myelin basic protein promotes functional recovery from spinal cord injury. *The Journal of Neuroscience*, Vol.23, No.25, (September 2003), pp. 8808-8819, ISSN 0270-6474

Hauben, E.; Ibarra, A.; Mizrahi, T.; Barouch, R.; Agranov, E. & Schwartz, M. (2001). Vaccination with a Nogo-A-derived peptide after incomplete spinal-cord injury promotes recovery via a T-cell-mediated neuroprotective response: comparison with other myelin antigens. *Proceedings of the National Academy of Sciences of the United States of America*, Vol.98, No.26, (December 2001), pp. 15173-15178, ISSN 0027-8424

Hauben, E.; Nevo, U.; Yoles, E.; Moalem, G.; Agranov, E.; Mor, F.; Akselrod, S.; Neeman, M.; Cohen, I.R. & Schwartz, M. (2000). Autoimmune T cells as potential neuroprotective therapy for spinal cord injury. *Lancet*, Vol.355, No.9200, (January 2000), pp. 286-287, ISSN 0140-6736

Hauben, E.; Roncarolo, M.G.; Nevo, U. & Schwartz, M. (2005). Beneficial autoimmunity in Type 1 diabetes mellitus. *Trends in immunology*, Vol.26, No.5, (May 2005), pp. 248-253, ISSN 1471-4906

Hendrix, S. & Nitsch, R. (2007). The role of T helper cells in neuroprotection and regeneration. *Journal of Neuroimmunology*, Vol.184, No.1-2, (March 2007), pp. 100-112, ISSN 0165-5728

Ibarra, A.; Correa, D.; Willms, K.; Merchant, M.T.; Guizar-Sahagun, G.; Grijalva, I. & Madrazo, I. (2003). Effects of cyclosporin-A on immune response, tissue protection and motor function of rats subjected to spinal cord injury. *Brain Research*, Vol.979, No.1-2, (July 2003), pp. 165-178, ISSN 0006-8993

Ibarra, A.; Garcia, E.; Flores, N.; Martinon, S.; Reyes, R.; Campos, M.G.; Maciel, M. & Mestre, H. (2010). Immunization with neural-derived antigens inhibits lipid peroxidation after spinal cord injury. *Neuroscience Letters*, Vol.476, No.2, (May 2010), pp. 62-65, ISSN 0304-3940

Ibarra, A.; Hauben, E.; Butovsky, O. & Schwartz, M. (2004). The therapeutic window after spinal cord injury can accommodate T cell-based vaccination and methylprednisolone in rats. *The European Journal of Neuroscience*, Vol.19, No.11, (June 2004), pp. 2984-2990, ISSN 0953-816X

Jameson, S.C. & Bevan, M.J. (1995). T cell receptor antagonists and partial agonists. *Immunity*, Vol.2, No.1, (January 1995), pp. 1-11, ISSN 1074-7613

Kersh, G.J. & Allen, P.M. (1996). Essential flexibility in the T-cell recognition of antigen. *Nature*, Vol.380, No.6574, (April 1996), pp. 495-498, ISSN 0028-0836

Kidd, P.M. (1997). Glutathione: systemic protectant against oxidative and free radical damage. *Alternative Medicine Review.*, Vol.1, (n.d.), pp. 155-176, ISSN 1089-5159

Kipnis, J.; Nevo, U.; Panikashvili, D.; Alexandrovich, A.; Yoles, E.; Akselrod, S.; Shohami, E. & Schwartz, M. (2003). Therapeutic vaccination for closed head injury. *Journal of Neurotrauma*, Vol.20, No.6, (June 2003), pp. 559-569, ISSN 0897-7151

Kipnis, J. & Schwartz, M. (2002). Dual action of glatiramer acetate (Cop-1) in the treatment of CNS autoimmune and neurodegenerative disorders. *Trends in Molecular Medicine*, Vol.8, No.7, (July 2002), pp. 319-323, ISSN 1471-4914

Kipnis, J.; Yoles, E.; Schori, H.; Hauben, E.; Shaked, I. & Schwartz, M. (2001). Neuronal survival after CNS insult is determined by a genetically encoded autoimmune response. *The Journal of Neuroscience*, Vol.21, No.13, (July 2001), pp. 4564-4571, ISSN 0270-6474

Kreutzberg, G.W. (1996). Microglia: a sensor for pathological events in the CNS. *Trends in Neurosciences*, Vol.19, No.8, (August 1996), pp. 312-318, ISSN 0166-2236

Kumpfel, T.; Schwan, M.; Pollmacher, T.; Yassouridis, A.; Uhr, M.; Trenkwalder, C. & Weber, F. (2007). Time of interferon-beta 1a injection and duration of treatment affect clinical side effects and acute changes of plasma hormone and cytokine levels in multiple sclerosis patients. *Multiple Sclerosis*, Vol.13, No.9, (November 2007), pp. 1138-1145, ISSN 1352-4585

Laurie, C.; Reynolds, A.; Coskun, O.; Bowman, E.; Gendelman, H.E. & Mosley, R.L. (2007). CD4+ T cells from Copolymer-1 immunized mice protect dopaminergic neurons in the 1-methyl-4-phenyl-1,2,3,6-tetrahydropyridine model of Parkinson's disease. *Journal of Neuroimmunology*, Vol.183, No.1-2, (February 2007), pp. 60-68, ISSN 0165-5728

Lee, K.H.; Yun, S.J.; Nam, K.N.; Gho, Y.S. & Lee, E.H. (2007). Activation of microglial cells by ceruloplasmin. *Brain Research*, Vol.1171, (September 2007), pp. 1-8, ISSN 0006-8993

Li, L.; Lu, J.; Tay, S.S.; Moochhala, S.M. & He, B.P. (2007). The function of microglia, either neuroprotection or neurotoxicity, is determined by the equilibrium among factors released from activated microglia in vitro. *Brain Research*, Vol.1159, (July 2007), pp. 8-17, ISSN 0006-8993

Liu, Z. & Martin, L.J. (2001). Isolation of mature spinal motor neurons and single-cell analysis using the comet assay of early low-level DNA damage induced in vitro and in vivo. *The Journal of Histochemistry and Cytochemistry*, Vol.49, No.8, (August 2001), pp. 957-972, ISSN 0022-1554

Lopez-Vales, R.; Garcia-Alias, G.; Fores, J.; Udina, E.; Gold, B.G.; Navarro, X. & Verdu, E. (2005). FK 506 reduces tissue damage and prevents functional deficit after spinal cord injury in the rat. *Journal of Neuroscience Research*, Vol.81, No.6, (September 2005), pp. 827-836, ISSN 0360-4012

Lopez-Vales, R.; Garcia-Alias, G.; Guzman-Lenis, M.S.; Fores, J.; Casas, C.; Navarro, X. & Verdu, E. (2006). Effects of COX-2 and iNOS inhibitors alone or in combination with olfactory ensheathing cell grafts after spinal cord injury. *Spine*, Vol.31, No.10, (May 2006), pp. 1100-1106, ISSN 0362-2436

Lublin, F.D. & Reingold, S.C. (2001). Placebo-controlled clinical trials in multiple sclerosis: ethical considerations. National Multiple Sclerosis Society (USA) Task Force on Placebo-Controlled Clinical Trials in MS. *Annals of Neurology*, Vol.49, No.5, (May 2001), pp. 677-681, ISSN 0364-5134

Ludolph, A.C.; Meyer, T. & Riepe, M.W. (2000). The role of excitotoxicity in ALS--what is the evidence? *Journal of Neurology*, Vol.247 Suppl 1, (March 2000), pp. I7-16, ISSN 0340-5354

Martin, L.J.; Price, A.C.; Kaiser, A.; Shaikh, A.Y. & Liu, Z. (2000). Mechanisms for neuronal degeneration in amyotrophic lateral sclerosis and in models of motor neuron. *International Journal of Molecular Medicine*, Vol.5, No.1, (January 1999), pp. 3-13, ISSN 1107-3756

Martinon, S.; Garcia, E.; Flores, N.; Gonzalez, I.; Ortega, T.; Buenrostro, M.; Reyes, R.; Fernandez-Presas, A.M.; Guizar-Sahagun, G.; Correa, D. & Ibarra, A. (2007). Vaccination with a neural-derived peptide plus administration of glutathione improves the performance of paraplegic rats. *The European Journal of Neuroscience*, Vol.26, No.2, (July 2007), pp. 403-412, ISSN 0953-816X

Meek, P.D.; McKeithan, K. & Schumock, G.T. (1998). Economic considerations in Alzheimer's disease. *Pharmacotherapy*, Vol.18, No.2, (March-April 1998), pp. 68-73, ISSN 0277-0008

Meininger, V.; Lacomblez, L. & Salachas, F. (2000). What has changed with riluzole? *Journal of Neurology*, Vol.247, (December 2001), pp. 19-22, ISSN 0340-5354

Moalem, G.; Leibowitz-Amit, R.; Yoles, E.; Mor, F.; Cohen, I.R. & Schwartz, M. (1999). Autoimmune T cells protect neurons from secondary degeneration after central nervous system axotomy. *Nature Medicine*, Vol.5, No.1, (January 1999), pp. 49-55, ISSN 1078-8956

Nel, A.E. & Slaughter, N. (2002). T-cell activation through the antigen receptor. Part 2: role of signaling cascades in T-cell differentiation, anergy, immune senescence, and development of immunotherapy. *The Journal of Allergy and Clinical Immunology*, Vol.109, No.6, (June 2002), pp. 901-915, ISSN 0091-6749

Nicoll, J.A.; Wilkinson, D.; Holmes, C.; Steart, P.; Markham, H. & Weller, R.O. (2003). Neuropathology of human Alzheimer disease after immunization with amyloid-beta peptide: a case report. *Nature Medicine*, Vol.9, No.4, (April 2003), pp. 448-452, ISSN 1078-8956

Nimmerjahn, A.; Kirchhoff, F. & Helmchen, F. (2005). Resting microglial cells are highly dynamic surveillants of brain parenchyma in vivo. *Science*, Vol.308, No.5726, (May 2005), pp. 1314-1318, ISSN 0036-8075

Orgogozo, J.M.; Gilman, S.; Dartigues, J.F.; Laurent, B.; Puel, M.; Kirby, L.C.; Jouanny, P.; Dubois, B.; Eisner, L.; Flitman, S.; Michel, B.F.; Boada, M.; Frank, A. & Hock, C. (2003). Subacute meningoencephalitis in a subset of patients with AD after Abeta42 immunization. *Neurology*, Vol.61, No.1, (July 2003), pp. 46-54, ISSN 0028-3878

Pan, W.; Zhang, L.; Liao, J.; Csernus, B. & Kastin, A.J. (2003). Selective increase in TNF alpha permeation across the blood-spinal cord barrier after SCI. *Journal of Neuroimmunology*, Vol.134, No.1-2, (January 2003), pp. 111-117, ISSN 0165-5728

Partidos, C.D.; Beignon, A.S.; Briand, J.P. & Muller, S. (2004). Modulation of immune responses with transcutaneously deliverable adjuvants. *Vaccine*, Vol.22, No.19, (June 2004), pp. 2385-2390, ISSN 0264-410X

Petrovsky, N. & Aguilar, J.C. (2004). Vaccine adjuvants: current state and future trends. *Immunology and Cell Biology*, Vol.82, No.5, (October 2004), pp. 488-496, ISSN 0818-9641

Popovich, P.G.; Guan, Z.; Wei, P.; Huitinga, I.; van Rooijen, N. & Stokes, B.T. (1999). Depletion of hematogenous macrophages promotes partial hindlimb recovery and neuroanatomical repair after experimental spinal cord injury. *Experimental Neurology*, Vol.158, No.2, (August 1999), pp. 351-365, ISSN 0014-4886

Popovich, P.G.; Stokes, B.T. & Whitacre, C.C. (1996). Concept of autoimmunity following spinal cord injury: possible roles for T lymphocytes in the traumatized central nervous system. *Journal of Neuroscience Research*, Vol.45, No.4, (August 1996), pp. 349-363, ISSN 0360-4012

Popovich, P.G.; Wei, P. & Stokes, B.T. (1997). Cellular inflammatory response after spinal cord injury in Sprague-Dawley and Lewis rats. *The Journal of Comparative Neurology*, Vol.377, No.3, (January 1997), pp. 443-464, ISSN 0021-9967

Raivich, G. (2005). Like cops on the beat: the active role of resting microglia. *Trends in Neurosciences*, Vol.28, No.11, (November 2005), pp. 571-573, ISSN 0166-2236

Rapalino, O.; Lazarov-Spiegler, O.; Agranov, E.; Velan, G.J.; Yoles, E.; Fraidakis, M.; Solomon, A.; Gepstein, R.; Katz, A.; Belkin, M.; Hadani, M. & Schwartz, M. (1998). Implantation of stimulated homologous macrophages results in partial recovery of paraplegic rats. *Nature Medicine*, Vol.4, No.7, (July 1998), pp. 814-821, ISSN 1078-8956

Resnick, D.K.; Graham, S.H.; Dixon, C.E. & Marion, D.W. (1998). Role of cyclooxygenase 2 in acute spinal cord injury. *Journal of Neurotrauma*, Vol.15, No.12, (December 1999), pp. 1005-1013, ISSN 0897-7151

Sanna, A.; Fois, M.L.; Arru, G.; Huang, Y.M.; Link, H.; Pugliatti, M.; Rosati, G. & Sotgiu, S. (2006). Glatiramer acetate reduces lymphocyte proliferation and enhances IL-5 and IL-13 production through modulation of monocyte-derived dendritic cells in multiple sclerosis. *Clinical and Experimental Immunology*, Vol.143, No.2, (February 2006), pp. 357-362, ISSN 0009-9104

Santoscoy, C.; Rios, C.; Franco-Bourland, R.E.; Hong, E.; Bravo, G.; Rojas, G. & Guizar-Sahagun, G. (2002). Lipid peroxidation by nitric oxide supplements after spinal cord injury: effect of antioxidants in rats. *Neuroscience Letters*, Vol.330, No.1, (September 2002), pp. 94-98, ISSN 0304-3940

Schmid, C.D.; Melchior, B.; Masek, K.; Puntambekar, S.S.; Danielson, P.E.; Lo, D.D.; Sutcliffe, J.G. & Carson, M.J. (2009). Differential gene expression in LPS/IFNgamma activated microglia and macrophages: in vitro versus in vivo. *Journal of Neurochemistry*, Vol.109 Suppl 1, (May 2009), pp. 117-125, ISSN 0022-3042

Schori, H.; Kipnis, J.; Yoles, E.; WoldeMussie, E.; Ruiz, G.; Wheeler, L.A. & Schwartz, M. (2001). Vaccination for protection of retinal ganglion cells against death from glutamate cytotoxicity and ocular hypertension: implications for glaucoma. *Proceedings of the National Academy of Sciences of the United States of America*, Vol.98, No.6, (March 2001), pp. 3398-3403, ISSN 0027-8424

Schwartz, M. & Cohen, I.R. (2000). Autoimmunity can benefit self-maintenance. *Immunology Today*, Vol.21, No.6, (June 2000), pp. 265-268, ISSN 0167-5699

Schwartz, M.; Shaked, I.; Fisher, J.; Mizrahi, T. & Schori, H. (2003). Protective autoimmunity against the enemy within: fighting glutamate toxicity. *Trends in Neurosciences*, Vol.26, No.6, (June 2003), pp. 297-302, ISSN 0166-2236

Sendtner, M.; Gotz, R.; Holtmann, B.; Escary, J.L.; Masu, Y.; Carroll, P.; Wolf, E.; Brem, G.; Brulet, P. & Thoenen, H. (1996). Cryptic physiological trophic support of motoneurons by LIF revealed by double gene targeting of CNTF and LIF. *Current Biology*, Vol.6, No.6, (June 1996), pp. 686-694, ISSN 0960-9822

Shaked, I.; Porat, Z.; Gersner, R.; Kipnis, J. & Schwartz, M. (2004). Early activation of microglia as antigen-presenting cells correlates with T cell-mediated protection and repair of the injured central nervous system. *Journal of Neuroimmunology*, Vol.146, No.1-2, (January 2003), pp. 84-93, ISSN 0165-5728

Sospedra, M. & Martin, R. (2005). Immunology of multiple sclerosis. *Annual Review of Immunology*, Vol.23, (n.d.), pp. 683-747, ISSN 0732-0582

Stuve, O.; Youssef, S.; Weber, M.S.; Nessler, S.; von Budingen, H.C.; Hemmer, B.; Prod'homme, T.; Sobel, R.A.; Steinman, L. & Zamvil, S.S. (2006). Immunomodulatory synergy by combination of atorvastatin and glatiramer acetate in treatment of CNS autoimmunity. *The Journal of Clinical Investigation*, Vol.116, No.4, (April 2006), pp. 1037-1044, ISSN 0021-9738

Terando, A.; Sabel, M.S. & Sondak, V.K. (2003). Melanoma: adjuvant therapy and other treatment options. *Current Treatment Options in Oncology*, Vol.4, No.3, (June 2003), pp. 187-199, ISSN 1534-6277

Turrin, N.P. & Rivest, S. (2006). Molecular and cellular immune mediators of neuroprotection. *Molecular Neurobiology*, Vol.34, No.3, (December 2007), pp. 221-242, ISSN 0893-7648

Vanegas, H. & Schaible, H.G. (2001). Prostaglandins and cyclooxygenases [correction of cycloxygenases] in the spinal cord. *Progress in Neurobiology*, Vol.64, No.4, (July 2001), pp. 327-363, ISSN 0301-0082

Vidovic, D. & Matzinger, P. (1988). Unresponsiveness to a foreign antigen can be caused by self-tolerance. *Nature*, Vol.336, No.6196, (November 1988), pp. 222-225, ISSN 0028-0836

Vieira, P.L.; Heystek, H.C.; Wormmeester, J.; Wierenga, E.A. & Kapsenberg, M.L. (2003). Glatiramer acetate (copolymer-1, copaxone) promotes Th2 cell development and increased IL-10 production through modulation of dendritic cells. *Journal of Immunology*, Vol.170, No.9, (May 2003), pp. 4483-4488, ISSN 0022-1767

Xu, J.Q.; Kochanek, K.D.; Murphy, S.L. & Tejada-Vera, B. (2007). *Deaths: Final data for 2007.* Hyattsville, MD: National Center for Health Statistics. 2010.

Yin, Y.; Cui, Q.; Li, Y.; Irwin, N.; Fischer, D.; Harvey, A.R. & Benowitz, L.I. (2003). Macrophage-derived factors stimulate optic nerve regeneration. *The Journal of Neuroscience*, Vol.23, No.6, (March 2003), pp. 2284-2293, ISSN 0270-6474

Yoles, E.; Hauben, E.; Palgi, O.; Agranov, E.; Gothilf, A.; Cohen, A.; Kuchroo, V.; Cohen, I.R.; Weiner, H. & Schwartz, M. (2001). Protective autoimmunity is a physiological response to CNS trauma. *The Journal of Neuroscience*, Vol.21, No.11, (June 2001), pp. 3740-3748, ISSN 0270-6474

Ziemssen, T.; Kumpfel, T.; Klinkert, W.E.; Neuhaus, O. & Hohlfeld, R. (2002). Glatiramer acetate-specific T-helper 1- and 2-type cell lines produce BDNF: implications for multiple sclerosis therapy. Brain-derived neurotrophic factor. *Brain*, Vol.125, No.Pt 11, (November 2002), pp. 2381-2391, ISSN 0006-8950

Ziemssen, T.; Kumpfel, T.; Schneider, H.; Klinkert, W.E.; Neuhaus, O. & Hohlfeld, R. (2005). Secretion of brain-derived neurotrophic factor by glatiramer acetate-reactive T-helper cell lines: Implications for multiple sclerosis therapy. *Journal of the Neurological Sciences*, Vol.233, No.1-2, (June 2005), pp. 109-112, ISSN 0022-510X

Ziv, Y.; Finkelstein, A.; Geffen, Y.; Kipnis, J.; Smirnov, I.; Shpilman, S.; Vertkin, I.; Kimron, M.; Lange, A.; Hecht, T.; Reyman, K.G.; Marder, J.B.; Schwartz, M. & Yoles, E. (2007). A novel immune-based therapy for stroke induces neuroprotection and supports neurogenesis. *Stroke*, Vol.38, No.2 Suppl, (February 2007), pp. 774-782, ISSN 0039-2499

# 7

# Quantification of Volumetric Changes of Brain in Neurodegenerative Diseases Using Magnetic Resonance Imaging and Stereology

Niyazi Acer[1], Ahmet Tuncay Turgut[2],
Yelda Özsunar[3] and Mehmet Turgut[4]
*[1]Dept. of Anatomy, Erciyes University School of Medicine, Kayseri,*
*[2]Dept. of Radiology, Ankara Training and Research Hospital, Ankara,*
*[3]Dept. of Radiology, Adnan Menderes University School of Medicine, Aydın,*
*[4]Dept. of Neurosurgery, Adnan Menderes University School of Medicine, Aydın,*
*Turkey*

## 1. Introduction

In this chapter, we review the different magnetic resonance imaging (MRI)-based methods used to quantify whole and subcortical brain structures volume, and discuss the relevance of the brain atrophy in different neurodegenerative disseases. Although there are a lot of studies for multiple sclerosis (MS) and dementia of Alzheimer's type (AD) for the brain atrophy using different methods, the optimal method for quantifying atrophy has not been established to date.

In recent years, computed tomography (CT) scanning has been replaced with MRI scanning due to its enhanced soft-tissue resolution, especially for cerebrospinal fluid (CSF)-filled spaces, such as ventricular enlargement in patients with AD. Thus, a transition has occurred from CT to MRI in longitudinal studies investigating the human brain. As a result of development of new neuroimaging methods in clinical practice, volumetric methods started to be more sophisticated depending on various imaging methods (Lim et al., 2000). There are numerous reasons for the aforementioned transition; first of all, unlike CT, MRI has no inherent radiation effect, and secondly, CT underestimates cortical sulcal volume relative to MRI due to poorer resolution and spectral shift artifact on CT (Lim et al., 2000). Due to higher contrast resolution, MRI can better characterize the brain morphology including the size, tissue composition such as gray (or grey) matter and white matter, and shape of different cortical or subcortical neuroanatomic structures (Lim et al., 2000). Nowadays, it is possible to use MRI to visualize and quantify the directional coherence of white matter fibers, called diffusion tensor imaging (DTI), for investigation of connectivity and disconnectivity between different brain regions (Basser et al., 1994). Additionally, MRI equipments are also used to provide functional brain responses with functional MRI (fMRI) and perfusion MRI as in some nuclear medicine neuroimaging methods such as positron emission tomography (PET) and single photon emission computed tomography (SPECT). These methods can provide pathognomonic data of certain structural lesions in AD, as they can demonstrate neuronal activity or receptor characteristics (Small, 2002). High field MRI has started to further depict the regional atrophy patterns AD and other neurodegenerative disorders.

In this chapter, we aim to overview the challenging and exciting radiological methods used for the diagnosis of various neurodegenerative diseases. Specifically, we focus on the neuroimaging techniques in the first part of the chapter, their clinical applications in the second part, and methods for volume estimation including stereological techniques on the last part of the text.

## 2. Neuroimaging techniques

Primary neuroimaging techniques that are widely used clinically are CT, PET, SPECT, conventional MRI, fMRI, magnetic resonance spectroscopy (MRS), and tractography or DTI. These techniques enlighten different aspects of brain structures or functions (Frey et al., 1999; Small, 2002). An overview of the neuroimaging techniques is following:

### 2.1 Computed tomography (CT)

CT is the first imaging modality to provide *in vivo* evidence of the brain atrophy in different neurodegenerative diseases. CT images are generated by passing an x–ray beam through the skull or other object (e.g. spine and vertebral column) and it measures the attenuation of an x-ray beam through different body tissues e.g. brain, bone and CSF. Therefore, tissue's appearance will vary according to degree of its attenuation (Frey et al., 1999). The degree of attenuation can be measured numerically as a tissue density number for each voxel (volume element) and then these numbers can be converted to gray scale values and presented visually as pixels (Frey et al., 1999). Among different body tissues, the bone has the highest attenuation and appears white on CT images (Small, 2002). On the other hand, CT study has some limitations such as radiation hazards, inability to differentiate gray and white matter due to low contrast resolution and visualization of the posterior fossa structures, particularly brain stem and cerebellum. Despite to these limitations, quantitative CT still can demonstrate the presence of greater brain atrophy and ventricular dilatation in patients with AD compared with controls (Creasey et al., 1986).

### 2.2 Single photon emission computed tomography (SPECT)

In SPECT, the scanner determines the site of the photon source following adminstration of an unstable isotope or inhaled/injected tracer and thus an image reflecting cerebral blood flow or receptor distribution is produced (Schuckit et al., 1992). Unfortunately, its spatial resolution is not high enough for imaging deep structures and determination of the source of single photon emitters is difficult (Small, 2002).

### 2.3 Positron emission tomography (PET)

A PET scanner determines the line along which the photons travel, by recording the simultaneous arrival of two different photons at different detectors, and an image is then constructed from information received by the scanner. Importantly, PET study demonstrates receptor characteristics like density and affinity following injection of receptor ligands labeled with nuclides, in addition to cerebral blood flow. In patients with AD, PET studies using fluorodeoxyglucose have revealed characteristic alterations in cerebral blood flow and metabolism in the parietal, temporal and prefrontal cortices (Mazziotta et al., 1992).

## 2.4 Conventional magnetic resonance imaging (MRI)

The MRI scanner detects the radiofrequency energy emitted and energy level changes represent different brain structures. Typically, T1-weighted images differentiate gray and white matter, while T2-weighted images delineate white matter hyperintensities. It is reported that spatial resolution for MRI is 1 to 2 mm, less than that of CT (Small, 2002). Fortunately, patients can have multiple MRI scans because it does not involve ionizing radiation. In MRI study, the object is placed in a high field strength magnetic field varying from 0.5 to 3 Tesla (T). Technically, different relaxation times, in addition to proton density, are measured and further manipulations by using various pulse sequences are possible. Today, various MRI techniques such as fast spin echo, high performance gradients, echo planar and diffusion weighted imaging are available for clinical use, in addition to MRI contrast agents, CSF velocity analysis, and interventional MRI (Bradley & Bydder, 1997). Recently, some technical improvements regarding the acquisition and processing of structural data have provided vivid visual representations of the external surface and internal structures of the human brain (Lim et al., 2000). Clinically, the progressive neuronal loss leading to atrophy in neurodegenerative disease increases the value of MRI (Loewe et al., 2002).

## 2.5 Functional magnetic resonance imaging (fMRI)

With recent developments in MRI techniques, it is also possible to measure brain activity and tissue signal changes, reflecting local changes in oxygenation of haemoglobin, which depend on regional blood perfusion. Technical point of view, the signal intensity of deoxygenated hemoglobin differs from that of oxygenated hemoglobin (Belliveau et al., 1992). This MRI method also called BOLD technique. As a rule, the brain tissue during brain activity does not use this excess oxygen, causing high concentration of oxygenated blood, greater levels of magnetic field homogeneity and higher MRI signal intensity (Wagner et al., 1998). Thus, brain regions receiving greater blood flow during brain activity produce a stronger MRI signal than do other regions and areas of relative brain activity can be easily detected (Small, 2002).

## 2.6 Diffusion tensor imaging (DTI)

DTI provides detailed information concerning the anatomy of white matter structure in the central nervous system. With use of DTI, visualizations of projections of axonal fibers, i.e. neuronal connectivity, is possible by quantitative evaluation on the anisotropy of water diffusion, local fiber orientation and integrity of white matter tracks (Jones et al., 1999). Technically, DTI visualizes diffusional anisotropy within each voxel as three-dimensional projections of axonal fibers. In patients with AD and other neuropsychiatric disorders, the degree of neuronal connectivity loss is a useful marker in the progression of the disease (Buchsbaum et al., 1998; Ewers et al., 2011). Moreover, recent studies revealed the presence of loss of myelin and axons in patients with AD, particularly periventricular areas (Hanyu et al., 1997; Ewers et al., 2011).

## 2.7 Magnetic resonance spectroscopy (MRS)

From the technical view, the magnetic resonance spectrum display according to frequency shows different chemical forms of the element such as characteristic peaks, thus reflecting tissue metabolite concentrations (Weiner, 1987; Bothwell & Griffin 2011). As a noninvasive study, MRS provides quantitative regional biochemical and physiologic features of the tissue. To determine *N*-acetylaspartate (NAA) content of hippocampus in patients with AD, some authors used proton MRS (1H MRS) and volumetric MRI (Weiner, 1987; Schuff et al. 1997).

## 2.8 Improvements in magnetic resonance imaging
### 2.8.1 Mechanisms of tissue contrast: Pulse sequences

By varying elements of the image acquisition sequence of MRI, it is possible to manipulate the amount of contrast between various tissues. It is well-known that hydrogen atoms are the most important element of the tissue and MRI device demonstrate signals related with free water. Based on proton density and relaxation time of any tissue, different structures will appear in an acquired image. T1 means the time taken for excited nuclei to return to equilibrium, while T2 is an xponential time constant related with the time for the excited nuclei to lose signal (Lim et al., 2000). Technical view of point, the time between radiofrequency pulses (TR) and the amount of time after the pulse called echo time (TE) are important parameters; a long TR and a long TE give T2-weighted image, while a short TR and a short TE gives T1-weighted image. Although T1-weighted spin-echo and inversion recovery sequences have poor definition of CSF/skull margins for reliably measuring intracranial volume, they are used for morphometric studies because they provide good white-gray contrast (Lim et al., 2000).

Sources of contrast other than that based on manipulation of T1, T2, fluid-attenuated inversion recovery (FLAIR) and proton density are used to obtain further information. T1-weighted images are superior to T2-weighted images for the evaluation of atrophy, because T2-weighted ones overestimate the dimensions of ventricles and sulci (Kucharczyk & Henkelman, 1994). On the other hand, T1-weighted imaging gives a clear distinction between grey matter, white matter and CSF; therefore, they are used for quantitative MRI studies of brain morphology, particularly of individual brain structures (Keller & Roberts, 2009) (Fig. 1).

Fast spin echo T2 sequences has been usually used in brain imaging due to their short acquisition time and increased robustness to motion artifacts. In imaging of neurodegenerative disorders like Parkinson-like syndromes, however, gradient echo T2-weighted spin-echo sequences are preferred because they increase the sensitivity for paramagnetic materials (ferritin, melanin etc.). Also, proton-density or FLAIR sequences identify gliosis owing to result of progressive neuronal loss (Loewe et al., 2002). Therefore, T2-weighted imaging may be used for determination of intracranial volume as the increased signal intensity of CSF provides better determination of CSF and the parenchyma of the brain (Keller & Roberts, 2009). Therefore, the type of MRI sequence used is important for volume estimation.

### 2.8.2 Two-dimensional multi-slice and three-dimensional imaging

Two-dimensional (2D) images are obtained in axial, sagittal and coronal planes (Fig. 1). Image orientation, giving a different view of the brain with optimal visualization of different structures, is described according to radiofrequency pulse excitations and the magnetic gradients in three orthogonal axes. Basically, a mid-sagittal section provides an image of the corpus callosum and the prefrontal cortex, coronal section gives an image of the limbic structures including hippocampus, and axial section gives an image of basal ganglia structures and the lateral ventricular system.

It is important to know that 2D image has a limitation so that only selected slices imaged and therefore a comparison across subjects is difficult, although it may be possible by orienting each slice acquisition relative to a specific anatomic plane. On the other hand, three-dimensional (3D) volume acquisition protocols include the entire brain and they are widely used in psychiatric neuroimaging. Using T1-weighted MRI sections with a good gray/white matter differentiation, the entire brain with 1.5 mm or thinner slices are obtained in 10 minutes or less. As a rule, an in-plane resolution of 1 mm means that each pixel in the image matrix represents 1 mm$^2$ (Lim et al., 2000).

Quantitative investigations of the brain using MRI may reveal important information about the function and organisation of the brain being studied, recently. MRI has become the method of choice for the examination of macroscopic neuroanatomy in vivo due to excellent levels of image resolution and between tissue contrasts. Estimation of brain compartment volume needs high resolution MRIs for the delineation of anatomical boundaries. With the use of higher magnetic field strength, a better image quality with can be obtained using thinner slices and shorter imaging time. For this reason, many researchers frequently use MRI scanners which are either with 1.5 T or 3 T systems (Fig. 2). Although 3 T systems offer increased resolution of between-tissue contrast (i.e. increased visualisation of the borders between gray matter, white matter and CSF), MRI scans on 1.5 T systems are sufficient for the quantification of relatively small brain structures, such as the hippocampus, amygdala, and deep gray matter nuclei (Keller & Roberts, 2009).

## 3. Clinical applications

### 3.1 Dementia syndromes

A number of studies reported that patients with MS have smaller volumes of the parenchyma than in age-matched control subjects (Bermel et al., 2003; Sanfilipo et al., 2005, 2006). The first method used for the estimation of brain atrophy is linear measurement of ventricles or other brain structural dimensions (Smith et al., 2002). In general, MRI studies reveal some differences in the volume of the brain structures in certain neurodegenerative diseases, an inhomogeneous group of neurological diseases with unknown etiology, such as demantia. In such diseases, multiple systems or one system or one group of nuclei may partly or totally be involved (Loewe et al., 2002). Basically, there are two principal pathological processes which determine imaging findings: neuronal or white matter loss and deposition of different compounds. The loss of neurons leads to progressive atrophy associated with white matter loss and gliosis (Kern & Behl, 2009).

Nowadays, dementia is a well-known illness with a high incidence in the aged population. Clinically, there are a number of neurodegenerative diseases causing dementia, including AD, dementia with Lewy bodies, and frontotemporal dementia. Furthermore, dementia picture is also present in some neurodegenerative illnesses including Creutzfeldt–Jakob disease, Huntington's disease, progressive supranuclear palsy, multiple system atrophy, amyotrophic lateral sclerosis, and Parkinson's disease (Loewe et al., 2002; Vitali et al., 2008).

### 3.1.1 Alzheimer disease (AD)

AD is well-known progressive neurodegenerative pathology, accounting for around 60% of all cases dementia. Clinically, patients with AD have serious cognitive findings related with memory, language, such as confusion, poor judgment, language disturbance, agitation, withdrawal, and hallucinations (Mohs & Haroutunian, 2002).

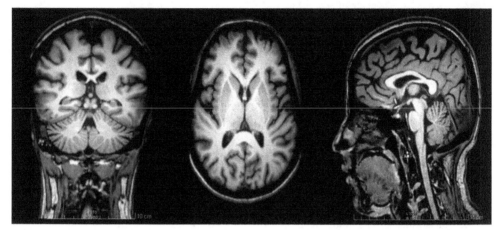

Fig. 1. T1-weighted MRI scans acquired in coronal (left), axial (center) and sagittal (right) planes with 3 T. All images were acquired with a field of view of 25 cm and 256 x 256 matrix, 1-mm slice thickness. Image was acquired using a turbo field echo sequence, gated to achieve an effective TR of >8 ms and TE of 4 ms. Left: Coronal image passing through lateral ventricles and temporal lobes. Center: Axial image passing through the lateral ventricles and basal ganglia. Right: Mid-sagittal image highlighting the corpus callosum, brain stem and cerebellum

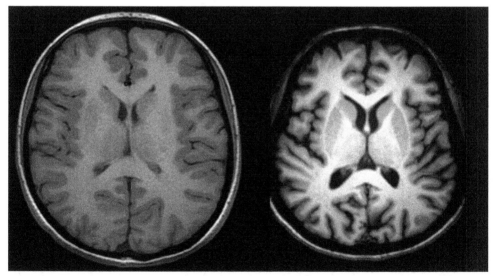

Fig. 2. T1-weighted axial MRIs acquired with 1.5 T (left) and 3T (right) MRI scanners. 3T MRI was acquired with a field of view of 25 cm and 256 x 256 matrix, 1-mm slice thickness. Image was acquired using a turbo field echo sequence, gated to achieve an effective TR of >8 ms and TE of 4 ms. 1.5T MRI was acquired with field of view of 24 cm, 1.5 mm slice thickness. Image was acquired using a spoiled gradient recalled acquisition sequence, gated to achieve an effective TR of >35 ms and TE of 15 ms

Gross examination of the brain in patients with AD demonstrated an obvious atrophy, widening of the sulci, and erosion of the gyri. Histologically, the atrophy of the cortex is associated with significant reductions in the numbers of neurons. Macroscopically, the weight of the brain is decreased compared to normal controls (Masliah et al., 1991). In a previous study using unbiased stereologic sampling techniques, about 50% loss in neurons of the superior temporal gyrus has been reported (Gomez-Isla et al., 1996, 1997). In another study, 40-46% loss of large neurons in the frontal and temporal cortices of specimens has been reported in patients with AD (Terry et al., 1981). In fact, neuronal loss and degeneration are not restricted to the cortex; it may be observed in subcortical nuclei such as the locus ceruleus, raphe aminergic nuclei (Zweig et al., 1988; Chan-Palay & Asan, 1989), and the nucleus basalis of Meynert (Whitehouse et al., 1982). In such cases, synaptic markers such as synaptophysin are significantly reduced in the cerebral cortex, especially the frontal and parietal cortices and in the hippocampus, with increasing age (Nagy et al., 1995).

Radiologically, MRI provides understanding of disease progression in AD and other dementias. Recently, it has been reported that patients with AD have atrophy in parietal lobes, medial temporal lobe and hippocampus on MRI (Loewe et al., 2002, Vitali et al., 2008). The parietal lobe atrophy is observed on axial or coronal T1-weighted or FLAIR sequences with thinning of the posterior part of the body of the corpus callosum on T1-weighted sagittal sequences (Yamauchi et al., 2000). In some studies, decreased hippocampal and entorhinal cortex (ERC) volumes in patients with AD were noted (Appel et al., 2009). Hippocampal atrophy is observed with thin coronal T1-weighted or FLAIR tomographic slices through the medial temporal lobes (Teipel et al., 2003). A lot of quantitative MRI studies indicate that white matter hyperintensities correlate with neuropsychological functioning in both healthy elderly persons and demented patients (Boone et al., 1992; Lopez et al., 1992). Other studies indicate loss of cerebral gray matter (Rusinek et al., 1991), hippocampal and parahippocampal atrophy (Kesslak et al., 1991), and lower left amygdala and ERC volumes in patients with AD (Pearlson et al., 1992; Obrien, 2007).

Recently, a longitudinal study demonstrated that most common neuropathologic findings in elderly patients are neuritic plaques and neurofibrillary tangles (Mohs &Haroutunian, 2002). The presence of these findings before clinical AD diagnosis suggests that *in vivo* methods that directly image these pathognomonic lesions would be useful presymptomatic detection technologies (Mohs & Haroutunian, 2002).

### 3.1.2 Frontotemporal demantia (FTD)

Frontotemporal demantia (FTD) is as common a cause of dementia. In particular, volumes of some regions of the frontal lobe (the ventromedial and posterior orbital regions of the frontal lobe), the cingulate cortex, and the insula are reduced in patients with the FTD, compared with those of both AD patients and age-matched controls. This feature differentiates this illness from AD as these areas are relatively spared in the latter disease (Rosen et al., 2002). In patients with the semantic variant of FTD, there is a relative preservation of frontal lobe volumes but marked loss of volumes in the temporal lobes (Rosen et al,. 2005, 2006). In clinical practice, FTD includes a group of neurodegenerative diseases characterized by focal atrophy of frontal and anterior temporal lobes and non-AD pathology (Neary et al., 1998; McKhann, 2001; Ratnavalli, 2002).

### 3.1.3 Dementia with Lewy bodies (DLB)

Dementia with Lewy bodies results a diffuse, irreversible and destructive atrophy (Seppi & Schocke, 2005). Measurement of brain volume to predict atrophy using MRI may be used as a predicter for outcome in different neurodegenerative diseases such as AD. There are a lot of biologic factors influencing cerebral volume measurement such as inflammation and edema, cerebrovascular disease, chronic alcoholism and normal aging (Ron et al., 1982; Molyneux et al., 2000).

### 3.2 Multiple Sclerosis (MS)
In cases with MS, various measurement techniques revealed atrophy of brain and spinal cord, axonal loss, and Wallerian degeneration (Sharma et al., 2004). Recent studies show that the MS is a destructive disease process and whole-brain atrophy is a valuable marker for the progression of the disease (Sharma et al., 2004).

### 3.3 Medial temporal lobe epilepsy (MTLE)
In patients with medial temporal lobe epilepsy (MTLE), the atrophy of the hippocampus is often observed on routine MRI. Recently, it has been reported that automatic morphometry can be used as a clinical tool to provide a quantifiable estimation of of hippocampal atrophy in patients with MTLE (Bonilha et al., 2009). Most recently, Henry et al. (2011) suggested that ultrahigh-field-strength MRI revealed prominent atrophy of Ammon horn in patients with MTLE and hippocampal sclerosis.

### 3.4 Ageing
With increasing age, there are some volumetric changes in the gray matter structures of the temporal lobe, amygdale, and hippocampus, a critical structure for memory in AD, but they are heterogenous, with some regions showing more atrophic changes than others (O'Sullivan, 2009). Recently, it has been reported that it is possible to differentiate ageing from AD with 87% accuracy (Likeman et al., 2005; O'Sullivan, 2009). Some volumetric studies demonstrated that changes in white matter regions provide an early and accurate diagnosis (Davatzikos et al., 2008).

## 4. Methods for volume estimation

### 4.1 Manual, automated and semiautomated methods for volume estimation
Use of imaging methods for quantitive volume estimation such as manual, semi-automated and automated methods can provide the capability to reliably detect and identify general and specific structural abnormalities of the brain. Use of these methods can aid to diagnose some specific neurological diseases and facilitate monitoring of the progression of the disease. Quantative measures of the brain atrophy can be clinically relevant and much work has been carried out to establish diagnosis of AD (Furlong, 2008).

At present, a number of manual, semi-automated and automated methods based on conventional MRI are available for measuring whole or regional brain volume. Ideally, the technique for measuring tissue volume should be reproducible, sensitive to subtle modifications, practical, fast and correct. Theoretically, many factors may affect the quantification of brain atrophy using segmentation methods, such as the pulse sequence and the resolution parameters chosen for the acquisition (Horsfield et al., 2003; Sharma et al., 2004).

One of these most important factors is slice thickness. The use of thin slice helps to reduce the partial volume effect and consequently permits a better estimation of tissue volumes. Moreover, high contrast makes segmentation between the different cerebral compartments easier. Depending on the compartment of interest, tissue contrast can be chosen such as CSF/parenchyma or gray/white matter (Grassiot et al., 2009). There are many different segmentation methods for estimating brain volume using manual or automated techniques. Flippi et al. (1998) used manual technique for whole brain volume with MS. Although the manual tracing of brain structure allows brain volume to be estimated, this technique is a time consuming method (Flippi et al., 1998).

Semi-automated techniques, quicker and more reproducible, use various algorithms of brain segmentation from 3D volume (Horsfield et al., 2003). For both semi-automated and automated methods, however, manual defining of brain structures is necessary. In semi-automated methods, manual marking of some anatomical landmarks and an automatic segmentation of the region of interest (ROI) are required, while automated methods are completely user-independent in the determination of various parameters such as brain size and shape. Importantly, experienced raters with detailed knowledge of neuroanatomy are necessary for manual techniques and correct estimations related to the neuroanatomical ROI are possible (Keller & Roberts, 2009).

Automated and semi-automated methods for segmentation and quantification of the brain are used in most studies. More recently, various image analysis tools have been developed, including both automated and semi-automated algorithms, relying on either raw or normalized brain volume assessments (Pelletier et al., 2004). Several previous studies have described automatic segmentation methods using MRIs. Calmon & Roberts (2000) reported a segmentation method for the lateral ventricles on coronal MR images. Stokking et al. (2000) described the development of a morphology-based brain segmentation method for fully automatic segmentation of the brain using T1-weighted MRI data. Webb et al. (1999) reported a method of automatic detection of the hippocampus with atrophy. These methods each segmented one target object on each MRI obtained by different sequences. Therefore, these methods could not segment two or more objects simultaneously on MRIs obtained by a single sequence.

There are two primary methods for manual quantification of brain compartment volume from MRIs, namely stereology in conjunction with point counting and planimetric methods or manual tracing (Acer et al., 2007; Keller & Roberts, 2009). Authors used manual tracing of brain boundaries from MRI scans using various softwares such as Analyze (Biomedical Imaging Resource, Mayo Foundation), BRAINS (Iowa Mental Health Clinical Research Center 2008), and FreeSurfer (Dale et al., 1999; Fischl et al., 1999; Fischl et al., 2002). Manual techniques such as planimetry or tracing methods require the investigator to delineate a brain region based on reliable anatomical landmarks, whilst the software package provides information on volume. Tracing methods require the investigator to trace the brain ROI using a mouse driven cursor throughout a defined number of MRI sections (Keller & Roberts, 2009). The cut surface areas, determined by pixel counting within the traced region, are summed and multiplied by the distance between the consecutive sections traced to estimate the total volume. Although tracing methods represent the most commonly used tool to estimate brain structure volume on MRIs, there are some drawbacks associated this technique (Geuze et al., 2005). Firstly, the time taken to perform manual tracing or manual segmentation methods is significantly longer than stereological point counting methods (Acer et al., 2007, 2008; Keller & Roberts, 2009). Secondly, tracing and manual segmentation methods suffer from the risk of "hand wobble" during the delineation of ROI boundaries on MRI sections (Keller & Roberts, 2009).

The measurement of rates of change requires volume quantification. In general, manual or semi-automated methods have been employed for volume quantification on structural brain

MRIs, but they are generally severely limited in practicality and reliability. For example, a high-resolution 3D brain MRI data set can contain more than 100 slices to cover an entire brain (Keller & Roberts, 2009). Manually delineating tissue boundaries for volumetric measurement can be a tedious and demanding process because of the presence of the extremely complex convoluted structures of the brain. Manual tracing is also well-known to be associated with large subjective variability and low reproducibility. As a result, methods with better reproducibility and higher precision are required for measuring subtle neuro-anatomic changes and these methods are likely to be based on computerized approaches. FreeSurfer is freely available on the World Wide Web (www or commonly known as the Web), it has been widely used in the neuroimaging field. At present, fully automated methods are most often used. Fully automated or semi-automated methods can be applied to a specific ROI (such as the thalamus or the hippocampus) to obtain a regional brain volume (Houtchens et al., 2007).

## 4.2 Brain segmentation

Brain tissue segmentation of MRIs means to specify the tissue type for each pixel or voxel in a 2D or 3D data set, respectively, on the basis of information available from both MRIs and the prior knowledge of the brain. It is an important preprocessing step in many medical research and clinical applications, such as quantification of tissue volume, visualization and analysis of anatomical structures, multimodality fusion and registration, functional brain mapping, detection of pathology, surgical planning, surgical navigation, and brain substructure segmentation (Suri et al., 2002). So far, various segmentation techniques such as Gaussian mixture models (Ashburner & Friston, 2005), discriminant analysis (Amato et al., 2003), k-nearest neighbor classification (Mohamed et al., 1999), and fuzzy c-means clustering (Pham & Prince, 1999; Suckling et al., 1999; Ahmed et al., 2002; Zhou & Bai, 2007) were used to determine gray and white matter volume. Most recently, it has been reported that "fuzzy" cluster or classifier approaches were found to have a high reliability, accuracy, and validity (Herndon, 1998).

## 4.3 Image processing and segmentation

Today, medical image processing and segmentation are used to improve the quality of diagnosis. We can calculate the cortical volume and surface area using the Fuzzy C-Means algorithm as a semi-automated segmentation method as described in Figure 3.
Firstly, T1-weighted MRIs are normalized using registration algorithms. Following normalization process, we obtain brain contour to calculate volume and surface area of the brain using image working algorithms. Images of brain are cleared brain contour using morphological image processing. This method involves two major steps and final segmented images result from separation of parenchyma for brain volume and surrounding line for cortical surface area of the brain (Tosun et al., 2004; Ueda et al., 2009; Brouwer et al., 2010; Lui et al., 2010) (Fig. 4).

## 4.4 Stereological approaches

In general, stereological methods provide quantitative data on 3D structures using 2D images. Stereological methods have been widely applied on MRIs to estimate geometric variables, such as volume and surface area, and various internal brain compartments. The volume of internal brain structure can be obtained using the Cavalieri principle of stereologic approaches.

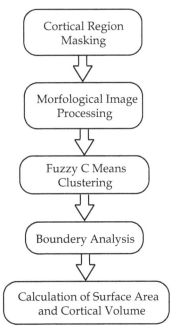

Fig. 3. Brain image segmentation blocks (Nakamura & Fisher, 2009)

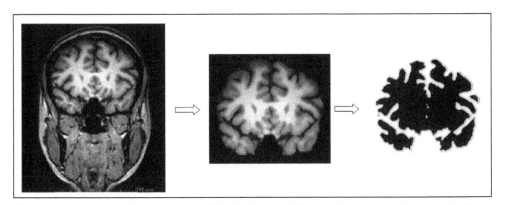

Fig. 4. Segmentation called the Fuzzy C. Left: Original T1-weighted image. Center: Masking and removal of artifacts the outer contour of the brain. Right: Contour of segmented image is outlined

### 4.4.1 Point-counting method

The Cavalieri method in combination with point counting requires beginning from a uniform random starting within the sectioning interval, a structure of interest is exhaustively sectioned with a series of parallel plane probes a constant distant apart. An unbiased estimate of volume is obtained by multiplying the total area of all sections through the structure by sectioning interval $t$ as following:

$$estV = t \times \left( a_1 + a_2 + .. + a_n \right) \qquad (1)$$

where $a_1, a_2 ... a_n$ show the section areas and $t$ is the sectioning interval (Roberts et al., 2000; García-Fiñana et al., 2003).

The point counting method involves overlying each MRI with a regular grid of test points. After each superimposition, the number of test points hitting the structure of interest is counted on each section and we can estimate volume following formula:

$$estV = t \times \left( \frac{a}{p} \right) \times \left( p_1 + p_2 + .. + p_n \right) \qquad (2)$$

where $p_1$, $p_2$,.....$p_n$ show point counts and $a/p$ represent the area associated with each test point. To avoid bias, the position of the test system should be uniform randomly (Roberts et al., 2000; García-Fiñana et al., 2003).

In any case, the following formula (Eq.3) can be used for volume estimation from MRIs of the brain (Şahin & Ergür, 2006; Acer et al., 2008):

$$V(pc) = t \times \left[ \frac{su \times d}{sl} \right]^2 \times \sum p \qquad (3)$$

where '$t$' is the section thickness, '$su$' the scale unit of the printed film, '$d$' the distance between the test points of the grid, '$sl$' the measured length of the scale printed on the film and '$\Sigma p$' is the total number of points hitting the sectioned cut surface areas of the related structures such as the cerebrum.

From stereological point of view, planimetry and point-counting are two different methods for estimating volume based on the Cavalieri principle. The Cavalieri principle may be used for estimating the volume of brain and substructures such as hypocampus, amygdale and thalamus. Therefore, a random beginning is necessary and the object is cut into slices of a known and fixed thickness. The volume is estimated by multiplying the distance between the slices by the total cut area of the structures are under investigation. The cut area of the structures may be estimated by point-counting or planimetry. Nevertheless, the Cavalieri principle in combination with point-counting is ideal for estimating total volumes of various brain and any compartments. Keller et al. (2002, 2007, 2008) and Acer et al. (2008, 2010) have previously applied this technique to obtain volume estimations of various brain structures such as Broca's area, hippocampus, ventricles, cerebral hemisphere, and cerebellum. In these studies, a set of parallel and equidistant MRIs of the brain is randomly selected, and the ROI is directly estimated on each image by randomly superimposing a grid of points, and subsequently, counting the number of points that fall within the ROI (Keller et al., 2002, 2007, 2008; Acer et al., 2008, 2010).

Stereology in combination with point counting has an advantage related with the time taken to estimate volume of brain structures on MRIs. Compared with manual tracing or segmentation methods, this technique is much more time efficient. Another advantage of stereology in combination with point counting is the prediction of the coefficient of error (CE) so that it may be used to identify the optimal parameters of sampling needed to achieve a given precision such as we need the number of MRI sections and the density of the point grid.

Importantly, the stereological approach provides an opportunity for the investigator making appropriate changes on their sampling or estimating procedures. Therefore, the Cavalieri method gives a CE of estimation for each volume assessment. Thus, an investigator may easily observe the potential variability in any given volume measurement. It may cause some problems in accuracy and hence interpretation in the presence of high CE for these measurements. If too few slices or too few points are taken for volume estimation, it is possible to encounter with such problems. The investigator is eligible to change the spacing of points in the grid or the number of slices available in any CT or MR study to provide a reasonable CE value. More importantly, an appropriate grid size and the number of slices required for volume estimation of an object is crucial at the beginning, obviating the need to calculate the CE value for repeated sessions (Sahin et al., 2003; Acer et al., 2008).

In the stereological method, continuous investigator computer interaction is necessary because all points intersecting the cerebral hemispheres should be removed or marked on consecutive MRI sections. For the reliable measurement of each brain structure using stereology in conjunction with point counting, the stereological parameters like grid size and slice gap should be optimized by counting at least 200 points per structure. In a previous study investigating the cerebral hemispheres, a grid size of 15 and slice gap of every 15 sections results in approximately 200 points being counted per hemisphere on frequently acquired 3D T1-weighted images (Mackay et al., 1998; Cowell et al., 2007), and it achieves a CE lower than the optimal 5% (Roberts et al., 2000). It has been reported that stereological volume estimation of a cerebral hemisphere using the Windows based software packages (EASYMEASURE and MEASURE) takes approximately 10 minutes (Keller & Roberts, 2009).

Stereological point counting method involves the random placement of a grid with sufficient resolution in 2D or 3D over the structure of interest and counting the points overlying the ROI. For this method, the requirements are a grid encompassing the region or structure completely, the structure placed with a grid randomly, and an adequate number of points counted on an adequate number of slices. Thus, the stereological point counting approach is very efficient and statistically sound, in addition to providing a CE of the measurement of the volume of the structure of interest.

### 4.4.2 Worked example for point-counting technique

According to point-counting technique, a square grid of test points is positioned on each MRI section, and all points hitting the cerebrum are counted (Fig. 5).

T = 1.6cm, d = 0.8cm, SU=8 cm, SL=7.8 cm, $\sum P = 796$

$$V(pc) = t \times \left[ \frac{su \times d}{sl} \right]^2 \times \sum p$$

$$V = 1.6 \times \left[ \frac{8 \times 0.8}{7.8} \right]^2 \times 796 = 856.90 cm^3$$

(3)

In the Cavalieri method in combination with point-counting technique using MRI sections, relationship between numbers of section and counts is given in Table 1.

| Section number | 1 | 2 | 3 | 4 | 5 | 6 | 7 | 8 | Total Point Counts |
|---|---|---|---|---|---|---|---|---|---|
| Point number | 42 | 72 | 122 | 132 | 129 | 116 | 115 | 68 | 796 |

Table 1. Relationship between numbers of section and counts of point in point-counting technique

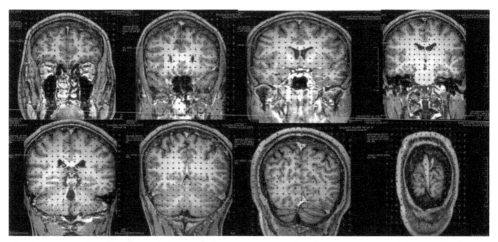

Fig. 5. Acoronal MRI series with a point-counting on it for the estimation of the cerebral volume from first to last section (T=1.6 cm)

### 4.4.3 Error prediction for point counting technique

The error predictors given below originate from the recent literature (García-Fiñana & Cruz-Orive, 2000; Garcia Finana, 2006; Garcia Finana et al., 2009). In particular, the estimation of volume and variance of the volume estimate for the cerebral volume are calculated as follows.

An unbiased estimator of $Q$ can be constructed from a sample of equidistant observations of $f$, with a distance $T$ apart, as follows:

$$\hat{Q}_T = T\sum_{k \in Z} f(x_0 + kT) = T(f_1 + f_2 + ...f_n) \tag{4}$$

where $x_0$ is a uniform random variable in the interval $[0,T)$ and $\{f_1, f_2, ... , f_n\}$ is the set of equidistant observations of $f$ at the sampling points which lie in $[a, b]$. In many applications, $Q$ represents the volume of a structure and $f(x)$ is the area of the intersection between the structure and a plane that is perpendicular to a given sampling axis at the point of abscissa $x$ (García-Fiñana & Cruz-Orive, 2000; Garcia Finana, 2006; Garcia Finana et al., 2009).

This data sample represents the area of cerebrum in cm² on a total of 8 MRI sections a distance $T = 1.6$ cm apart (Table 1).

To estimate Var ($\hat{Q}_T$) via Eq. (5) we have to calculate first $\alpha(q)$, $C_0$, $C_1$, $C_2$ and $C_4$ (Table 2).

$$\text{var}(\hat{Q}_T) = \alpha(q)(3C_0 - 4C_1 + C_2)T^2 \quad q \in [0,1] \tag{5}$$

From Eq. (6), we have:

$$C_k \sum_{i=1}^{n-k} f_i f_{i+k}, \quad k = 1, 2, ... n - 1 \tag{6}$$

Equation (5) is an extended version of the variance estimator given in (García-Fiñana & Cruz-Orive, 2004).

| Section (i) | $P_i$ | $P_i^2$ | $P_i.P_{i+1}$ | $P_i.P_{i+2}$ | $P_i.P_{i+4}$ |
|---|---|---|---|---|---|
| 1 | 42 | 1764 | 3024 | 5124 | 5418 |
| 2 | 72 | 5184 | 8784 | 9504 | 8352 |
| 3 | 122 | 14884 | 16104 | 15738 | 14030 |
| 4 | 132 | 17424 | 17028 | 15312 | 8976 |
| 5 | 129 | 16641 | 14964 | 14835 | 0 |
| 6 | 116 | 13456 | 13340 | 7888 | 0 |
| 7 | 115 | 13225 | 7820 | 0 | 0 |
| 8 | 68 | 4624 | 0 | 0 | 0 |
| | | 87202 | 81064 | 68401 | 36776 |
| Total | 796 | $C_0$ | $C_1$ | $C_2$ | $C_4$ |

Table 2. Calculation of the constants C0, C1, C2, C4

The smoothness constant can be estimated from Eq. (7) as follows:

$$q = \max\left\{0, \frac{1}{2\log 2}\log\left[\frac{(3C_0 - 4C_2 + C_4)}{(3C_0 - 4C_1 + C_2)}\right] - \frac{1}{2}\right\} \tag{7}$$

$$q = \left\{0, \frac{1}{2\log 2}\log\left[\frac{3 \times 87202 - 4 \times 68401 + 36776}{3 \times 87202 - 4 \times 81064 + 68401}\right] - \frac{1}{2}\right\} = 0.53$$

We apply Eq. (7) with $\alpha = 0.53$.
The coefficient $\alpha(q)$ has the following expression (Eq.8):

$$\alpha(q) = \frac{\Gamma(2q+2)\zeta(2q+2)\cos(\pi q)}{(2\pi)^{2q+2}\left(1 - 2^{2q-1}\right)} \quad q \in [0,1] \tag{8}$$

where $\Gamma$ and $\zeta$ denote the gamma function and the Riemann Zeta function, respectively.

$$a(0.53) = \frac{\Gamma(2.06)\zeta(2.06)\cos(1.66)}{(2\tau)^{2.06}(1 - 2^{0.06})} = 0.018$$

Therefore, the estimate of Var ($\hat{Q}_T$) obtained via Eq. (5) is:

$$\text{var}(Q_T) = a(q)(3C_0 - 4C_1 + C_2)T^2$$
$$\text{var}(Q_T) = 0.018 \times (3 \times 87202 - 4 \times 81064 + 68401) \times (1.6)^2 \tag{9}$$
$$\text{var}(Q_T) = 9.2$$

We predict the value of CE;

$$CE(Q_T) = \sqrt{9.2 / 856.9} = 0.0103 = 1.03\%$$

In our studies, we calculate the CE values as predictive using the R program. First, by using
the statistical package R, codes are developed to calculate the contribution to the predictive

CE (García-Fiñana & Cruze-Orive, 2004). A value of CE lower than 5% is in the acceptable range (Gundersen & Jensen, 1987, and 1999; Sahin et al., 2003). In addition, it is very important to note that an appropriate grid size and the number of slices required for volume estimation of an object is crucial at the beginning.

## 5. Conclusion

In conlusion, MRI may help to specify the cause of the disease such as the brain atrophy, if a kind of neurodegenerative dissease is present. Unfortunately, however, conventional MRI study not give subsutructural detailed information about cellular and molecular organisation of the brain tissue. On the other hand, it is also possible to define the etiologies of the pathologies using new functional MRI methods, such as diffusion weighted imaging and MRS. Future advances in functional and anatomic neuroimaging techniques provide further insights into certain neurodegenerative disseases of the brain. A combination of different neuroimaging techniques and atrophy correction through MRI, PET and SPECT superimposition may demonstrate functional and morphological features of the brain tissue. In similar to MRI, PET and SPECT are useful in the diagnosis of some neurodegenerative diseases.

By using MRI, the estimation of the brain volume is a well-known entity for the determination of the brain atrophy. Several different methods such as segmentation techniques are available for the estimation of the brain volume, but there are only a few stereological studies using point-counting and planimetric methods. Recently, the Cavalieri principle in combination with point-counting has become popular in the understanding of the pathologies of brain morphology. There is no doubt that determination of the brain atrophy using MRI will be useful in understanding of neurodegenerative diseases, monitoring of disease progression, and treatment of such patients. In conclusion, the Cavalieri principle in combination with point-counting is an ideal method for the estimation of total volume of the brain or any of its compartment for the diagnosis of atrophic neurodegenerative diseases.

Nevertheless, further combinations of new imaging techniques with different methods for volume estimation using a combination of different neuroimaging techniques are needed for early diagnosis and monitorization of course of the disease. It is important to know that these techniques for volume estimation must be reproducible and reliable. The greater accuracy of imaging methods in detection of early neurodegenerative disseases will result in early optimal treatment to delay further cognitive decline.

## 6. References

Acer, N.; Sahin, B.; Baş, O.; Ertekin, T. & Usanmaz, M. (2007). Comparison of three methods for the estimation of total intracranial volume: stereologic, planimetric, and anthropometric approaches. *Ann Plast Surg* Vol. 58, No. 1, (Jan 2007), pp. 48-53. ISSN 0148-7043

Acer, N.; Sahin, B.; Usanmaz, M., Tatoğlu, H. & Irmak, Z. (2008). Comparison of point counting and planimetry methods for the assessment of cerebellar volume in human using magnetic resonance imaging: a stereological study. *Surg Radiol Anat* Vol. 30, No. 4, (Jun 2008), pp. 335-9. ISSN 0930-1038

Acer, N.; Uğurlu, N.; Uysal, DD.; Unur, E.; Turgut, M. & Camurdanoğlu, M. (2010). Comparison of two volumetric techniques for estimating volume of intracerebral ventricles using magnetic resonance imaging: a stereological study. *Anat Sci Int* Vol. 85, No. 3, (Sep 2010), pp. 131-9. ISSN 1447-6959

Ahmed, MN.; Yamany, SM.; Mohamed, N.; Farag, AA. & Moriarty, T. (2002). A modified fuzzy c-means algorithm for bias field estimation and segmentation of MRI data. *EEE Trans Med Imag* Vol. 21, No. 3, (Mar 2002), pp. 193–199. ISSN 0278-0062

Amato, U.; Larobina, M.; Antoniadis, A. & Alfano, B. (2003). Segmentation of magnetic resonance brain images through discriminant analysis. *J Neurosci Methods* Vol. 131, No. 1-2, (Dec 2003), pp 65–74. ISSN 0165-0270

Appel, J.; Potter, E.; Shen, Q.; Pantol G.; Greig, MT.; Loewenstein, D. & Duara, R. (2009). A comparative analysis of structural brain MRI in the diagnosis of Alzheimer's disease. *Behav Neurol* Vol. 21, No. 1, (Oct 2009), pp. 13–19, ISSN 0953-4180

Ashburner, J. & Friston, KJ. (2005). Unified segmentation. *NeuroImage* Vol. 26, No. 3, (Jul 2005), pp. 839–851. ISSN 1053-8119

Belliveau JW, Kennedy DN, McKinstry RC, Buchinder, BR; Weiskoff, RM; Cohen, MS; Vevea, JM, Brady, TJ. & Rosen BR. (1992). Functional mapping of the human visual cortex by magnetic resonance imaging. *Science* Vol. 254, No. 5032, (Nov 1991), pp. 716–719. ISSN 0036-8075

Basser, PJ.; Mattiello, J. & LeBihan, D. (1994). MR diffusion tensor spectroscopy and imaging. *Biophysics Journal* Vol. 66, No. 1 (Jan 1994), pp. 259-267, ISSN 0006-3495/94/01/259/09

Bermel, RA.; Sharma, J.; Tjoa, CW.; Puli, SR. & Bakshi, R. (2003). A semiautomated measure of whole-brain atrophy in multiple sclerosis. *J Neurol Sci* Vol. 208, No. 1-2, (Apr 2003), pp. 57–65, ISSN 0022-510X

Bothwell, JH. & Griffin JL. (2011). An introduction to biological nuclear magnetic resonance spectroscopy. *Biol Rev Camb Philos Soc* Vol. 86, No. 2, (May 2011), pp. 493-510, ISSN 0006-3231

Brouwer, RM.; Hulshoff, PHE. & Schnack, HG. (2010). Segmentation of MRI brain scans using non-uniform partial volume densities. *NeuroImage* Vol. 49, No. 1, (Jan 2010), pp. 467-477, ISSN 1053-8119

Bradley, WG. Jr. & Bydder, GM. (1997). *Advanced MR Imaging techniques.* Martin Dunitz Ltd, Informa Healthcare; 1 ed., , London. ISBN 978-1853170249

Boone, KB.; Miller, BL.; Lesser, IM.; Mehringer, CM.; Hill-Gutierrez, E.; Goldberg, MA. & Berman, NG. (1992). Neuropsychological correlates of white-matter lesions in healthy elderly subjects. A threshold effect. *Arch Neurol* Vol. 49, No. 5, (May 1992), pp. 549–554, ISSN 0003-9942

Bonilha, L.; Halford, JJ.; Rorden, C.; Roberts, DR.; Rumboldt, Z. & Eckert, MA. (2009). Automated MRI analysis for identification of hippocampal atrophy in temporal lobe epilepsy. *Epilepsia* Vol. 50, No. 2 (Feb 2009) pp. 228-233. ISSN 0013-9580

Buchsbaum, MS.; Tang, CY.; Peled, S.; Gudbjartsson, H.; Lu, D.; Hazlett, EA.; Downhill, J.; Haznedar, M.; Fallon, JH. & Atlas SW. (1998). MRI white matter dianffusion anisotropy and PET metabolic rate in schizophrenia. *Neuroreport* Vol. 9, No. 3 (Feb 1998), pp. 425–430, ISSN 0959-4965

Creasey, H.; Schwartz, M.; Frederickson, H.; Haxby, JV. & Rapoport, SI. (1986). Quantitative computed tomography in dementia of the Alzheimer type. *Neurology* Vol. 36, No. 12 (Dec 1986), pp. 1563-1568. ISSN 0811-8663

Chan-Palay, V. & Asan, E. (1989). Alterations in catecholamine neurons of the locus coeruleus in senile dementia of the Alzheimer type and in Parkinson's disease with and without dementia and depression. *J Comp Neurol* Vol. 287, No. 3, (Sep1989), pp. 373-392, ISSN 0021-9967

Calmon, G. & Roberts, N. (2000). Automatic measurement of changes in brain volume on consecutive 3DMR images by segmentation propagation. *Magn Reson Imaging* Vol. 18, No.4 (May 2000), pp. 439-453, ISSN 0730-725X

Cowell, PE.; Sluming, VA.; Wilkinson, ID.; Cezayirli, E.; Romanowski, CA.; Webb, JA.; Keller, SS.; Mayes, A. & Roberts, N. (2007). Effects of sex and age on regional prefrontal brain volume in two human cohorts. *Eur J Neurosci* Vol. 25, No. 1 (Jan 2007), pp. 307-318, ISSN 0953-816X

Dale, AM.; Fischl, B. & Sereno, MI. (1999). Cortical surface-based analysis I. Segmentation and surface reconstruction. *Neuroimage* Vol. 9, No. 2 (Feb 1999), pp. 179-194, ISSN 1053-8119

Davatzikos, C.; Fan, Y.; Wu, X.; Shen, D. & Resnick, SM. (2008). Detection of prodromal Alzheimer's disease via pattern classification of magnetic resonance imaging. *Neurobiol Aging* Vol. 29, No. 4 (Apr 2008), pp. 514-523, ISSN 0197-4580

Ewers M, Frisoni GB, Teipel SJ, Grinberg LT, Amaro E Jr, Heinsen H, Thompson PM. & Hampel H. (2011). Staging Alzheimer's disease progression with multimodality neuroimaging. *Prog Neurobiol* (in press). ISSN 0301-0082

Fischl, B.; Sereno, MI. & Dale, AM. (1999). Cortical surface-based analysis. II: Inflation, flattening, and a surface-based coordinate system. *Neuroimage* Vol. 9, No. 2 (Feb 1999), pp. 195-207, ISSN 1053-8119

Fischl, B., Salat, DH.; Busa, E.; Albert, M.; Dieterich, M.; Haselgrove, C.; van der Kouwe, A.; Killiany, R.; Kennedy, D.; Klaveness, S.; Montillo, A.; Makris, N.; Rosen, B. & Dale, AM. (2002). Whole brain segmentation: automated labeling of neuroanatomical structures in the human brain. *Neuron* Vol. 33, No. 3 (Jan 2002), pp. 341-355, ISSN 0896-6273

Flippi, M.; Masrtonardo, G.; Rocca, MA.; Pereira, C. & Comi, G. (1998). Quntative volumetric analysis of brain magnetic resonance imaging from patients with multiple sclerosis. *J Neurol Sci* Vol. 158, No. 2 (Jun 1998), pp. 148-153. ISSN 0022-510X

Frey, H.; Lahtinen, A.; Heinonen, T. & Dastidar, P. (1999). Clinical Application of MRI Image Processing in Neurology *IJBEM* Vol. 1, No. 1 (May 1999), pp. 47-53, ISSN 1456-7865

Furlong, C. (2008) Investigation of the precision and accuracy of surface area and volume estimators of the human brain using stereology and magnetic resonance. *Liverpool University.* Doctorate Thesis, (March 2008), England

García-Fiñana, M.; Cruz-Orive, LM.; Mackay, CE.; Pakkenberg, B. & Roberts, N. (2003). Comparison of MR imaging against physical sectioning to estimate the volume of human cerebral compartments. *Neuroimage* Vol. 18, No. 2 (Feb 2003), pp. 505-516, ISSN 1053-8119

García-Fiñana, M. (2006). Confidence intervals in Cavalieri sampling. *J Microsc* Vol. 222, No. 3, (Jun 2006), pp. 146-157, ISSN 0022-2720

García-Fiñana, M.; Keller, SS. & Roberts, N. (2009). Confidence intervals for the volume of brain structures in Cavalieri sampling with local errors. *J Neurosci Methods* Vol. 179, No. 1 (Apr 2009), pp. 71-77, ISSN 0165-0270

García-Fiñana M. & Cruze-Orive LM. (2004). Improved variance prediction for systematic on R. *Statistics* Vol. 38, No. 3, pp. 243-272, ISSN 0233-1888

García-Fiñana, M. & Cruz-Orive, LM. (2000). New approximations for the variance in cavalieri sampling. *J Microsc* Vol. 199, No. 2 (Sep 2000), pp. 224–238, ISSN 0022-2720

Geuze, E.; Vermetten, E. & Bremner, JD. (2005). MR-based in vivo hippocampal volumetrics: 1. Review of methodologies currently employed. *Mol Psychiatry* Vol. 10, No. 2 (Feb 2005), pp. 147-159, ISSN 1359-4184

Gundersen, HJ. & Jensen, EB. (1987). The efficiency of systematic sampling in stereology and its prediction. *J Microsc* Vol. 147, No. 3 (Sep 1987), pp. 229-263, ISSN 0022-2720

Gomez-Isla, T.; Hollister, R.; West, H.; Mui, S.; Growdon, JH.; Petersen, RC.; Parisi, JE. & Hyman, BT. (1997). Neuronal loss correlates with but exceeds neurofibrillary tangles in Alzheimer's disease. *Ann Neurol* Vol. 41, No. 1 (Jan 1997), pp. 17–24, ISSN 0364-5134

Gomez-Isla, T.; Price, JL.; McKeel, DW Jr.; Morris, JC.; Growdon, JH. & Hyman, BT. (1996). Profound loss of layer II entorhinal cortex neurons occurs in very mild Alzheimer's disease. *J Neurosci* Vol. 16, No. 14 (Jul 1996), pp. 4491–4500, ISSN 0270-6474

Grassiot, B.; Desgranges, B.; Eustache, F. & Defer, G. (2009). Quantification and clinical relevance of brain atrophy in multiple sclerosis: a review. *J Neurol* Vol. 256, No. 9 (Sep 2009), pp. 1397-1412, ISSN 0340-5354

Gundersen, HJ.; Jensen, EB.; Kiêu, K. & Nielsen, J. (1999). The efficiency of systematic sampling in stereology reconsidered. *J Microsc* Vol. 193, No. 4 (Mar 1999), pp. 199–211, ISSN 0022-2720

Hanyu, H.; Shindo, H.; Kakizaki D.; Abe, K.; Iwamoto, T. & Takasaki M. (1997). Increased water diffusion in cerebral white matter in Alzheimer's disease. *Gerontology* Vol. 43, No. 6 (Oct 24, 1996), pp. 343–351, ISSN 0304-324X

Henry, TR.; Chupin, M.; Lehéricy, S.; Strupp, JP.; Sikora, MA.; Sha, ZY.; Ugurbil, K. & Van de Moortele, PF. (2011). Hippocampal sclerosis in temporal lobe epilepsy: findings at 7 T. *Radiology* (in press). [Epub ahead of print]. ISSN 0033-8419

Horsfield, MA.; Rovaris, M.; Rocca, MA.; Rossi, P.; Benedict, RH.; Filippi, M. & Bakshi, R. (2003). Whole-brain atrophy in multiple sclerosis measured by two segmentation processes from various MRI sequences. *Neurol Sci* Vol. 216, No. 1 (Dec 2003), pp. 169-177, ISSN 0020-510X

Houtchens, MK.; Benedict, RH.; Killiany, R.; Sharma, J.; Jaisani, Z., Singh, B.; Weinstock-Guttman, B.; Guttmann, CR. & Bakshi, R. (2007). Thalamic atrophy and cognition in multiple sclerosis. *Neurology* Vol. 69, No. 17 (Sep 2007), pp. 1213–1223, ISSN 0028-3878

Herndon, RC., Lancaster, JL., Giedd, JN. & Fox, PT. (1998). Quantification of white matter and gray matter volumes from three-dimensional magnetic resonance golume studies using fuzzy classifiers. *J Magn Reson Imaging* Vol. 8, No. 5 (Sep 1998), pp. 1097-1005, ISSN 1053-1807

Jones, EK.; Simmons, A.; Williams, SCR. & Horsfield, MA. (1999). Non-invasive assessment of axonal fiber connectivity in the human brain via diffusion tensor MRI. *Magn Reson Med* Vol. 42, No. 1 (July 1999), pp. 37–41, ISSN 1522-2594

Keller, SS. & Roberts, N. (2009). Measurement of brain volume using MRI: software, techniques, choices and prerequisites. *Journal of Anthropological Sciences* Vol. 87, pp. 127-151, ISSN 1827-4765

Keller, SS.; Mackay, CE.,; Barrick, TR.; Wieshmann, UC.; Howard, MA. & Roberts N. (2002). Voxel-based morphometric comparison of hippocampal and extrahippocampal abnormalities in patients with left and right hippocampal atrophy. *Neuroimage* Vol. 16, No. 1 (May 2002), pp. 23-31, ISSN 1053-8119

Keller SS.; Highley JR.; Garcia-Finana M.; Sluming V.; Rezaie R. & Roberts N. (2007). Sulcal variability, stereological measurement and asymmetry of Broca's area on MR images. *J Anat* Vol. 211, No. 4 (Oct 2007), pp. 534-555, ISSN 0021-8782

Keller, SS & Roberts, N. (2008). Voxel-based morphometry of temporal lobe epilepsy: An introduction and review of the literature. *Epilepsia* (May 2008), Vol. 49, No. 5, pp. 741-757, ISSN 0013-9580

Kern, A. & Behl, C. (2009). The unsolved relationship of brain aging and late-onset Alzheimer disease *Biochimica et Biophysica Acta (BBA)* Vol. 1790, No. 10, (Oct 2009), pp. 1124-1132, ISSN 0304-4165

Kesslak, JP.; Nalcioglu, O. & Cotman, CW. (1991). Quantification of magnetic resonance scans for hippocampal and parahippocampal atrophy in Alzheimer's disease. *Neurology* Vol. 41, No. 1 (Jan 1991), pp. 51–54, ISSN 0811-8663

Kucharczyk, W. & Henkelman, M. (1994). Visibility of Calcium on MR and CT: can MR show calcium that CT can not?. *AJNR Am J Neuroradiol.* Vol. 15, No. 6 (Jun 1994), pp. 1145–1148, ISSN 0195-6108

Likeman, M.; Anderson, VM.; Stevens, JM.; Waldman, AD.; Godbolt, AK.; Frost, C.; Rossor, MN. & Fox, NC. (2005). Visual assessment of atrophy on magnetic resonance imaging in the diagnosis of pathologically confirmed young-onset demantias. *Arch Neurol* Vol. 62, No. 9 (Sept 2005), pp. 1410-1415, ISSN 0003-9942

Lim, OK.; Rosenbloom, M. & Pfefferbaum, A. (2000). In Vivo Structural Brain Assessment: In: *Psychopharmacology-4th Generation of Progress,* Bloom FE, Kupfer DJ. (Ed.), Part II Clinic section, ISBN 978-0781701662.
http://www.acnp.org/g4/GN401000089/Default.htm

Liu, YS.; Yi, J.; Zhang, H.; Zheng, G. & Paul, JC. (2010). Surface area estimation of digitized 3D objects using quasi-Monte Carlo methods. *Pattern Recogn.* Vol. 43, No. 11 (November 2010), pp. 3900-3909, ISSN 0031-3203

Loewe, C.; Oschatz, E. & Prayer, D. (2002). Imaging of Neurodegenerative Disorders of the Brain in Adults. *Imaging Decisions* Vol. 6, Suplement 1 (Dec 2002), pp. 4-18, ISSN 1617-0830

Lopez, OL.; Becker, JT.; Rezek, D.; Wess, J.; Boller F.; Reynolds CF, 3rd. & Panisset, M. (1992). Neuropsychiatric correlates of cerebral white-matter radiolucencies in probable Alzheimer's disease. *Arch Neurol* Vol. 49, No. 8 (Aug 1992), pp. 828–834, ISSN 0003-9942

Mackay, CE.; Roberts, N.; Mayes, AR.; Downes, JJ.; Foster, JK. & Mann, D. (1998). An exploratory study of the relationship between face recognition memory and the volume of medial temporal lobe structures in healthy young males. *Behav Neurol* Vol. 11, No. 1 (Jan 1998), pp. 3-20, ISSN 0953-4180

Masliah, E.; Terry, R.; Alford, M.; DeTeresa, R. & Hansen, LA. (1991). Cortical and subcortical patterns of synaptophysin-like immunoreactivity in Alzheimer's disease. *Am J Pathol* Vol. 138, No. 1 (Jan 1991), pp. 235–246, ISSN 0002-9440

Mazziotta, JC.; Frackowiak, RSJ. & Phelps, ME. (1992). The use of positron emission tomography in the clinical assessment of dementia. *Semin Nucl Med* Vol. 22, No. 4 (Oct 1992), pp. 233–246, ISSN 0001-2998

McKhann, GM.; Albert, MS.; Grossman, M.; Miller, B.; Dickson, D. & Trojanowski, JQ. (2001). Clinical and pathological diagnosis of frontotemporal dementia: Report of the Work Group on Frontotemporal Dementia and Pick's Disease. *Arch Neurol* Vol. 58, No. 11 (Nov 2001), pp. 1803-1809, ISSN 0003-9942

Mohamed, FB.; Vinitski, S.; Faro, SH.; Gonzalez, CF.; Mack, J. & Iwanaga, T. (1999). Optimization of tissue segmentation of brain MR images based on multispectral 3D feature maps. *Magn. Reson. Imaging* Vol.17, No. 3 (Apr 1999), pp. 403–409, ISSN 0730-725X

Mohs, RC. & Haroutunian, V. (2002) Chapter 82: Alzheimer Disease: From Earliest Symptoms to End Stage, *Neuropsychopharmacology*: pp. 1189-1197. Edited by Kenneth L. Davis, Dennis Charney, Joseph T. Coyle, and Charles Nemeroff. American College of Neuropsychopharmacology The Fifth Generation of Progress

Molyneux, PD.; Kappos, L.; Polman, C.; Pozzilli, C.; Barkhof, F.; Filippi, M.; Yousry, T; Hahn, D.; Wagner, K.; Ghazi, M.; Beckmann, K.; Dahlke, F.; Losseff, N.; Barker, GJ.; Thompson, AJ. & Miller, DH. (2000). The effect of interferon beta-1b treatment on MRI measures of cerebral atrophy in secondary progressive multiple sclerosis. European Study Group on Interferon Beta-1b in Secondary Progressive Multiple Sclerosis. *Brain* Vol. 123, No. 11 (Nov 2000), pp. 2256-2263, ISSN 0006-8950

Nagy, Z.; Esiri, MM.; Jobst, KA.; Morris, JH.; King, EM.; McDonald, B.; Litchfield, S.; Smith, A.; Barnetson, L. & Smith, AD. (1995). Relative roles of plaques and tangles in the dementia of Alzheimer's disease: correlations using three sets of neuropathological criteria. *Dementia* Vol. 6, No. 1 (Jan 1995), pp. 21–31, ISSN 1013-7424

Nakamura, K. & Fisher, E. (2009). Segmentation of brain magnetic resonance iamges for measuremnt of gray matter atrophy in multple sclerosis patients. *Neuroimage* Vol. 44, No. 3 (Feb 2009), pp. 796-776, ISSN 1053-8119

Neary, D,; Snowden, JS.; Gustafson, L.; Passant, U.; Stuss, D.; Black, S.; Freedman, M.; Kertesz, A.; Robert, PH.; Albert, M.; Boone, K.; Miller, BL.; Cummings, J. & Benson, DF. (1998). Frontotemporal lobar degeneration: A consensus on clinical diagnostic criteria. *Neurology* Vol. 51, No. 6 (Dec 1998), pp. 1546-1554, ISSN 0811-8663

Obrien, JT. (2007). Role of imaging techniques in the diagnosis of dementia. *Br J Radiol* Vol. 80, No. 2 (Dec 20074), pp. 71-77, ISSN 0007-1285

O'Sullivan, M. (2009). Patterns of brain atrophy on magnetic resonance imaging and the boundary between ageing and Alzheimer's disease. *Rev Clin Gerontol* Vol. 19, No. 4 (Nov 2009), pp. 295-307, ISSN 0959-2598

Pearlson, GD.; Harris, GJ.; Powers, RE.; Barta, PE.; Camargo, EE.; Chase, GA.; Noga, JT. & Tune, LE. (1992). Quantitative changes in mesial temporal volume, regional cerebral blood flow, and cognition in Alzheimer's disease. *Arch Gen Psychiatry* Vol. 49, No. 5 (May 1992), pp. 402–408. ISSN 0003-990X

Pelletier, D.; Garrison, K. & Henry, R. (2004). Measurement of whole brain atrophy in multiple sclerosis. *J Neuroimaging* Vol. 14, No. 3 (Jul 2004), pp.11S–19S, ISSN 1051-2284

Pham, DL. & Prince, JL. (1999). Adaptive fuzzy segmentation of magnetic resonance images. *IEEE Trans Med Imag* Vol. 18, No. 9 (Sep 1999), pp. 737–752, ISSN 0278-0062

Ratnavalli, E.; Brayne, C.; Dawson, K. & Hodges, JR. (2002). The prevalence of frontotemporal dementia. *Neurology* Vol. 58, No. 11 (Jun 2002), pp. 1615-1621. ISSN 0811-8663

Rusinek, H.; de Leon, MJ.; George, AE.; Stylopoulos, LA.; Chandra, R.; Smith, G.; Rand, T.; Mourino, M. & Kowalski, H. (1991). Alzheimer disease: measuring loss of cerebral gray matter with MR imaging. *Radiology* Vol. 178, No. 1 (Jan 1991), pp. 109–114. ISSN 0033-8419

Rosen, HJ.; Gorno-Tempini, ML.; Goldman, WP.; Perry, RJ.; Schuff, N.; Weiner, M.; Feiwell, R.; Kramer, JH. & Miller, BL. (2002). Patterns of brain atrophy in frontotemporal dementia and semantic dementia. *Neurology* Vol. 58, No. 2 (Jan 2002), pp. 198–208. ISSN 0811-8663

Rosen, HJ.; Allison, SC.; Schauer, GF.; Gorno-Tempini, ML.; Weiner, MW. & Miller, BL. (2005). Neuroanatomical correlates of behavioural disorders in dementia. *Brain* Vol. 128, No. 11 (Nov 2005), pp. 2612–2625. ISSN 0006-8950

Rosen, HJ.; Wilson, MR.; Schauer, GF.; Allison S.; Gorno-Tempini ML.; Pace-Savitsky C.; Kramer JH.; Levenson RW.; Weiner M. & Miller BL. (2006). Neuroanatomical correlates of impaired recognition of emotion in dementia. *Neuropsychologia* Vol. 44, No. 3 (Sep 2005), pp. 365–373, ISSN 0028-3932

Ron, MA.; Acker, W.; Shaw, GK. & Lishman, WA. (1982). Computerized tomography of the brain in chronic alcoholism: a survey and follow-up study. *Brain* Vol. 105, No. 3 (Sep 1982), pp. 497-514. ISSN 0006-8950

Roberts, N.; Puddephat, MJ. & McNulty, V. (2000). The benefit of stereology for quantitative radiology. *Br J Radiol* Vol. 73, No. 871 (Jul 200), pp. 679-697, ISSN 0007-1285.

Sahin, B. & Ergur, H. (2006). Assessment of the optimum section thickness for the estimation of liver volume using magnetic resonance images: a stereological gold standard study. *Eur J Radiol* Vol. 57, No. 1 (Jan 2006), pp. 96-101. ISSN 0720-04X

Sahin, B.; Emirzeoglu, M.; Uzun, A.; Incesu, L.; Bek, Y.; Bilgic, S. & Kaplan, S. (2003). Unbiased estimation of the liver volume by the Cavalieri principle using magnetic resonance images. *Eur J Radiol* Vol. 47, No. 2 (Aug 2003), pp. 164– 170, ISSN 0720-04X

Sanfilipo, MP.; Benedict, RH.; Sharma, J.; Weinstock-Guttman, B. & Bakshi, R. (2005). The relationship between whole brain volume and disability in multiple sclerosis: a comparison of normalized gray vs white matter with misclassification correction. *Neuroimage* Vol. 26, No. 4 (July 2005), pp. 1068–1077. ISSN 1053-8119

Sanfilipo, MP.; Benedict, RH.; Weinstock-Guttman, B. & Bakshi, R. (2006). Gray and white matter brain atrophy and neuropsychological impairment in multiple sclerosis. *Neurology* Vol. 66, No. 5 (Mar 2006), pp. 685–692, ISSN 0811-8663

Schuckit, MA. (1992). An introduction and overview of clinical applications of NeuroSPECT in psychiatry. *J Clin Psychiatry* Vol. 53, Suppl (November 1992), pp. 3–6, ISSN 0160-6689

Schuff, N.; Amend, D.; Ezekiel, F.; Steinman, SK.; Tanabe, J.; Norman, D.; Jagust, W.; Kramer, JH.; Mastrianni, JA.; Fein, G. & Weiner, MW. (1997). Changes of hippocampal N-acetyl aspartate and volume in Alzheimer's disease: a proton MR spectroscopic imaging and MRI study. *Neurology* Vol. 49, No. 6, pp. 1513–1521. ISSN 0811-8663

Seppi, K. & Schocke, MF. (2005). An update on conventional and advanced magnetic resonance imaging techniques in the differential diagnosis of neurodegenerative parkinsonism. *Curr Opin Neurol* Vol. 18, No. 4 (Aug 2005), pp. 370–375. ISSN 1350-7540

Sharma, J.; Sanfilipo , MP.; Benedict, RH.;Weinstock-Guttman, B.; Munschauer, FEIII.. & Bakshi, R. (2004). Whole-brain atrophy in multiple sclerosis measured by automated versus semiautomated MR imaging segmentation. *AJNR Am J Neuroradiol* Vol. 25, No. 6 (Jun 2004), pp. 985–996, ISSN 0195-6108

Small, GW. (2002). Structural And Functional Brain Imaging of Alzheimer Disease. *Neuropsychopharmacology: The Fifth Generation of Progress,* Davis, KL.; Charney, D.; Joyle, J. (Ed). pp. 1232-1242. ISBN 978-0781728379.

Smith, SM.; Zhang, Y.; Jenkinson, M.; Chen, J.; Matthews, PM.; Federico, A. & De Stefano, N. (2002). Accurate, robust, and automated longitudinal and cross-sectional brain change analysis, *Neuroimage* Vol. 17, No. 1 (Sep 2002), pp. 479–489, ISSN 1053-8119

Stokking, R.; Vincken, KL. & Viergever, MA. (2000). Automatic morphology-based brain segmentation (MBRASE) from MRI-T1 data. *Neuroimage* Vol. 12, No. 6 (Dec 2000), pp. 726–738, ISSN 1053-8119

Suckling, J.; Sigmundsson, T.; Greenwood, K. & Bullmore, ET. (1999). A modified fuzzy clustering algorithm for operator independent brain tissue classification of dual echo MR images. *Magn Reson Imaging* Vol. 17, No. 7 (Sep 1999), pp. 1065–1076, ISSN 0730-725X

Suri, JS.; Setarehdan, SK. & Singh, S. (2002). Advanced Algorithmic Approaches to Medical Image Segmentation: *State-of-the-Art Applications in Cardiology, Neurology, Mammography and Pathology.* Spring- Verlag, London/Berlin/Heidelberg, ISBN 978-1-85233-389-8

Terry, RD.; Peck, A.; DeTeresa, R.; Schechter, R. & Horoupian, DS. (1981). Some morphometric aspects of the brain in senile dementia of the Alzheimer type. *Ann Neurol* Vol. 10, No. 2 (Aug 1981), pp. 184–192, ISSN 0364-5134

Teipel, SJ.; Bayer, W.; Alexander, GE.; Bokde, AL.; Zebuhr, Y.; Teichberg, D.; Müller-Spahn, F.; Schapiro, MB.; Möller, HJ.; Rapoport, SI. & Hampel, H. (2003). Regional pattern of hippocampus and corpus callosum atrophy in Alzheimer's disease in relation to dementia severity: evidence for early neocortical degeneration. *Neurobiol Aging* Vol. 24, No. 1 (Jan 2003), pp. 85–94, ISSN 0197-4580

Tosun, D.; Rettmann, ME.; Han, X.; Tao, X., Xu, C.; Resnick, SM., Dzung, LP. & Prince, JL. (2004). Cortical surface segmentation and mapping, *NeuroImage* Vol. 23, Suppl. 1, pp. 108-118, ISSN 1053-8119

Ueda, K.; Fujiwara, H.; Miyata, J.; Hirao, K.; Saze, T.; Kawata, R.; Fujimoto, S., Tanaka, Y., Sawamoto, N.; Fukuyama, H. & Murai T. (2009). Investigating association of brain volumes with intracranial capacity in schizophrenia. *Neuroimage* Vol. 19, No. 3, (Sep 2009), pp. 2503-2508, ISSN 1053-8119

Vitali, P.; Migliaccio, R.; Agosta, F.; Rosen, HJ. & Geschwind, MD. (2008). Neuroimaging in dementia. *Semin Neurol* Vol. 28, No. 4, pp. 467-483. ISSN 0271-8235

Wagner, AD.; Schacter, DL.; Rotte, M.; Koutstaal, W.; Maril, A.; Dale, AM.; Rosen, BR. & Buckner, RL. (1998). Building memories: remembering and forgetting of verbal experiences as predicted by brain activity. *Science* Vol. 281, No. 5380 (Aug 1998), pp.1188-1191, ISSN 0036-8075

Webb, J.; Guimond, A., Eldridge, P.; Chadwick, D.;   Meunier, J. & Thirion, JP. (1999). Automatic detection of hippocampal atrophy on magnetic resonance images. *Magn Reson Imaging* Vol. 17, No. 8 (Oct 1999), pp. 1149–1161, ISSN 0730-725X

Weiner, MW. (1987). NMR spectroscopy for clinical medicine, animal models, and clinical examples. *Ann NY Acad Sci* Vol. 508, (November 1987), pp. 287–289, ISSN 1749-6632

Whitehouse, PJ.; Price, DL.; Struble, RG.; Clark, AW.; Coyle, JT. & Delon, MR. (1982). Alzheimer's disease and senile dementia: loss of neurons in the basal forebrain. *Science* Vol. 215, No. 4537 (Mar 1982), pp. 1237–1239, ISSN 0036-8075

Yamauchi, H.; Fukuyama, H.; Nagahama, Y.; Katsumi, Y.; Hayashi, T.; Oyanagi, C.; Konishi, J. & Shio, H. (2000). Comparison of the pattern of atrophy of the corpus callosum in frontotemporal dementia, progressive supranuclear palsy, and Alzheimer's disease. *J Neurol Neurosurg Psychiatry* Vol. 69, No. 5, (Nov 2000), pp. 623–629, ISSN 0022-3050

Zweig, RM.;  Ross, CA.; Hedreen, JC.; Steele, C.; Cardillo, JE.; Whitehouse, PJ.; Folstein, MF. & Price, DL. (1988). The neuropathology of aminergic nuclei in Alzheimer's disease. *Ann Neurol* Vol. 24, No. 2, (Aug 1988), pp. 233–242, ISSN 0364-5134

Zhou, Y. & Bai, J. (2007). Atlas-based fuzzy connectedness segmentation and intensity nonuniformity correction applied to brain MRI. *IEEE Trans. Biomed Eng* Vol. 54, No. 1, pp. 122–129, ISSN 0278-0062

# 8

# Genome Profiling and Potential Biomarkers in Neurodegenerative Disorders

Luca Lovrečić, Aleš Maver and Borut Peterlin

*Clinical Institute of Medical Genetics, University Medical Center Ljubljana,*
*Slovenia*

## 1. Introduction

Neurodegenerative disorders (NDG) are incurable, progressive and debilitating conditions resulting from progressive degeneration and death of nerve cells. They are among the most serious health problems faced by modern society. Most of these disorders become more common with advancing age, including Alzheimer's disease and Parkinson's disease. The burden of these neurodegenerative diseases is growing inexorably as the population ages, with incalculable economic and human costs. According to the Global Burden of Disease Study, a collaborative study of the World Health Organization, the World Bank and the Harvard School of Public Health, dementia and other neurodegenerative diseases will be the eighth cause of disease burden for developed regions in 2020 [1, 2]. Also, according to the WHO, neurodegenerative diseases will become the world's second leading cause of death by 2050, overtaking cancer [2]. True, such estimates and predictions need to be taken with caution, but they definitely confirm that neurodegenerative diseases are of an increasing public concern.

Most NDG diseases are characterized by the aggregation of intracellular proteins. Majority of neurodegenerative disorders occur sporadically and are believed to arise through interactions between genetic and environmental factors. Only a small minority belong to familial forms where certain disease occurs due to a mutation of the gene coding for the abnormally aggregating protein.

We differentiate many types of NDG disease, but the lines that separate one from another are often unclear. For instance, symptoms such as motor impairment and dementia may occur in many different types of NDG disease. Motor impairment similar to that seen in Parkinson's disease is not enough to rule out other diagnoses, especially when both motor and cognitive impairment are present. At the time being, there is no such diagnostic test that can clearly indicate the presence, absence, or category of a NDG disease. Individual diagnosis is based on clinical evaluation of the symptoms, with the exception of monogenic NDG diseases, such as Huntington's disease (HD). HD is a single gene disorder and cause is invariably trinucleotide expansion mutation [3].

Definitive diagnosis of certain NDG diseases still relies on neuropathological evaluation. But it has been demonstrated that brain pathology can show marked overlap among the syndromes of age-related cognitive and motor impairment [4]. Also, previous research reports have shown that pathological markers do not always correlate optimally with clinical findings. Some individuals with extensive neuropathology may retain relatively intact neurological function while others with less extensive pathology may be significantly impaired [5, 6]. The neuropathological findings may be the response to other antecedent disease processes and are not necessarily the cause of the underlying disease at the early disease stages. Later, as disease progresses, they probably contribute to disease progression in a positive feedback loop.

Analysis of whole genome transcriptome in brain might give us insights into the disturbed pathways and processes involved in disease onset and progression. Many different mechanisms have been proposed to be dysregulated in NDG diseases. We collected all reported studies to date on brain transcriptome in Parkinson's disease, Alzheimer disease, Huntington disease and Down syndrome and performed an integrated meta-analysis.

## 2. Background

### 2.1 Common neurodegenerative disorders – Alzheimer and Parkinson disease

Two most common neurodegenerative diseases, Parkinson's disease (PD) and Alzheimer disease(AD) are believed to be heterogeneous based on the causes - combination of genetic and environmental factors, vast variety in the age at onset, variability in leading symptoms and presenting clinical manifestations, disease progression and responses to different therapies employed. Definitive diagnosis of both, AD and PD still relies on a 'gold standard' post mortem neuropathological evaluation, although a number of clinical and neuropsychological tests are often employed when making a clinical diagnosis. AD is detected with approximately 85–90% accuracy and PD with approximaly 75% accuracy. The pathogenesis of both AD and PD are complex and still remain unexplained in worldwide research community.

It has been recently estimated [7] that 24 million people have dementia worldwide and majority is attributable to AD. The authors emphasized the urgency of better understanding of pathophysiology of the disease in order to improve development of disease-modifying treatment. Due to the age-dependent incidence rate of AD and due to the population ageing, it is foreseen that more than 80 million people will have AD by 2040 [8]. It is a progressive neurologic disease affecting particularly cortical and hippocampal neurons, leading to their irreversible loss [9]. Major clinical signs and symptoms are progressive impairment in memory, judgment, decision making, orientation to physical surroundings, and language. The key pathological characteristics are neuronal loss, β amyloid containing extracellular senile plaques, and neurofibrillary tangles, which are composed of a hyperphosphorylated form of the microtubular protein tau.

PD is the second most prevalent NDG disease after AD. According to available data of European Parkinson's Disease Association (EPDA), there are 6.3 million people with PD worldwide. Prevalence is age-dependent - there are approximately 0.5 to 1 percent of individuals with PD in the age group 65 to 69 years, and 1 to 3 percent of individuals with PD in the group of people older than 80 years [10]. Typical clinical sign is parkinsonism - resting tremor, bradykinesia, rigidity, and postural instability. Neuropathological characteristics are the loss of neurons in the substantia nigra and the presence of neuronal inclusions termed Lewy bodies and Lewy neurites whose main component is aggregated and phosphorylated alpha-synuclein [11].

Important futuristic challenge in the management AD and PD remains the establishment of early diagnosis or even identification of individuals prior to the onset of dementia in AD or resting tremor in PD. This implicates advancement in understanding disease pathogenesis and development of diagnostic approaches, including disease/process specific biomarkers.

## 2.2 Huntington disease – A model of genetic neurodegenerative disorder

Huntington disease is a late onset, single gene disorder and its cause is invariably trinucleotide expansion mutation, known for almost 2 decades [3]. Clinical characteristics of the disease include progressive motor impairment, cognitive decline and various psychiatric symptoms with the typical age of onset in the third to fifth decade. The disease is fatal after 15-20 years of progressive neurodegeneration [12]. So far, no effective treatment has been available to cure the disease or to slow its progression. Hyperkinesias and psychiatric symptoms may respond well to pharmacotherapy, but neuropsychological deficits and dementia remain untreatable [13]. We are unable to predict the age at onset and to follow the disease progression over short time periods due to the unsensitivity of rating scales. Even more, no useful measures to follow response to symptomatic treatment over short time periods are known. In addition, in the presymptomatic period when preventive treatment and slowing of neurodegeneration might be most effective, we have no measures/markers to monitor those responses and benefits.

Although the responsible gene and mutation were already identified and characterized in 1993, the function of normal huntingtin and the mutation mechanism that leads to neurodegeneration are still not clear. Basic research has demonstrated that the pathogenesis of HD involves recruitment of multiple biochemical pathways like protein degradation, apoptosis, accumulation of misfolded mutated proteins, intracelular signaling, oxidative stress, mitochondrial involvement and in the last years also transcription [14, 15].

## 2.3 Dementia and Down syndrome

Dementia, common symptom of all three already mentioned neurodegenerative diseases is also a common symptom in individuals with Down syndrome (DS). Most of individuals with DS after about age of 30 have the characteristic plaques and neurofibrillary tangles, associated with AD. As in general population, the prevalence of AD in people with DS increases significantly with age. On the other hand, age-related cognitive decline and dementia in people with DS occurs 30–40 years earlier than in the general population, reaching almost 40% in the 50s [16]. Life expectancy of people with DS continues to increase and therefore, dementia is becoming an important issue.

## 2.4 Biomarkers

Research in the field of biomarkers is a rapidly growing and developing area in medicine. Everyday advances in genomic, proteomic, metabolomic and epigenomic knowledge and technologies have made their way also in the neuroscientific research area. Biomarkers are very important indicators of normal and abnormal biological processes. By definition, biological marker or biomarker is a characteristic that is objectively measured and evaluated as an indicator of normal biological processes, pathogenic processes, or pharmacologic responses to a therapeutic intervention [17]. Despite the fact that enormous effort and extensive research have been concentrated on this area, there is still a major lack of biomarkers for diagnosis, progression monitoring, response to treatment evaluation, etc. in neurodegenerative disorders such as Alzheimer's disease (AD), Parkinson's disease (PD) and Huntington's disease (HD).

Biomarkers have many valuable applications, such as identification of major neuropathological processes in specific disease, disease detection and monitoring of health status, early efficacy and safety evaluations in *in vitro* studies in tissue samples, *in vivo* studies in animal models, and early-phase clinical trials. They are invaluable as a diagnostic tool for identification of patients with a disease or abnormal condition, as a tool in staging the disease or classification of the extent of disease, as an indicator of disease prognosis and in predicting and monitoring of a clinical response to treatment.

Biomarkers are of extreme relevance in chronic NDG diseases - there are no cures for these diseases, as neurons of the central nervous system cannot regenerate on their own after cell death or damage. Tremendous efforts have been made in recent years to identify the neuropathological, biochemical, and genetic biomarkers of these diseases aiming to establish the diagnosis in earlier stages, to survey the rate of progression, or response to treatment. Currently, the neuropathologic diagnosis is a gold standard, but it can only be made in the form of an autopsy after the patient's death. On the other hand, biomarkers may improve the early diagnosis at a stage when disease-modifying therapies are likely to be most effective, the monitoring of disease progression and the efficacy of any therapeutic intervention [18].

## 2.5 Brain transcriptome in neurodegenerative disorders

Many different research groups have tried to solve the neuropathophysiological puzzle in PD, AD, HD and DS. Human brain has been extensivelly studied using many approaches, in the last decade also variety of »omic« technologies. Whole-genome gene expression studies in brain of each of four diseases individually have shown changes in transcription of number of genes when compared to normal human brain.

We investigated, reviewed and collected data from all reported studies to date on brain transcriptome in Parkinson's disease, Alzheimer disease, Huntington disease and Down syndrome and performed integrated meta-analysis.

## 3. Methods

In an attempt to present the alterations consistently reported by studies of brain transcriptome in neurodegenerative diseases, we initially searched for such reports in literature databases, then obtained raw and processed experimental data from microarray data repositories, after which we performed probe level meta-analyses of datasets originating from various studies. In addition, to reveal possible commonalities and shared pathways across various neurodegenerative diseases, we inspected the similarities and differences in gene expression dysregularities occurring in these conditions.

## 3.1 Study inclusion

Initially, we have searched Medline database (http://www.ncbi.nlm.nih.gov/pubmed) for reports from studies of interest using the search string (transcriptom* OR microarray OR profiling OR Affymetrix OR Agilent OR Illumina OR array) AND (Parkinson's disease OR Parkinsons disease OR Parkinson disease AND Alzheimer's disease OR Alzheimers disease OR Alzheimer disease OR dementia OR Down's syndrome OR Downs syndrome OR Down syndrome OR trisomy 21 OR Huntington's disease OR Huntingtons disease OR Huntington disease) to obtain the complete list of studies reporting results relating to transcriptional alterations in brain tissues affected by neurodegenerative processes.

As we were primarily interested in the studies with microarray experimental results accessible from biological repositories, we then searched Gene Expression Omnibus (GEO) repository (*http://www.ncbi.nlm.nih.gov/geo/*), ArrayExpress database (*http://www.ebi.ac.uk/arrayexpress/*) and Stanford Microarray database (*http://smd.stanford.edu*) for studies with data available in the raw or processed form. As most of the gene expression profiling experiments were performed on Affymetrix platform and to avoid difficulties due to different probe annotations utilized by different microarray manufacturers, only results from experiments performed on the Affymetrix U133 platform were included to facilitate further steps in probe level meta-analysis of microarray data. The detailed information on datasets included in the analyses may be observed in Table 1.

### 3.2 Microarray data pre-processing and preparation for meta-analysis
All the integration and statistical steps described were performed in R statistical environment version 2.13.1 (http://cran.r-project.org), using Bioconductor version 2.8 packages (available at http://bioconductor.org) [19]. Raw data from all microarray experiments listed in Table 1 was obtained directly from Gene Expression Omnibus (GEO) repository (http://www.ncbi.nlm.nih.gov/geo/) utilizing the GEOquery package for R [20, 21].

Before the meta-analysis of data from selected studies was performed, all the datasets obtained in such manner were inspected for significant inter-array differences in distribution of probe intensities. For this reason, raw datasets were initially examined using arrayQualityMetrics package and where necessary the straightforward quantile normalization functions in the affyPLM package was utilized [30, 31]. Non-specific intensity and interquartile variation filters were applied using methods in genefilter package [19]. $Log_2$ transformations were applied where discrepancies in data reporting format were observed.

Data collections for each individual neurodegenerative disease were then merged using probeset annotations as the common denominator. Using this approach we avoided potential statistical issues originating from averaging probe intensity values to obtain a single mean intensity value for each gene, possibly disregarding distinct expression of different transcripts from the same gene.

These steps resulted in generation of 4 separate data matrices, each carrying data for a single disease, originating from multiple studies – Alzheimer disease (AD), Down syndrome (DS), Huntington disease (HD) and Parkinson disease (PD) datasets.

### 3.3 Meta-analysis
Summarized differential expression of genes in each merged dataset was calculated using meta-analysis algorithms incorporated in the RankProd package for R [32]. RankProd uses a non-parametric statistical algorithm that facilitates detection of genes that are consistently highly ranked across microarray datasets originating from various microarray experiments in various studies perfomed on the same condition (ie. disease). As this approach is based on rank statistics in contrast to approaches requiring analyzing absolute intensity values, it allows for inclusion of data originating from different laboratories, differing platforms and potentially studies performed under differing conditions [32].

For analyses of such multi-study data, RPadvance function was utilized in our analyses, with origin parameter set to account for data originating from number of different sources corresponding to the number of different originating study [32]. Here it is important to

| GEO Accession | Disease name | Platform | Number of probesets* | Number of array experiments | | Tissue | Ref |
|---|---|---|---|---|---|---|---|
| | | | | Affected tissue | Unaffected tissue | | |
| GSE5281 | Alzheimer's disease | Affymetrix HG-U133Plus2 | 54,675 | 87 | 74 | Entorhinal cortex Hippocampus Medial temporal gyrus Posterior cingulate cortex Primary visual cortex Superior frontal gyrus | [22] |
| GSE1297 | Alzheimer's disease | Affymetrix HG-U133A | 22,283 | 22 | 9 | Hippocampus | [23] |
| †GSE16759 | Alzheimer's disease | Affymetrix HG-U133Plus2 | 54,675 | 4 | 4 | Parietal lobe tissue | [24] |
| †GSE7307 | Parkinson's disease | Affymetrix HG-U133Plus2 | 54,675 | 22 | 45 | Caudate Gloubus pallidum Putamen Substantia nigra Subthalamic nucleus Thalamus lateral nuclei Thalamus subthalamic nucleus | NA‡ |
| GSE8397 | Parkinson's disease | Affymetrix HG-U133A and Affymetrix HG-U133B | 22,283 and 22,645 | 29 and 29 | 18 and 18 | Substantia nigra Frontal cortex | [25] |
| GSE7621 | Parkinson's disease | Affymetrix HG-U133Plus2 | 54,675 | 16 | 9 | Substantia nigra | [26] |
| GSE3790 | Huntington's disease | Affymetrix HG-U133A and Affymetrix HG-U133B | 22,283 and 22,645 | 114 | 87 | Cerebellum Frontal cortex Caudate nucleus | [27] |
| †GSE1397 | Down syndrome | Affymetrix HG-U133A | 22,283 | 9 | 9 | Cerebrum Cerebellum Astrocyte samples | [28] |
| GSE5390 | Down Syndrome | Affymetrix HG-U133A | 22,283 | 7 | 8 | Dorsolateral prefrontal cortex | [29] |

* According to data obtained from the GEO site
† The dataset included some microarray experiments not related to the scope of this study and those were omitted from the analyses
‡ The study related to listed GEO entry was not yet published

Table 1. Detailed information on studies included in meta-analysis

stress that we have faced the issue of multiple studies simultaneously reporting differential expression in several different anatomical brain parts. As we wanted to facilitate the discovery of differentially expressed genes in diseased tissue in comparison to control samples, we set the origin parameter to take into account these considerations and regard such data as originating from different sources, thereby avoiding comparisons of gene expression between different brain regions rather than between affected and unaffected samples. Afterwards, P-values and q-values were obtained by performing 100 permutation cycles of complete originating datasets. An arbitrary P-value cut-off for significance of differential gene expression was then set at $P<0.05$.

### 3.4 Investigating intersections between datasets and gene set enrichment analyses
Resulting ordered lists of differentially expressed probesets were subsequently investigated for overlap between AD, DS, HD and PD datasets. Top 1000 genes from each dataset were used and intersections between combinations of two, three and four datasets were obtained. Venn diagrams in the results section were produced using Venny utility available at *http://bioinfogp.cnb.csic.es/tools/venny/index.html*. Furthermore, to gain insight in functional properties of genes in the intersections, gene set enrichment analyses (GSEA) were performed, utilizing GOstats package for R and investigating significant (uncorrected $p<0.05$) over- or underrepresentation of GeneOntology (GO) and KEGG terms annotating genes occurring in the intersections [33-36]. Additionally, DAVID tool (http://david.abcc.ncifcrf.gov/) was used to reveal the functional annotation clusters related to intersecting genes [37]. Required annotation conversions were performed using the hgu133plus.db package from Bioconductor annotation package collection and using biomaRt package for R in combination with Ensembl Biomart service (http://www.biomart.org/) [38, 39].

## 4. Results

Alltogether, our data collection comprised of data from 9 whole-genome expression studies, performed on samples from 4 neurodegenerative conditions (AD, DS, HD and PD). Collectively, 200, 33, 201, and 186 microarray analysed samples were included in the investigations of AD, DS, HD and PD, respectively, which accounted for 620 separate experiments included overall. A slight predominance of experiments performed on case tissues was noted in most of the experiments with summary case:control ratio amounting to 1,2:1 (339 affected tissues and 281 unaffected tissues included).

Separate analyses of datasets for each NDG disorder have revealed significant perturbances in expression profiles of several genes. When arbitrary permutation p-value cut-off was set at 0.05 for upregulated genes, 5701 probesets attained significance in the AD dataset, 3291 in DS dataset, 4174 in the HD dataset and 3043 in the PD dataset. In the downregulated gene group the $p<0.05$ significance was reached for 5496 probesets in the AD dataset, 2983 probesets in the DS dataset, 4079 in the HD dataset and 3410 in the PD dataset. A detailed view of the distribution of significance values of the top 10,000 ordered differentially expressed genes may be observed in Figure 1 for each of the NDG disorders.

The resulting numbers of significant results are inflated by the effect of multiple testing and therefore the q- values were also estimated as described in the article by Breitling et al [40]. The numbers of upregulated probesets with estimated q-values below 0.05 were 3775 for AD, 1496 for DS, 3182 for HD and 1894 for PD datasets. The numbers of downregulated probesets meeting this criterion were 3624 in AD, 652 in DS, 3065 in HD and 2541 probesets in the PD dataset.

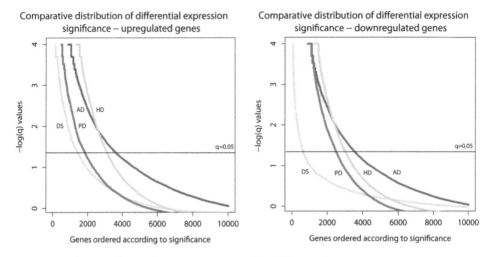

Fig. 1. Distribution of significance estimations for differential expression in 4 neurodegenerative disorders

An extent of global perturbation of the transciptome may be compared, with AD displaying the greatest extent of differentially expressed genes (blue line) and DS displaying the lowest extent, especially in the case of genes displaying downregulation.

## 4.1 Common patterns of differential expression in neurodegenerative disorders

Comparisons of comformity between profiles of transcriptome perturbations in four neurodegenerative diseases was initially performed by inspecting lists of top 1000 DE (differentially expressed) probesets for each condition and subsequently obtaining probesets (and genes) found to be differentially expressed simultaneously in several conditions.

The numbers of overlapping probesets may be observed in Figure 2. The largest overlap was observed between between the PD and HD lists, with altogether 338 (33.8%) upregulated and 267 (26.7%) downregulated genes differentially expressed in both conditions. Detailed overview of the extent of overlap between pairs of top DE gene list may be observed in Figure 3. A notable number of probesets was DE in all four conditions: 44 upregulated and 16 downregulated as presented in Figure 2a and 2b.

## 4.2 Comparative functional analyses of differential expression profile in neurodegenerative diseases

Calculations of gene set enrichment profile of upregulated and downregulated sets of genes presented here, were performed using hypergeometric test in the GOstats package. The profiles of DE genes were first calculated for each disorder separately, and afterwards every intersection between combinations of four sets of DE genes was evaluated.

Results of interests from separate GSEA analyses are presented in Table2(a-d) for top 1000 downregulated DE gene sets (the data for upregulated GSEA are not shown). Several GO biological process annotations appeared in all of the four analyses, most notably terms related to synaptic transmission and to cognitive processes.

We have also investigated the extent of similarity of GSEA profiles across four diseases. Top 200 enriched GO terms were inspected in each neurodegenerative disorder and compared for matching terms in pair with other three disorders. Greatest similarity was observed between GSEA terms annotating downregulated genes in all four disorders, which may be observed in more detail in Figure 4. As previously observed for overlapping genes, greatest overlap was observed between PD and HD GO profiles in the upregulated (40.0% overlap) and downregulated sets (59.5% overlap).

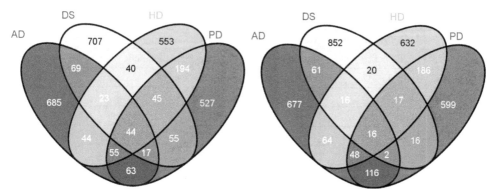

Fig. 2. Number of probesets overlapping between four sets of top 1000 DE upregulated (2a) and of top 1000 DE downregulated (2b) genes

Please note the abbreviations: Alzheimer disease (AD), Down syndrome (DS), Huntington disease (HD) and Parkinson disease (PD).

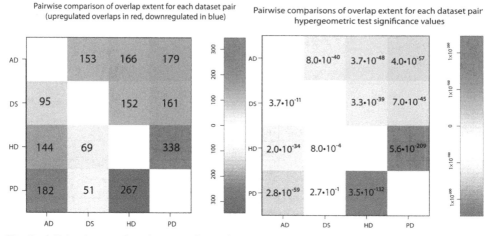

Fig. 3. a) Pairwise overlaps between lists of top DE upregulated (in red) and downregulated genes (in blue). Color intensiy of each square is proportional to size of overlap between a pair of DE gene lists. b) Pairwise overlaps between lists of top DE upregulated (in red) and downregulated genes (in blue). Color intensiy of each square is proportional to the value of –logp value obtained by performing hypergeometric test

| GOBPID Accession | P-value | Count of genes annotated | Term |
|---|---|---|---|
| GO:0007268 | 1,01E-10 | 61 | synaptic transmission |
| GO:0019226 | 1,49E-09 | 63 | transmission of nerve impulse |
| GO:0035637 | 1,49E-09 | 63 | multicellular organismal signaling |
| GO:0044282 | 2,61E-07 | 68 | small molecule catabolic process |
| GO:0051443 | 5,09E-07 | 17 | positive regulation of ubiquitin-protein ligase activity |
| GO:0019752 | 9,12E-07 | 70 | carboxylic acid metabolic process |
| GO:0009144 | 1,82E-06 | 46 | purine nucleoside triphosphate metabolic process |
| GO:0051438 | 5,03E-06 | 17 | regulation of ubiquitin-protein ligase activity |
| GO:0007017 | 9,55E-06 | 35 | microtubule-based process |
| GO:0007611 | 1,65E-05 | 18 | learning or memory |
| GO:0030330 | 4,23E-05 | 16 | DNA damage response, signal transduction by p53 class mediator |
| GO:0031398 | 4,70E-05 | 17 | positive regulation of protein ubiquitination |

Table 2a Alzheimer disease (downregulated genes). GOBPID stands for GeneOntology biological process ID

| GOBPID Accession | P-value | Count of genes annotated | Term |
|---|---|---|---|
| GO:0007268 | 3,47E-37 | 90 | synaptic transmission |
| GO:0019226 | 2,02E-35 | 93 | transmission of nerve impulse |
| GO:0007267 | 5,12E-29 | 110 | cell-cell signaling |
| GO:0007399 | 8,47E-15 | 113 | nervous system development |
| GO:0007611 | 6,38E-13 | 25 | learning or memory |
| GO:0007610 | 1,09E-12 | 46 | behavior |
| GO:0050890 | 5,29E-12 | 25 | cognition |
| GO:0048666 | 2,05E-10 | 59 | neuron development |
| GO:0006836 | 2,24E-10 | 23 | neurotransmitter transport |
| GO:0006811 | 9,51E-10 | 73 | ion transport |
| GO:0001505 | 1,00E-09 | 21 | regulation of neurotransmitter levels |
| GO:0031175 | 3,23E-09 | 52 | neuron projection development |
| GO:0032940 | 9,52E-09 | 50 | secretion by cell |
| GO:0048667 | 1,66E-08 | 46 | cell morphogenesis involved in neuron differentiation |
| GO:0022008 | 3,13E-08 | 67 | neurogenesis |

Table 2b Huntington's disease (downregulated genes). GOBPID stands for GeneOntology biological process ID

| GOBPID Accession | P-value | Count of genes annotated | Term |
|---|---|---|---|
| GO:0007268 | 4,16E-17 | 68 | synaptic transmission |
| GO:0051234 | 1,99E-16 | 229 | establishment of localization |
| GO:0019226 | 1,34E-15 | 70 | transmission of nerve impulse |
| GO:0035637 | 1,34E-15 | 70 | multicellular organismal signaling |
| GO:0006836 | 9,40E-14 | 29 | neurotransmitter transport |
| GO:0009259 | 8,03E-13 | 58 | ribonucleotide metabolic process |
| GO:0009144 | 1,47E-12 | 55 | purine nucleoside triphosphate metabolic process |
| GO:0007399 | 8,20E-11 | 115 | nervous system development |
| GO:0001505 | 8,41E-11 | 24 | regulation of neurotransmitter levels |
| GO:0072521 | 9,91E-11 | 69 | purine-containing compound metabolic process |
| GO:0007269 | 1,05E-10 | 20 | neurotransmitter secretion |
| GO:0006753 | 2,95E-10 | 73 | nucleoside phosphate metabolic process |
| GO:0009117 | 2,95E-10 | 73 | nucleotide metabolic process |
| GO:0007267 | 3,23E-10 | 82 | cell-cell signaling |
| GO:0015980 | 9,19E-10 | 39 | energy derivation by oxidation of organic compounds |

Table 2c Parkinson's disease (downregulated genes). GOBPID stands for GeneOntology biological process ID

| GOBPID Accession | P-value | Count of genes annotated | Term |
|---|---|---|---|
| GO:0048856 | 6,65E-11 | 173 | anatomical structure development |
| GO:0007267 | 2,83E-08 | 65 | cell-cell signaling |
| GO:0050877 | 6,86E-07 | 69 | neurological system process |
| GO:0050789 | 1,60E-06 | 318 | regulation of biological process |
| GO:0022008 | 3,01E-06 | 58 | neurogenesis |
| GO:0030182 | 3,71E-06 | 53 | neuron differentiation |
| GO:0007399 | 4,91E-06 | 82 | nervous system development |
| GO:0048839 | 8,26E-06 | 14 | inner ear development |
| GO:0009887 | 1,69E-05 | 42 | organ morphogenesis |
| GO:0007186 | 1,76E-05 | 41 | G-protein coupled receptor protein signaling pathway |
| GO:0051716 | 2,70E-05 | 194 | cellular response to stimulus |
| GO:0003001 | 4,34E-05 | 24 | generation of a signal involved in cell-cell signaling |
| GO:0010903 | 5,15E-05 | 3 | negative regulation of very-low-density lipoprotein particle remodeling |
| GO:0007268 | 7,44E-05 | 35 | synaptic transmission |
| GO:0048667 | 7,44E-05 | 35 | cell morphogenesis involved in neuron differentiation |
| GO:0007165 | 9,36E-05 | 165 | signal transduction |
| GO:0048666 | 1,73E-04 | 41 | neuron development |

Table 2d Down's syndrome (downregulated genes). GOBPID stands for GeneOntology biological process ID

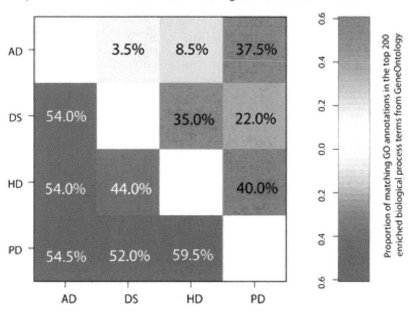

Fig. 4. Pairwise comparison of GO terms between pairs of datasets representing four neurodegenerative diseases. Percentages were calculated by dividing the number of GO terms overlapping by the number of all GO terms included in the overlapping analysis (N=200). GO terms annotating upregulated genes are presented in shades of red color and those annotating downregulated genes in blue

## 5. Conclusion

We have shown that whole-genome transcription analysis might be useful for identification and clarification of pathophysiological mechanisms in neurodegenerative diseases. We have used innovative approach of comparing and integrating experiment results from different NDG diseases and provided new important insights into the common NDG processes. Elucidation of these mechanisms holds important potential for future prediction and development of new useful treatments as well as for identification of biomarkers of neurodegeneration.

When comparisons of intersections between groups of top DE genes were performed, the greatest overlap was found between DE genes in brain samples of patients with HD and PD, which is possibly in accordance with their primary manifestation in movement disturbances related to function of basal ganglia. On the other hand, this similarity is surprising, as the known etiological agents in HD and PD differ significantly, one disorder being a consequence of monogenic disruption and other being a complex disorder with heterogeneous combination of genetic and environmental factors [41]. Surprisingly high is also the profile overlap between AD and PD, which present as clinically somewhat distinct entities. Recently however, it has been becoming progressively more obvious that the two disorders share not only a significant proportion of clinical elements (movement disorder, cognitive decline, mood and psychiatric disorders) but also share common pathophysiological pathways [42]. These results potentially suggest that clinical distinction between disease entities may not be perfect projection of actual processes at cellular and molecular level. Additionally, in contrast to expectation, however, the lowest overlap was observed between samples from patients with DS and AD, especially as these conditions have been known to share NDG pathways related to amyloid beta deposition in neurons. Reasons for lower extent of overlap may be found in significant differences in the age of patients from whom the brain samples were obtained for studies of DS in comparison with AD. Additionally, it is important that in most instances, a complete triplication of genes located on chromosome 21 may dominate genes commonly dysregulated in DS and AD [29]. Also, the number of brain tissue samples samples profiled in microarray experiments was by far the lowest among other types of NDG diseases investigated in our survey. Therefore, before final answer regarding this finding is obtained, more studies investigating transcriptional alterations in DS brain samples must be performed.

Several GO categories appeared to be consistently singled out in GSEA analyses of separate and overlapping genes DE in NDG disorders. Interestingly several terms were related to processes previously associated with neuron degeneration [42], most prominently GO terms: synaptic transmission (GO:0007268), neurogenesis (GO:0022008) and terms related to higher cognitive processes (GO:0007611). Dysfunctional synaptic transmission (as in glutamate exitotoxicity) and defects in neurogenesis have been previously repeatedly shown to be related to various NDG diseases [42-44]. It is interesting that although disturbances in neuroinflammatory mechanisms have been proposed as a possible causative factor in a number of NDG diseases, our analysis of intersecting genes dysregulated in brain samples of these conditions did not single out a particular common inflammatory pathogenetic pathway. This notion may be interpreted in the light of previously recognized differences in complement-activating immunogenic activity of plaques in different NDG diseases, resulting in absence of commonly overlapping inflammatory genes and GO terms [42].

When we investigated the compatibility of functional profiles between four NDG diseases, we have found greatest overlaps between sets of GO terms annotating genes characterized by downregulation in NDG diseases, where an overlap greater than 40% was observed in all of the pairwise comparisons of the sets of top 200 enriched GO terms. Again, the greatest functional conformance was noted between top downregulated genes in HD and PD as well as AD and PD dataset pairs. Notable overlap was also observed in the functional profiles of upregulated genes, where we noted good functional conformity between DS and HD datasets in addition to HD-PD and AD-PD functional overlaps.

It is important to stress that genome-wide expression studies included in this survey are inherently burdened by important statistical issues that predominantly originate from the issue of testing a large number of variables on a relatively small population of biological replicates (ie. study subjects) [45]. For this reason we attempted to gain a more complete account of biological alterations in neurodegenerative diseases by merging data from several different studies investigating transcriptional changes in brain samples of distinct neurological conditions (AD, DS, HD and PD) [46]. This increased the number of biological replicates considerably, allowing for potentially more reliable calling of DE genes in these conditions. There are, however, important downsides to this approach: the studies included were performed under differing conditions in different institutions and by different research staff. Even more important is the great heterogeneity between brain tissue samples investigated. We have attempted to circumvent these issues by using appropriate RankProd meta-analysis methods, nevertheless these results must be interpreted in light of these considerations.

Nevertheless it is still difficult to differentiate between the causal changes in transcriptome in contrast to changes resulting from previous damage to neural tissue. It is possible, however, that the similarities in transcriptome profile between clinically and pathologically distinct entities suggest a common response to an unknown initial damaging stimulus. We propose that in future, integration of various data such as genomic in combination with transcriptomic data should provide a way to delineate possible mechanisms, where genetic predisposition results in manifestation of transcriptional imbalances, consequently resulting in observed phenotype. Genome-wide expression profiling may however direct further research attempts into a particular direction. Also, there are other "omics" approaches besides transcriptomics and integrating all of them is future challenge.

## 6. References

[1] C.J.L. Murray ADL, *The Global Burden of Disease*. 1996, World Health Organisation: Geneva.

[2] Menken M, Munsat TL, Toole JF. The global burden of disease study: implications for neurology. *Arch Neurol* 2000; 57(3): p: 418-20.

[3] A novel gene containing a trinucleotide repeat that is expanded and unstable on Huntington's disease chromosomes. The Huntington's Disease Collaborative Research Group. *Cell* 1993; 72(6): p: 971-83.

[4] Schneider JA, Arvanitakis Z, Bang W, Bennett DA. Mixed brain pathologies account for most dementia cases in community-dwelling older persons. *Neurology* 2007; 69(24): p: 2197-204.

[5] Pathological correlates of late-onset dementia in a multicentre, community-based population in England and Wales. Neuropathology Group of the Medical Research Council Cognitive Function and Ageing Study (MRC CFAS). *Lancet* 2001; 357(9251): p: 169-75.

[6] Prohovnik I, Perl DP, Davis KL, et al. Dissociation of neuropathology from severity of dementia in late-onset Alzheimer disease. *Neurology* 2006; 66(1): p: 49-55.

[7] Ballard C, Gauthier S, Corbett A, et al. Alzheimer's disease. *Lancet*; 377(9770): p: 1019-31.

[8] Forlenza OV, Diniz BS, Gattaz WF. Diagnosis and biomarkers of predementia in Alzheimer's disease. *BMC Med*; 8: p: 89.

[9] McKhann G, Drachman D, Folstein M, et al. Clinical diagnosis of Alzheimer's disease: report of the NINCDS-ADRDA Work Group under the auspices of Department of Health and Human Services Task Force on Alzheimer's Disease. *Neurology* 1984; 34(7): p: 939-44.

[10] Nussbaum RL, Ellis CE. Alzheimer's disease and Parkinson's disease. *N Engl J Med* 2003; 348(14): p: 1356-64.

[11] Spillantini MG, Schmidt ML, Lee VM, et al. Alpha-synuclein in Lewy bodies. *Nature* 1997; 388(6645): p: 839-40.

[12] Harper PS. Huntington's disease. Major Problems in Neurology. 1996, London: W.B. Saunders Company Ltd.

[13] Bonelli RM, Hofmann P. A systematic review of the treatment studies in Huntington's disease since 1990. *Expert Opin Pharmacother* 2007; 8(2): p: 141-53.

[14] Harjes P, Wanker EE. The hunt for huntingtin function: interaction partners tell many different stories. *Trends Biochem Sci* 2003; 28(8): p: 425-33.

[15] Sugars KL, Rubinsztein DC. Transcriptional abnormalities in Huntington disease. *Trends Genet* 2003; 19(5): p: 233-8.

[16] Holland AJ, Hon J, Huppert FA, Stevens F, Watson P. Population-based study of the prevalence and presentation of dementia in adults with Down's syndrome. *Br J Psychiatry* 1998; 172: p: 493-8.

[17] Biomarkers and surrogate endpoints: preferred definitions and conceptual framework. *Clin Pharmacol Ther* 2001; 69(3): p: 89-95.

[18] Henley SM, Bates GP,Tabrizi SJ. Biomarkers for neurodegenerative diseases. *Curr Opin Neurol* 2005; 18(6): p: 698-705.

[19] Gentleman RC, Carey VJ, Bates DM, et al. Bioconductor: open software development for computational biology and bioinformatics. *Genome Biol* 2004; 5(10): p: R80.

[20] Barrett T, Edgar R. Gene expression omnibus: microarray data storage, submission, retrieval, and analysis. *Methods Enzymol* 2006; 411: p: 352-69.

[21] Sean D, Meltzer PS. GEOquery: A bridge between the Gene Expression Omnibus (GEO) and BioConductor. *Bioinformatics* 2007; 23(14): p: 1846-7.

[22] Liang WS, Dunckley T, Beach TG, et al. Gene expression profiles in anatomically and functionally distinct regions of the normal aged human brain. *Physiol Genomics* 2007; 28(3): p: 311-22.

[23] Blalock EM, Geddes JW, Chen KC, et al. Incipient Alzheimer's disease: microarray correlation analyses reveal major transcriptional and tumor suppressor responses. *Proc Natl Acad Sci U S A* 2004; 101(7): p: 2173-8.

[24] Nunez-Iglesias J, Liu CC, Morgan TE, Finch CE, Zhou XJ. Joint genome-wide profiling of miRNA and mRNA expression in Alzheimer's disease cortex reveals altered miRNA regulation. *PLoS One* 2010; 5(2): p: e8898.

[25] Moran LB, Duke DC, Deprez M, et al. Whole genome expression profiling of the medial and lateral substantia nigra in Parkinson's disease. *Neurogenetics* 2006; 7(1): p: 1-11.

[26] Lesnick TG, Papapetropoulos S, Mash DC, et al. A genomic pathway approach to a complex disease: axon guidance and Parkinson disease. *PLoS Genet* 2007; 3(6): p: e98.

[27] Hodges A, Strand AD, Aragaki AK, et al. Regional and cellular gene expression changes in human Huntington's disease brain. *Hum Mol Genet* 2006; 15(6): p: 965-77.

[28] Mao R, Wang X, Spitznagel EL, Jr., et al. Primary and secondary transcriptional effects in the developing human Down syndrome brain and heart. *Genome Biol* 2005; 6(13): p: R107.

[29] Lockstone HE, Harris LW, Swatton JE, et al. Gene expression profiling in the adult Down syndrome brain. *Genomics* 2007; 90(6): p: 647-60.

[30] Kauffmann A, Gentleman R, Huber W. arrayQualityMetrics--a bioconductor package for quality assessment of microarray data. *Bioinformatics* 2009; 25(3): p: 415-6.

[31] Heber S,Sick B. Quality assessment of Affymetrix GeneChip data. *OMICS* 2006; 10(3): p: 358-68.

[32] Hong F, Breitling R, McEntee CW, et al. RankProd: A bioconductor package for detecting differentially expressed genes in meta-analysis. *Bioinformatics* 2006; 22(22): p: 2825-7.

[33] Falcon S, Gentleman R. Using GOstats to test gene lists for GO term association. *Bioinformatics* 2007; 23(2): p: 257-8.

[34] Ashburner M, Ball CA, Blake JA, et al. Gene ontology: Tool for the unification of biology. The Gene Ontology Consortium. *Nat Genet* 2000; 25(1): p: 25-9.

[35] Ogata H, Goto S, Sato K, et al. KEGG: Kyoto Encyclopedia of Genes and Genomes. *Nucleic Acids Res* 1999; 27(1): p: 29-34.

[36] Mootha VK, Lindgren CM, Eriksson KF, et al. PGC-1alpha-responsive genes involved in oxidative phosphorylation are coordinately downregulated in human diabetes. *Nat Genet* 2003; 34(3): p: 267-73.

[37] Huang da W, Sherman BT, Lempicki RA. Systematic and integrative analysis of large gene lists using DAVID bioinformatics resources. *Nat Protoc* 2009; 4(1): p: 44-57.

[38] Durinck S, Spellman PT, Birney E, Huber W. Mapping identifiers for the integration of genomic datasets with the R/Bioconductor package biomaRt. *Nat Protoc* 2009; 4(8): p: 1184-91.

[39] Durinck S, Moreau Y, Kasprzyk A, et al. BioMart and Bioconductor: A powerful link between biological databases and microarray data analysis. *Bioinformatics* 2005; 21(16): p: 3439-40.

[40] Breitling R, Armengaud P, Amtmann A, Herzyk P. Rank products: A simple, yet powerful, new method to detect differentially regulated genes in replicated microarray experiments. *FEBS Lett* 2004; 573(1-3): p: 83-92.

[41] Feany MB. ASIP Outstanding Investigator Award Lecture. New approaches to the pathology and genetics of neurodegeneration. *Am J Pathol* 2010; 176(5): p: 2058-66.

[42] Grunblatt E. Commonalities in the genetics of Alzheimer's disease and Parkinson's disease. *Expert Rev Neurother* 2008; 8(12): p: 1865-77.

[43] Palomo T, Archer T, Beninger RJ, Kostrzewa RM. Gene-environment interplay in neurogenesis and neurodegeneration. *Neurotox Res* 2004; 6(6): p: 415-34.

[44] Shankar GM, Walsh DM. Alzheimer's disease: synaptic dysfunction and Abeta. *Mol Neurodegener* 2009; 4: p: 48.

[45] Allison DB, Cui X, Page GP, Sabripour M. Microarray data analysis: from disarray to consolidation and consensus. *Nat Rev Genet* 2006; 7(1): p: 55-65.

[46] Cahan P, Rovegno F, Mooney D, et al. Meta-analysis of microarray results: challenges, opportunities, and recommendations for standardization. *Gene* 2007; 401(1-2): p: 12-8.

# 9

# Neurodegenerative Disease Monitoring Using a Portable Wireless Sensor Device

Paul Bustamante[1,2],
Gonzalo Solas[1] and Karol Grandez[1]
*[1]CEIT University of Navarra*
*[2]Tecnun University of Navarra*
*Spain*

## 1. Introduction

Neurodegenerative diseases are characterized by progressive loss of neurons in the central nervous system. The disorders are clinically well-defined as a disease-related dementia, Alzheimer's disease the most typical case, or as a movement disorder, Parkinson's disease (PD). The risk of developing these diseases increases significantly with age: Parkinson's disease affects 1% of the population over 65 years of age, rising to 2% for those over 80 years.

Parkinson's disease is a common neurodegenerative disorder that often impairs motor skills and speech of the patient. PD is characterized by muscle rigidity, tremor, slowing of physical movement (bradykinesia) and in extreme cases, loss of physical movement (akinesia). In particular, PD is due to a loss of dopaminergic neurons (related to the neurotransmitter dopamine), and subcortical neurons in the brain. Replacement therapy with dopaminergic drugs (levodopa, pramipexole) effectively reverses all the symptoms and signs of the disease. After a changeable period of time, however, this excellent initial response to dopaminergic treatment is complicated by the appearance of disorders known as motor response complications (MRC). These complications are divided into two main categories: (i) fluctuations in motor response and (ii) the emergence of abnormal involuntary movements known as levodopa-induced dyskinesias (LID) (Konitsiotis, 2005).

Generally, motor fluctuations appear first as a shortening of the initially soft and lasting dopaminergic response. For patients with advanced PD, a few hours after the administration of medication the patient begins to notice the reappearance of signs and symptoms of the disease. This is known as "end of dose deterioration" or "wearing off". This may happen several times a day, so the patient can actually spend several hours per day in an "off" state. During the short visit with the neurologist, the patient may appear to be well and thus the neurologist misses the symptoms related to wearing off. As a result, changes in the recent drug treatment availability do not take place in time. It is now well known that early treatment of wearing-off fluctuations delay the onset of more severe complications in the future, as well as the appearance of LID. Therefore any strategy that can detect early changes associated with wearing off would provide a valuable clinical tool that would allow early treatment interventions.

The quantitative assessment of the human body and motor movement disorders has been a topic of great interest for decades. Advanced equipment has been used to study various pathologies of the motor performance of the human body. However, sophisticated equipment alone is not a guarantee for success in the detection and analysis of motor disorders. In many situations, deficiencies in motor performance are not always frequent and motor disorders can occur only in very specific situations that are difficult to imitate or reproduce in a laboratory. The underlying testing and monitoring processes have not experienced the innovation and advancement required to fulfil the needs that such detection and analysis present.

Amyotrophic lateral sclerosis (ALS), often referred to as "Lou Gehrig's Disease," is a progressive neurodegenerative disease that affects nerve cells in the brain and the spinal cord. Motor neurons reach the spinal cord from the brain, and from the spinal cord to the muscles throughout the body. The progressive degeneration of the motor neurons in ALS causes these motor neurons to die and when this happens the ability of the brain to initiate and control muscle movement is lost. With voluntary muscle action progressively affected, patients in the later stages of the disease may become totally paralyzed.

The cases for Parkinson disease and ALS are expected to double worldwide by the year 2020 (Von Campenhausen et al., 2005). Proper medical care of these patients is becoming increasingly complex and expensive. Lengthy hospital stays for monitoring and adjustment of the patients' treatment and the problems related with it, contribute to cost increase and morbidity due to the hospitalization itself. But there is a clinical deficit of objective data on which neurologists can base the assessment and care of patients with chronic neurologically-based movement disorders.

## 2. Patient monitoring

The patient monitoring is a technique that has become popular in recent years in the field of research, and soon the number of actual implementations in clinics and hospitals will begin to increase. Monitoring of patients is not new, in fact, today there are many hospitals that supply devices (thermometers, gauges, pulse and blood pressure, pulse oximetry, electrocardiogram, electro-devices, etc). The disadvantage of these devices is their large size and weight, and the little mobility they offer. The key innovation lies in one word: continuous monitoring. It consists of a series of devices and techniques designed to monitor, continuously and for a period of time established by the specialists, the physiological parameters of the patient. The specific values and the time evolution of these parameters allow a more precise analysis of the evolution of the disease, and therefore more effective treatment.

There are two main factors that have contributed to the rise of this technology. On one hand, the development of new physiological sensors that allow the measurement of more and more parameters related to the human body. Advances in biological, chemical, electrical and mechanical sensor technologies have led to their wider use as wearable sensors or implants. Improvements in the manufacture of sensors and techniques for nano-engineering, along with parallel advances in technology of microelectromechanical systems (MEMS) offer the potential for implantable or attachable sensors getting smaller.

On the other hand, the popularization of wireless sensor networks (WSN) and the recent advances in their use as body sensor networks (BSN), has been another key development for recent continuous monitoring of patients (Yick et al., 2008). The human body is a complex interior environment that responds and interacts with its external environment, but is somehow "independent." The monitoring of the human body using a wireless sensor network can be achieved by attaching the sensors to the body (or even implanted in the tissues).

The wireless sensor networks are formed by a group of sensor nodes with certain capacity for sensing environment variables and transmitting them wirelessly. These nodes allow forming ad-hoc networks without an established physical infrastructure or a centralized management. These kinds of networks are known for being easy to deploy and for being auto configurable.

The majority of the researches carried out in the field of wireless sensor networks are focused on the network architecture, as well as on the communication protocols within the network. But few advances have been made in the development of novel sensor node architectures. The efforts are focused on the miniaturization of the nodes and the reduction of the energy consumption (Anastasi et al., 2009).

The objective of the work described in this chapter is to develop a single device which could be used in several application fields, due to its capability of being able to acquire signals coming from different types of sensors. Apart from that, the treatment of the data can be carried out in multiple ways, as the device is equipped with an SD card, a RF transceiver (IEEE 802.15.4 specification compliant) and a USB connector, for communication as well as for charging functions.

In order to test its versatility, an application field has been chosen and several tests have been carried out related to that field. More concretely, the application field that has been selected the validity of the objectives proposed in this work has been e-Health, and thus, a continuous monitoring system has been developed.

## 3. System architecture

The study of the state of the art shows that the devices and methods developed so far for the testing activities in patients affected by PD and ALS lack the most important characteristics of the device described in this article:

- **Accuracy**: the data provided by the device show exact values for the parameters the doctors are interested in. They are not based on subjective appreciation of the performance of the tests carried out by the patients.
- **Ease of use**: both for the clinicians and for the patients. The patient can carry out the tests without having to move from their own homes. And the data is stored in a PC, which offers the possibility of sending it to the hospital via Internet, for the doctors to analyze the results.
- **Frequency**: the ease of use of the system makes it possible to carry out more frequent tests, so the tracking of the variations of the motor functions of the patients is more accurate.
- **Versatility**: using the devices presented in this article, several different tests can be performed, and in each test, several parameters can be measured. For example, for the finger tapping case, both the speed and the regularity (periodicity) can be obtained, which enriches the results of the test and enhances the analysis and the conclusions obtained with it.

In order to comply with this characteristics or requirements, in this work we describe the system developed, which is based on the architecture shown in Fig. 1.

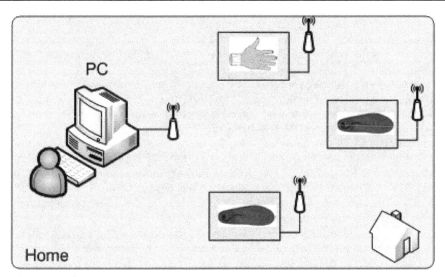

Fig. 1. System architecture

The whole system architecture is composed of four main building blocks:

- **Sensorized glove**: this glove is equipped with five sensors, which are attached to it. Each sensor is a FSR sensor and is connected to the circuit with a simple interface, done with a division resistor. When the user presses the FSR sensor, its resistance varies, and it is converted in voltage, in order to be acquired by the A/D converter.
- **Sensorized insole**: each insole is designed with five FSR sensors, in order to measure the area where the patient puts more pressure and to analyse the way he/she walks.
- **Hardware device**: this is the main development of the present research work. It consists of a tiny electronic circuit, based on a low cost and low energy microprocessor (PIC), protected by a case specifically designed for it. Its main functions are the acquisition and processing of the signals coming from the sensors, and transmitting them to the PC via the USB connection. The selected microprocessor has an 8 channel 10 bit A/D converter and an USB interface, which can be easily programmed and this allows saving space with another chip converter.
- **PC application**: the fourth component of the system architecture is in charge of receiving the data sent by the hardware device via the USB connection, storing and visualizing them, using a graphical user interface. This application was done in Windows with Visual C++ environment.

## 4. Device architecture

The main aim of the system is to gather data from any kind of sensor in order to store those data in an SD card or transmit them to Base Central Unit (BCU), connected to PC through USB connection. The SD card gives the system the possibility of having longer recording periods which allows the device to be used at a further distance from the BCU.

The data gathered and stored in the SD by the system is downloaded to a PC, by USB connection or by the radio transceiver, which operates in the 2.4GHz ISM band, using the BCU.

## 4.1 FSR sensors

The sensors used in this work have been Force Sensitive Resistors (FSR). A force-sensitive resistor (alternatively called a force-sensing resistor) has a variable resistance as a function of applied pressure. In this sense, the term "force-sensitive" is misleading – a more appropriate one would be "pressure-sensitive", since the sensor's output is dependent on the area on the sensor's surface to which force is applied.

The sensors used in this work are manufactured by Tekscan, and are constructed of two layers of substrate film. On each layer, a conductive material (silver) is applied, followed by a layer of pressure-sensitive ink (Vecchi et al., 2000). Adhesive is then used to laminate the two layers of substrate together to form the force sensor. The active sensing area is defined by the silver circle on top of the pressure-sensitive ink. Silver extends from the sensing area to the connectors at the other end of the sensor, forming the conductive leads. Fig. 2 shows a picture of the Tekscan FSR sensor.

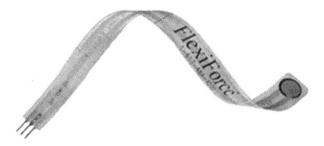

Fig. 2. Tekscan FSR sensor

After choosing Force Sensitive Resistors (FSR) as transducers, both a sensorized glove and an insole have been designed, and then used to carry out several tests related to Parkinson Disease (PD) and Amyotrophic lateral sclerosis (ALS).

## 4.2 Hardware architecture

The design of the device was related to its main functionality explained above. Measurements obtained from sensors are transmitted through wires to an IDC connector located at one edge of the device. This connector allows these inputs to be connected to A/D channels extended from the CPU. An interface stage is needed for each input due to sensors, done basically with some operational amplifiers and passive filters.

The architecture of the approach presented in this work is shown in Fig. 3. The CPU of the portable wireless device is the 18LF4550, a Microchip PIC18 Microcontroller with nanoWatt technology. It is an 8-bit System On-chip mainly featured by USB and SPI communication interfaces; it has a maximum number of 13 input A/D channels; each with a 10-bit resolution. It is also characterized for its low power consumption in deep-sleep mode, ideal to work as sensor node in monitoring applications. Also, this CPU has an RTC (Real Timer Clock), ideal for use in applications where is necessary to store the data sample time.

Analogical input signals attached to the IDC connector are converted into digital values which are put in an established frame structure according to a particular protocol. The frame arranged is ready to be transmitted via USB or RF.

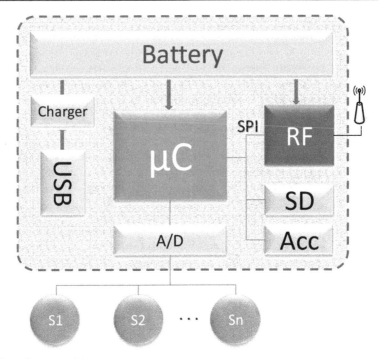

Fig. 3. Wireless device architecture

The USB device module is a mini-USB 2.0 compliant allowing fast transmission of data. It allows also charging the battery using a standard chip with a LED to monitor the charging action.

The device has also 3 more LEDs, whose main functionality is to indicate states in the program or can be programmed for different functions.

The device is designed also to use a 3-axis accelerometer in case it was needed; it also offers the option to record data in a micro-SD card placed in the bottom side. In order to increase the time access to the SD card, which means saving power, a proprietary system files access was implemented, based on the standard FAT32.

The wireless device has a radio frequency chip, the MRF24J40, from Microchip, which works in the 2.4GHz and has a SPI interface to communicate with the CPU. This chip was mainly chosen due to its IEEE 802.15.4 specification compliant (Hardware CSMA-CA mechanism, Automatic ACK response and support RSSI/LQI), additionally it has a hardware security engine and offers a low power consumption: 2uA in sleep mode, 22mA in TX mode (at +0dBm) and 18mA in RX mode.

The distribution of the device's components is illustrated in Fig. 4, where the left side shows the layout of the PCB and the distribution of the chips on the device. On the right side the connection procedure of the device with different kinds of sensors through a sensor interface is shown. This connection is possible by using the IDC connector, which includes pins for a VCC signal, the GND and 10 signals which are directed to the A/D converter. That was done due the fact that the main functionality of this device is to be a multifunctional wireless device.

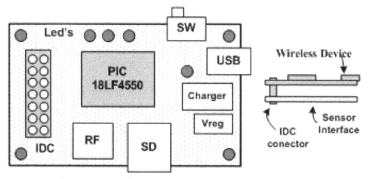

Fig. 4. PCB layout and sensor interface

## 4.3 Embedded software
The developed software to be embedded into the device has a modular scheme. This design allows the software to be independent from the platform and also gives flexibility.

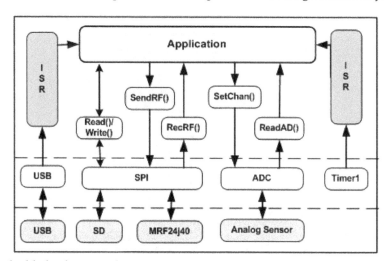

Fig. 5. Embedded software architecture

The whole software structure is divided in 4 layers as depicted in Fig. 5. The layers are separated by dotted lines and a short description for each one is given below:

- **Physical level**: is the lowest level and it depends on the hardware directly. The modules present in this level correspond to the physical modules of the node; these are the force sensors, accelerometer (not mounted), the USB port, the mini-SD slot (optional) and the RF module, which is controlled by the CPU using the SPI bus.
- **Controller level**: the functions developed in this level permit the application level to invoke controller functions. The ADC module converts analogical signals from the force sensors to digital, and the SPI allows communications of the CPU with the accelerometer and the mini-SD card and the RF chip. In this layer the set of USB and RTC (Real Time Clock) functions are also included.

- **Interface level**: this layer is the interface between controller and application; it contains the main functions that the device performs during its duty cycle. These functions range from reading ADC channels or communicating through the SPI interface, to sending and receiving data from the USB, the SD card and the RF chip. Interruption routines are also developed in this layer.
- **Application level**: this is the top level layer and executes related actions according to received interruptions (external switches or internal interruptions).

## 4.4 Data frame

The structure of the data frame, which is sent by RF or USB, is composed of a header which contains the ID of the device, followed by 4 bytes, indicating the measurement time, and a byte which indicates the length of the data.

Fig. 6 shows the data frame enclosed information of the measurements taken; the first two bytes give information about the frequency of sampling and the next byte gives the number of sensors measured. According to this last parameter, the rest of bytes corresponding to each sensor in groups of two bytes due to the 10-bit conversion configuration of the A/D converter.

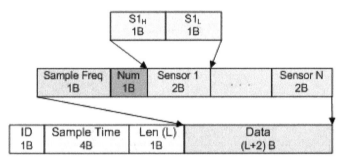

Fig. 6. Data frame

## 5. Device test in ALS disease

One of the ways of overcoming the lack of data in ALS disease is to develop new easy-to-use testing devices, which can be left in the patient's own home and used to carry out periodic tests without having to go to hospital to do so. The comfortable testing processes and devices make the patients more willing to wear them outside the home, and this leads to a wider amount of data available for the doctors.

Two of the more widely used tests with neurodegenerative disease patients are the Finger Tapping Test (FTT) (Jobbágy et al., 2005) and the Hand-grip Strength Test (Long, 1970). In the case of the FTT, the patient is asked to tap two of the fingers of one hand as quick as possible, and the main parameter measured by the doctors is the tapping frequency. On the other hand, in the hand grip strength test the measured parameter is the force the patient is capable of apply when grabbing an object.

The Finger Tapping Test (FTT), originally developed as part of the Halstead Reitan Battery (HRB) of neuropsychological tests, is a simple measure of motor speed and motor control and is used in neuropsychology as a sensitive test for brain damage (Christianson & Leathem, 2004). Although motor functioning in humans is controlled by many areas of the brain, the motor strip rostral to the central sulcus is the most important, and the functioning of this area is reflected directly in the FTT. As well as direct motor effects, the speed, co-ordination, and pacing requirements of finger tapping can be affected by levels of alertness, impaired ability to focus attention, or slowing of responses. Tapping frequency can distinguish patients with motor dysfunctions of cerebella, basal ganglia, and cerebral origins from normal subjects.

At the onset of ALS the symptoms may be so slight that they are frequently overlooked. With regard to the appearance of symptoms and the progression of the illness, the course of the disease may include muscle weakness. Muscle weakness is a hallmark initial sign in ALS, occurring in approximately 60% of patients. The hands and feet may be affected first, causing difficulty in lifting, walking or using the hands for the activities of daily living such as dressing, washing and buttoning clothes.

ALS is a very difficult disease to diagnose. To date, there is no one test or procedure to ultimately establish the diagnosis of ALS. Methods for the evaluation of strength in people with ALS include a clinical neurological exam, manual muscle testing (MMT) (Aitkens et al., 1989), and rating scales. These methods are subjective and lack sensitivity to detect small changes. The purpose of the Hand Grip Strength Test is to measure the maximum isometric strength of the hand and forearm muscles.

The devices and methods used so far for the proposed tests have not had any significant improvement or innovation for many years. Traditional ways of performing the tests are still used.

For the finger tapping test, several methods have been proposed and used. The standard method consists of asking the patients to start with the finger tapping process and an examiner using a stopwatch to keep track of the 10-second trial interval. Electronic devices which are based on the same testing methodology have been marketed. The electronic device has an internal timer that starts on the first tap and stops counting taps when the 10 seconds have elapsed. The use of automatic timing is intended to increase the accuracy of testing (McDermid, 2000).

Other devices used, which can be found in the literature, include precision image-based motion analyzer and passive marker-based movement analyzer (Jobbágy et al., 2005); the Halstead-Reitan finger tapping test (HRFTT), developed and manufactured by Reitan Neuropsychological Laboratory, which uses an electronic counter and a tapping key; finger tapping devices containing pressure sensors (Soichiro et al., 2004); systems consisting of accelerometers and touch sensor (Yokoe et a., 2009) (Okuno et al., 2007).

In the case of the hand-grip strength measurement, the innovations carried out in recent years have been even poorer. The most usual way to carry out this specific test is by using hand-grip and pinch-force dynamometers, which offer very poor information about the way the hand grabs objects. Electromyography has been also used in some studies (Long, 1970).

In this work we have used our wireless device to carry out both of the tests. It is integrated in a system consisting of the mentioned device, a sensorized glove (see Fig. 7) which is worn by the patient, and a PC or base station, which is in charge of receiving the data sent by the device, and visualizing them graphically in order to be analyzed by the doctors.

As mentioned before, the sensors used in this test have been Force Sensitive Resistors (FSR). The approach followed in this research work has been the one of attaching several sensors to a glove. This design allows complying with one of the key characteristics identified in the system architecture section: versatility. We consider that this design is more versatile in order to allow carrying out different type of tests and obtaining a wide range of results.

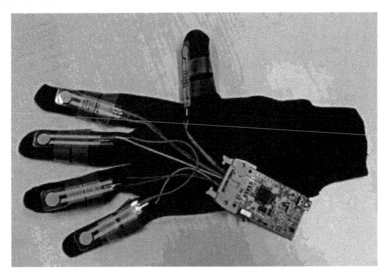

Fig. 7. Sensorized Glove attached to the wireless device

## 5.1 PC application

In order to gather the data and to be analyzed, a PC application was designed. It has been developed in Visual C++ using the Object Oriented Programming methodology (OOP), which is based in classes. The architecture is shown in Fig. 8. There are five blocks; the most important ones are the USB process and the graphical routines.

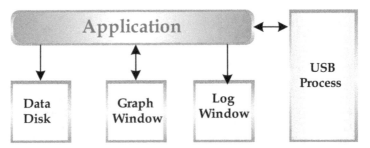

Fig. 8. PC application diagram

The data obtained by the hardware device after gathering and processing the signals coming from the FSR sensor, are sent via the USB connection to a PC, where an application is running. This application receives the data and visualizes and stores them.

Due the fact that the data rate of the device is low (less than 1KBps), the HID protocol has been implemented in the Sensor Device, providing the PC application an easier method of gathering the data, because most operating systems recognize standard USB HID devices, like keyboards and mice, without needing a special driver. In this way, the software can run in any compatible PC with Windows XP Operating System installed.

The application has some functionality that makes it easier for the doctors to analyze the data gathered by the hardware device. These functionalities are:

- **Start/Stop**: this button allows the exact moment in which the test starts and ends to be controlled. When the test starts, a new process is created in the application, which is constantly controlling the USB communications with the device, and passing the gathered data to the GUI window.
- **Zoom**: the zooming tool enables the signals corresponding to the force applied by the patient's each of the fingers to be visualised more accurately. It is also possible to analyze only one finger in the application or to compare with other tests carried out previously.
- **Log**: the application enables a registry or log with the messages corresponding to the events that appear during the testing process (communication states) to be visualised.
- **Files**: the application allows the data in files with ".csv" format to be saved, in order to edit and analyze later in a PC program such as Excel. Also, in the new version of the program, it is possible to save in a Matlab binary format, as some clinicians have experience with that mathematical tool.
- **Options**: in this option, the user can configure the device, by changing the sample frequency, the date of the device in order to maintain well synchronized, etc.

### 5.2 Hand-grip results

Fig. 9 shows a screen capture of the PC application, where a hand-grip force test is being carried out. As it can be seen in that figure, the force signal corresponding to each of the fingers is plotted using a different colour. That way the analysis of the graph is easier for the clinicians, where they can see for example that the patient has more force with one finger.

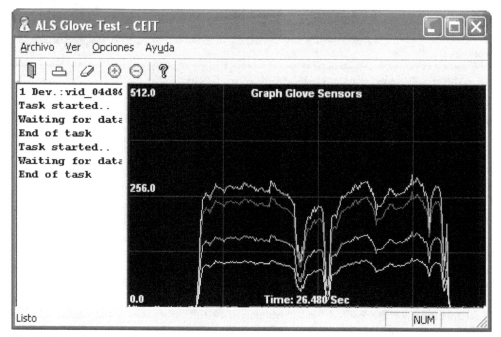

Fig. 9. PC application showing hand-grip force test results

### 5.3 Finger tapping results

The main innovation of this system is that it can measure both the frequency of the tapping and the force the patient applies when carrying out the test. Fig. 10 shows a screen capture of the PC application used to visualize the results in real-time, in which an ongoing finger tapping test can be seen.

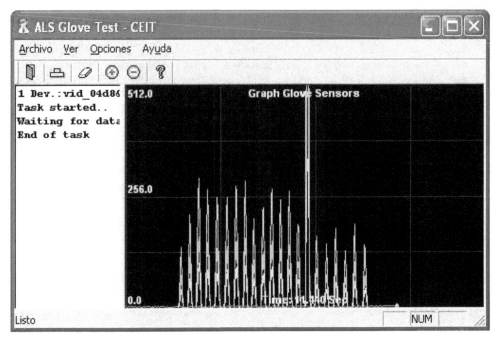

Fig. 10. PC application showing Finger-Tapping test results

Another key point of this finger-tapping test system compared to the existing ones is that the test can be performed using any of the five fingers of the hand. That way, two kinds of finger tapping tests can be carried out: one in which the fingers the patient uses most are involved in the testing process, and another one in which the patient uses the fingers that he or she is less likely to use.

## 6. Device's test in gait analysis

One of the ways of measuring and quantifying the movement disorders is performing gait analysis. Although several techniques and methods have been developed and used for years, all of them are based on hospitalizing patients and using in-hospital equipment.

Several interviews and meetings held with experts in neurology show that the most common way to carry out the gait analysis is by using sensorized ground platforms, as well as video cameras, in order to capture movement, where the two main disadvantages of these methods are the limited, and short period of time over which the patient can be monitored; and the fact of the monitoring process being carried out in a controlled environment, in which the patient may feel safe.

Recent advances on gait analysis of PD patients include portable digital monitoring systems. These systems allow gathering data by the patient themselves, wearing sensors at home and outside home. The developments performed to date are based on tiny electronic circuits which gather and transmit data coming from sensors, mainly accelerometers (Kauw-A-Tjoe et al., 2007).

Combining the advantages of both approaches used till date (sensorized ground platforms and portable monitoring devices) a gait monitoring system has been developed, using our wireless sensor device. For the approach presented in this test, Force Sensitive Resistors (FSR) sensors have also been selected. Regarding the location of the sensors on the insole, several medical considerations have to be taken into account. As shown in Fig. 11, the most interesting zones to place the sensors are three: the plantar area, the heel and one in the middle. These zones are the ones in which most of the force is applied and, thus, the zones from which more information can be obtained.

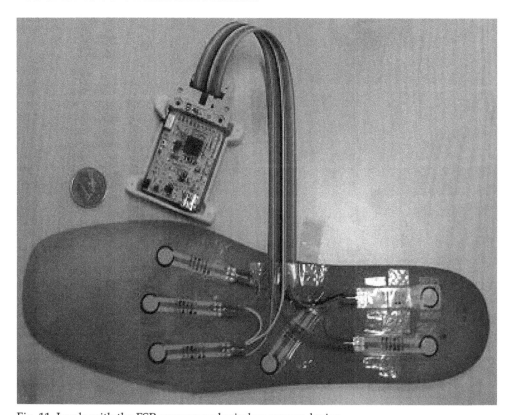

Fig. 11. Insole with the FSR sensors and wireless sensor device

## 6.1 Gait analysis results

The test methodology carried out consists of several tests performed on patients affected by PD and on healthy individuals. Two people from each group participated in the tests, and each of them carried out three repetitions, in order to avoid random results.

The parameters to be measured are the amplitude of the signal of each sensor (i.e., the force of the step) and the frequency of the signal, which gives an idea of the cadence of the gait. Table 1 shows the results obtained, where it can be seen that parkinsonian people has more frequency in their steps than healthy people. Fig. 11 shows the results for 2 sensors, gathered on the gait of a healthy person. The signal with the greater amplitude corresponds to a sensor located in the heel and the other one to the plantar area.

| Samples | | Results | |
|---|---|---|---|
| | | Amplitude(V) | Central frequency (Hz.) |
| Non-Parkinsonian | 1 | 2.64 | 0.88 |
| | 2 | 2.42 | 0.82 |
| Parkinsonian | 1 | 1.64 | 1.76 |
| | 2 | 1.76 | 1.85 |

Table 1. Results of the test in patients

A delay can be noted between the two signal in Fig. 12. This is due to the nature of the step in a normal gait. Another difference lies in the amplitude of the signals and this is because most of the weight rests on the heel. On the other hand, Fig. 13 shows the analogous results for a Parkinsonian individual.

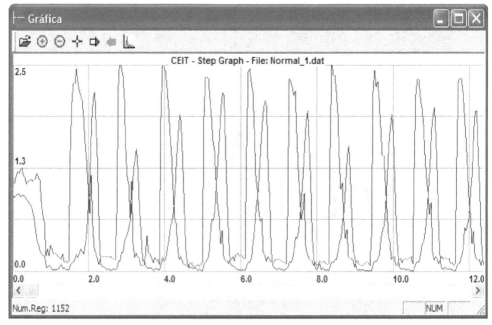

Fig. 12. Signal of a non-Parkinsonian individual over a temporal axis

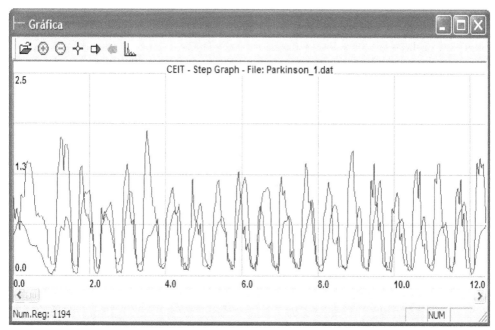

Fig. 13. Signal of a Parkinsonian patient

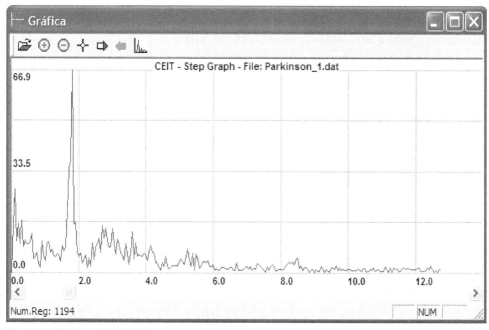

Fig. 14. FFT Signal of a Parkinsonian patient

As Fig. 13 shows, there is no delay between signals which suggests that this is due to the typical short steps of a Pakinsonian patient. Two more interesting conclusions are that the amplitude of these signals is lower than in the previous case, and the frequency is greater, around twice as much. This can be seen in Fig. 14, where the FFT of the Parkinsonian patient's signal is plotted.

## 7. Conclusion

The design of a tiny wireless sensor node platform has been carried out in this work. This device is mainly featured with its multifunctional functionality which has been proven in this paper on e-Health applications, specifically on tests related to patients affected by neurodegenerative diseases.

The presented work is based on the development of two specific tests for the treatment and analysis of Parkinson Disease (PD) and Amyotrophic Lateral Sclerosis (ALS). For each, the device has a different sensorized platform according to the nature of the performed test. Collected data from sensors can be either transmitted online through RF or downloaded via USB to a PC, or just stored in a card memory for a further download and analysis of data. A sensorized glove allows two tests to be carried out, mostly used on ALS patients; those are the hand-grip and the finger tapping tests. In the same way an insole with sensors located strategically is used to carry out a gait analysis which is one of the ways of measuring the movement disorders in parkinsonian people.

Results from both kinds of tests can be visualized and analyzed with the PC application developed in this work which also proves the versatility of the whole designed system. This application provides useful tools for the analysis of results; it was designed taking into account clinicians feedback as part of the work under the scope of the PERFORM project, acting as an interface between the clinician and the system.

The obtained results show and prove the viability and value of the multifunctional characteristics of the designed device. Additionally, by using the several tools provided by the PC application tools, important parameters can be obtained such as the frequency of a signal through the implemented FFT calculation function, the correlation among sensor signals in terms of phase and magnitude, the customization in the selection of specific signals and the zoom tool for a better appreciation of data.

These functionalities of the PC application allow clinician to obtain valuable conclusions like the stability of the gait (from the harmonics of the signals), the relation between air and ground time of the step (in PD analysis), the finger tapping frequency, the relation between the force applied by the different fingers, or the recording of the periods of time in which the patient is in "on" or "off" state.

Future work, which remains to be done is to focus on the accelerometer not mounted in this work. This component will provide relevant information for the gait analysis mainly helping to determine orientation and acceleration parameters of the patient.

## 8. Acknowledgement

This work is partly funded by the ICT programme of the European Commission (PERFORM Project: FP7-ICT-2007-1-215952)

# 9. References

Aitkens, S., Lord, J., Bernauer, E., Fowler, W.M. Jr, Lieberman, J.S., Berck, P. (1989). Relationship of manual muscle testing to objective strength measurements. *Muscle & Nerve.* Vol. 12, No. 3, (March 1989), pp. (173-177), ISSN 1097-4598.

Anastasi, G., Conti, M., Di Francesco, M., & Passarella, A. (2009). Energy conservation in wireless sensor networks: A survey. *Ad Hoc Networks.* Vol. 7, No. 3, (May 2009), pp. (537-568), ISSN 1570-8705.

Christianson, M. K., Leathem, J. M. (2004). Development and Standardisation of the Computerised Finger Tapping Test: Comparison with other finger tapping instruments. *New Zealand Journal of Psychology*, Vol. 33, No. 2, (July 2004), pp. (44-49), ISSN 0112-109X.

Jobbágy Á., Harcos, P., Karoly, R., & Fazekas, G. (2005). Analysis of finger-tapping movement. *Journal of Neuroscience Methods*, Vol. 141, No. 1, (January 2005), pp. (29–39), ISSN 0165-0270.

Kauw-A-Tjoe, R.G., Thalen, J., Marin-Perianu, M., & Havinga, P. (2007). SensorShoe: Mobile Gait Analysis for Parkinson's Disease Patients, *Proceedings of the 9th International Conference on Ubiquitous Computing (UbiComp 2007)*, ISBN: 3-540-74852-0, Innsbruck (Austria), September 2007.

Konitsiotis, S. (2005). Novel pharmacological strategies for motor complications in Parkinson's disease. *Expert Opinion on Investigational Drugs*, Vol. 14, No. 14, (April 2005), pp. (377-399), ISSN 1354-3784.

Long, C. (1970). Intrinsic-extrinsic muscle control of hand in power grip and precision handling - an electromyographic study. *Journal of bone and joint surgery - American volume.* Vol. 52, No. 5, (1970), pp. (853-859), ISSN 0021-9355.

McDermid, R. (2000). A comparison of alternative devices of the finger tapping test. *Archives of Clinical Neuropsychology*, Vol. 15, No. 8, (November 2000).

Okuno, R., Yokoe, M., Fukawa, K., Sakoda, S., & Akazawa, K. (2007). Measurement system of finger-tapping contact force for quantitative diagnosis of Parkinson's disease, *Proceedings of the 29th Annual International Conference of the IEEE Engineering in Medicine and Biology Society EMBS 2007*, ISBN 978-1-4244-0788-3, Lyon (France), August 2007

Soichiro, M., Hisayoshi, O., Akira, K., Hironori, S., & Ko, K. (2004). Quantitative analysis of cerebellar ataxia with a finger tapping device containing a pressure sensor. *Neurological Medicine*, Vol.61, No. 1, pp. (99-101), ISSN0386-9709.

Vecchi, F., Freschi, C., Micera, S., Sabatini, A. M., & Dario, P. (2000). Experimental evaluation of two commercial force sensors for applications in biomechanics and motor control, *Proceedings of the 5th IFESS Annual Conference*, ISBN 4-9980783-1-3, Aalborg (Denmark), June 2000.

Von Campenhausen, S., Bornschein, B., Wick, R., Bötzel, K., Sampaio, C., Poewe, W., Oertel, W., Siebert, U., Berger, K., & Dodel, R. (2005). Prevalence and incidence of Parkinson's disease in Europe. *European Neuropsychopharmacology*, Vol. 15, No. 4, (August 2005), pp. (473-490), ISSN 0924-977X.

Yick, J., Mukherjee, B., & Ghosal, D. Wireless sensor network survey. *Computer Networks (Elsevier).* Vol. 52, No. 12, (August 2008), pp. (2292-2330), ISSN 1389-1286.

Yokoe, M., Okuno, R., Hamasakib, T., Kurachic, Y., Akazawaf, K., & Sakoda, S. (2009). Opening velocity, a novel parameter, for finger tapping test in patients with Parkinson's disease. *Parkinsonism Related Disorders*, Vol. 15, No. 6, (July 2009), pp. (440-444), ISSN 1353-8020

# Permissions

The contributors of this book come from diverse backgrounds, making this book a truly international effort. This book will bring forth new frontiers with its revolutionizing research information and detailed analysis of the nascent developments around the world.

We would like to thank Raymond Chuen-Chung Chang, PhD, for lending his expertise to make the book truly unique. He has played a crucial role in the development of this book. Without his invaluable contribution this book wouldn't have been possible. He has made vital efforts to compile up to date information on the varied aspects of this subject to make this book a valuable addition to the collection of many professionals and students.

This book was conceptualized with the vision of imparting up-to-date information and advanced data in this field. To ensure the same, a matchless editorial board was set up. Every individual on the board went through rigorous rounds of assessment to prove their worth. After which they invested a large part of their time researching and compiling the most relevant data for our readers. Conferences and sessions were held from time to time between the editorial board and the contributing authors to present the data in the most comprehensible form. The editorial team has worked tirelessly to provide valuable and valid information to help people across the globe.

Every chapter published in this book has been scrutinized by our experts. Their significance has been extensively debated. The topics covered herein carry significant findings which will fuel the growth of the discipline. They may even be implemented as practical applications or may be referred to as a beginning point for another development. Chapters in this book were first published by InTech; hereby published with permission under the Creative Commons Attribution License or equivalent.

The editorial board has been involved in producing this book since its inception. They have spent rigorous hours researching and exploring the diverse topics which have resulted in the successful publishing of this book. They have passed on their knowledge of decades through this book. To expedite this challenging task, the publisher supported the team at every step. A small team of assistant editors was also appointed to further simplify the editing procedure and attain best results for the readers.

Our editorial team has been hand-picked from every corner of the world. Their multi-ethnicity adds dynamic inputs to the discussions which result in innovative outcomes. These outcomes are then further discussed with the researchers and contributors who give their valuable feedback and opinion regarding the same. The feedback is then collaborated with the researches and they are edited in a comprehensive manner to aid the understanding of the subject.

Apart from the editorial board, the designing team has also invested a significant amount of their time in understanding the subject and creating the most relevant covers. They scrutinized every image to scout for the most suitable representation of the subject and create an appropriate cover for the book.

The publishing team has been involved in this book since its early stages. They were actively engaged in every process, be it collecting the data, connecting with the contributors or procuring relevant information. The team has been an ardent support to the editorial, designing and production team. Their endless efforts to recruit the best for this project, has resulted in the accomplishment of this book. They are a veteran in the field of academics and their pool of knowledge is as vast as their experience in printing. Their expertise and guidance has proved useful at every step. Their uncompromising quality standards have made this book an exceptional effort. Their encouragement from time to time has been an inspiration for everyone.

The publisher and the editorial board hope that this book will prove to be a valuable piece of knowledge for researchers, students, practitioners and scholars across the globe.

# List of Contributors

**Alexander Shpakov, Oksana Chistyakova, Kira Derkach and Vera Bondareva**
Sechenov Institute of Evolutionary Physiology and Biochemistry, Russia

**Céline Domange**
Toulouse Nationale Veterinary School, Alimentation & Botanics, Toulouse, France

**Alain Paris**
INRA - Mét@risk Unit, AgroParisTech, Paris, France

**Henri Schroeder**
UR AFPA, INRA UC340, Nancy University, France Faculty of Sciences & Technologies, Nancy

**Nathalie Priymenko**
Toulouse Nationale Veterinary School, Alimentation & Botanics, Toulouse, France
UMR 1331 ToxAlim INRA INP, Toulouse, France

**Xuri Li, Anil Kumar, Chunsik Lee, Zhongshu Tang, Yang Li, Pachiappan Arjunan, Xu Hou and Fan Zhang**
National Eye Institute, National Institutes of Health, Rockville, Maryland, United States of America

**Anat Elmann, Alona Telerman, Sharon Mordechay, Hilla Erlank and Miriam Rindner**
Department of Food Science, Volcani Center, Agricultural Research Organization, Bet Dagan, Israel

**Rivka Ofir**
Dead Sea & Arava Science Center and Department of Microbiology & Immunology Ben-Gurion University of the Negev, Beer-Sheva, Israel

**Elie Beit-Yannai**
Department of Clinical Pharmacology, Faculty of Health Sciences, Ben-Gurion University of the Negev, Beer-Sheva, Israel

**Chu Xiang-Ping and Wang John Q**
Department of Basic Medical Science, University of Missouri-Kansas City, Kansas City, Missouri, USA

**Xiong Zhi-Gang**
Department of Neurobiology, Morehouse School of Medicine, Atlanta, Georgia, USA

**Niyazi Acer**
Dept. of Anatomy, Erciyes University School of Medicine, Kayseri, Turkey

**Ahmet Tuncay Turgut**
Dept. of Radiology, Ankara Training and Research Hospital, Ankara, Turkey

**Yelda Özsunar**
Dept. of Radiology, Adnan Menderes University School of Medicine, Aydın, Turkey

**Mehmet Turgut**
Dept. of Neurosurgery, Adnan Menderes University School of Medicine, Aydın, Turkey

**Luca Lovrečić, Aleš Maver and Borut Peterlin**
Clinical Institute of Medical Genetics, University Medical Center Ljubljana, Slovenia

**Gonzalo Solas and Karol Grandez**
CEIT University of Navarra, Spain

**Paul Bustamante**
Tecnun University of Navarra, Spain
CEIT University of Navarra, Spain

.

Printed in the USA
CPSIA information can be obtained
at www.ICGtesting.com
JSHW011412221024
72173JS00003B/521